Integrative, Complementary and Alternative Medicine (CAM) in Healthcare

Integrative, Complementary and Alternative Medicine (CAM) in Healthcare

Editors

Kavita Batra
Manoj Sharma

MDPI • Basel • Beijing • Wuhan • Barcelona • Belgrade • Manchester • Tokyo • Cluj • Tianjin

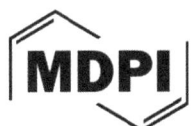

Editors
Kavita Batra
UNLV Medicine Trauma and
Critical Care, Kirk Kerkorian
School of Medicine
University of Nevada, Las Vegas
Las Vegas
United States

Manoj Sharma
Social and Behavioral Health
University of Nevada, Las Vegas
Las Vegas
United States

Editorial Office
MDPI
St. Alban-Anlage 66
4052 Basel, Switzerland

This is a reprint of articles from the Topical Collection published online in the open access journal *Healthcare* (ISSN 2227-9032) (available at: www.mdpi.com/journal/healthcare/special_issues/CAM_Health).

For citation purposes, cite each article independently as indicated on the article page online and as indicated below:

LastName, A.A.; LastName, B.B.; LastName, C.C. Article Title. *Journal Name* **Year**, *Volume Number*, Page Range.

ISBN 978-3-0365-3630-9 (Hbk)
ISBN 978-3-0365-3629-3 (PDF)

© 2022 by the authors. Articles in this book are Open Access and distributed under the Creative Commons Attribution (CC BY) license, which allows users to download, copy and build upon published articles, as long as the author and publisher are properly credited, which ensures maximum dissemination and a wider impact of our publications.

The book as a whole is distributed by MDPI under the terms and conditions of the Creative Commons license CC BY-NC-ND.

Contents

About the Editors vii

Preface to "Integrative, Complementary and Alternative Medicine (CAM) in Healthcare" . . . ix

Ram Lakhan, Manoj Sharma, Kavita Batra and Frazier B. Beatty
The Role of Vitamin E in Slowing Down Mild Cognitive Impairment: A Narrative Review
Reprinted from: *Healthcare* **2021**, *9*, 1573, doi:10.3390/healthcare9111573 1

Jian-An Liao, Shih-Chieh Shao, Chian-Ting Chang, Pony Yee-Chee Chai, Kok-Loon Owang, Tse-Hung Huang, Chung-Han Yang, Tsai-Jen Lee and Yung-Chih Chen
Correction of Breech Presentation with Moxibustion and Acupuncture: A Systematic Review and Meta-Analysis
Reprinted from: *Healthcare* **2021**, *9*, 619, doi:10.3390/healthcare9060619 13

Chan-Young Kwon, Boram Lee, Beom-Joon Lee, Kwan-Il Kim and Hee-Jae Jung
Comparative Effectiveness of Western and Eastern Manual Therapies for Chronic Obstructive Pulmonary Disease: A Systematic Review and Network Meta-Analysis
Reprinted from: *Healthcare* **2021**, *9*, 1127, doi:10.3390/healthcare9091127 27

Manoj Sharma, Matthew Asare, Erin Largo-Wight, Julie Merten, Mike Binder, Ram Lakhan and Kavita Batra
Testing Multi-Theory Model (MTM) in Explaining Sunscreen Use among Florida Residents: An Integrative Approach for Sun Protection
Reprinted from: *Healthcare* **2021**, *9*, 1343, doi:10.3390/healthcare9101343 45

Angela Martín-García, Ana-Isabel Corregidor-Sánchez, Virginia Fernández-Moreno, Vanesa Alcántara-Porcuna and Juan-José Criado-Álvarez
Effect of Doll Therapy in Behavioral and Psychological Symptoms of Dementia: A Systematic Review
Reprinted from: *Healthcare* **2022**, *10*, 421, doi:10.3390/healthcare10030421 57

Stephen D. Edwards, David J. Edwards and Richard Honeycutt
HeartMath as an Integrative, Personal, Social, and Global Healthcare System
Reprinted from: *Healthcare* **2022**, *10*, 376, doi:10.3390/healthcare10020376 71

Cristiano Scandurra, Selene Mezzalira, Sara Cutillo, Rosanna Zapparella, Giancarlo Statti, Nelson Mauro Maldonato, Mariavittoria Locci and Vincenzo Bochicchio
The Effectiveness of Neroli Essential Oil in Relieving Anxiety and Perceived Pain in Women during Labor: A Randomized Controlled Trial
Reprinted from: *Healthcare* **2022**, *10*, 366, doi:10.3390/healthcare10020366 81

Miri Kwon, Moon Joo Cheong, Jungtae Leem and Tae-hun Kim
Effect of Acupuncture on Movement Function in Patients with Parkinson's Disease: Network Meta-Analysis of Randomized Controlled Trials
Reprinted from: *Healthcare* **2021**, *9*, 1502, doi:10.3390/healthcare9111502 93

Jihye Kim, Jang-Kyung Park, Jung-Youn Park, Eun-Jin Lee and Soo-Hyun Sung
The Use of Traditional Korean Medicine (TKM) by Children: A Correlational Study between Parent's Perception and Their Children's Use Reported by Parents
Reprinted from: *Healthcare* **2021**, *9*, 385, doi:10.3390/healthcare9040385 113

Bonhyuk Goo, Min-gi Jo, Eun-Jung Kim, Hyun-Jong Lee, Jae-Soo Kim, Dongwoo Nam, Jung Won Kang, Tae-Hun Kim, Yeon-Cheol Park, Yong-Hyeon Baek, Sang-Soo Nam, Myeong Soo Lee and Byung-Kwan Seo
Korean Medicine Clinical Practice Guidelines for Lumbar Herniated Intervertebral Disc in Adults: Based on Grading of Recommendations Assessment, Development and Evaluation (GRADE)
Reprinted from: *Healthcare* **2022**, *10*, 246, doi:10.3390/healthcare10020246 . . . . **125**

About the Editors

Kavita Batra, BDS, MPH, Ph.D., serves as an Assistant Professor and Medical Research Biostatistician with the Kirk Kerkorian School of Medicine at the University of Nevada, Las Vegas (UNLV). Dr. Batra received her Ph.D. in Global and Environmental Health from UNLV. Her research interests include maternal and child health, the impact of COVID-19, and disparities among racial and gender minorities. Dr. Batra is an expert in qualitative and quantitative research and presented her work in several state and national public health conferences. She has published multiple peer-reviewed articles to investigate the impact of COVID-19 on mental health, social connectedness, and employment vulnerability among different demographic and workforce groups. Dr. Batra's recent work related to COVID-19 has been featured in reputed outlets, such as Medscape and Inside Higher Ed. Currently, she is editing three Special Issues with the Healthcare journal. She also serves as a key member to the Nevada Taskforce on Sexual Misconduct.

Manoj Sharma, MBBS, Ph.D., MCHES® is currently a tenured Full Professor and Chair of the Department of Social & Behavioral Health at the University of Nevada, Las Vegas, School of Public Health. He is a prolific researcher and has published 12 books, over 325 peer-reviewed research articles, and over 450 other publications and secured funding for over $8 million (h-index 44, i-10 index over 175, and over 10,000 citations). He has been awarded several prestigious honors including American Public Health Association's Mentoring Award, ICTHP Impact Award, and J. Mayhew Derryberry Award and William R. Gemma Distinguished Alumnus Award, from the College of Public Health Alumni Society (Ohio State University) among others. His research interests are in developing and evaluating theory-based health behavior change interventions, obesity prevention, stress-coping, community-based participatory research, and integrative mind-body-spirit interventions.

Preface to "Integrative, Complementary and Alternative Medicine (CAM) in Healthcare"

We have often seen words such as "alternative," "complementary," and "integrative," but it is important to decipher these terminologies in the context of the preventive medicine. In the evolving landscape of the medicine, "alternative," and "complementary" are not interchangeable terms; in fact, these are two different concepts. A complementary approach is used in conjunction with the conventional medicine, whereas "alternative" medicine replaces the conventional medicine. Integrative medicine, on the other hand, is a "functional" medicine that combines traditional practices with European health care approaches. The sole aim of the integrative medicine is focused on whole person health with interconnected domains of biological, behavioral, social, and environmental aspects. The potential of complementary and alternative medicine is yet to be understood. Its effects are more felt than being measured, and it may be challenging to convince patients about the science behind the complementary and alternative modalities. This underscores the need of promoting physicians' education about the complementary and alternative medicine to convince their patients. The research evidence plays a critical role in improving the uptake of these modalities in the preventive medicine, which may offer more personal autonomy and control over the healthcare decisions.

This collection of ten studies starts with a narrative review related to neuroprotective effects of vitamin E in preventing the progression of dementia among older adults with the Alzheimer disease. Following chapter provides a robust evidence from Taiwan, which reports the positive effects of moxibustion therapy (acupuncture type intervention) on correcting the breech presentation among Asian population groups. Another study from Korea performed a network meta-analysis to compare the effectiveness of Western and Eastern manual therapies for respiratory diseases, including the Chronic Obstructive Pulmonary Diseases. This study underscores the need of performing high-quality randomized controlled trials. Simple integrative approaches such as wearing sunscreen to prevent skin cancer can offer a cost-effective solution, which was highlighted by a Florida-based study grounded in a fourth-generation behavioral theory. Next, a Spain-based study described the effect of "Doll Therapy" in treating the behavioral and psychological symptoms of neurodegenerative diseases. The "Doll Therapy" offers an integrated solution based on the Attachment Theory, the Transitional Object Theory, and the Person-centered Theory. One study from South Africa explained an interesting yet new approach called as "HeartMath," which can serve as a global healthcare meditation model, particularly in the current COVID-19 era. Next, labor pain control remedies (using aromatherapies) were studied among an Italian sample of pregnant women. Following a chapter about a study, which was performed in Korea, that provided level 1 evidence related to the effects of acupuncture on mobility among patients with the Parkinson's disease. Another Korean study assessed the parental perception of the use of Traditional Korean Medicine among their children through a survey-based study. Last chapter of this collection attempts to provide and validate the information related to the Korean medicine clinical practice guidelines for Lumbar Herniated Intervertebral Disc in adults. To summarize, this compendium contains a plethora of information related to the evidence-based interventions in the realm of preventive medicine.

Kavita Batra, Manoj Sharma
Editors

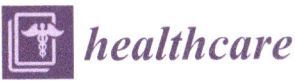

Review

The Role of Vitamin E in Slowing Down Mild Cognitive Impairment: A Narrative Review

Ram Lakhan [1], Manoj Sharma [2], Kavita Batra [3,*] and Frazier B. Beatty [4]

1. Department of Health and Human Performance, Berea College, Berea, KY 40404, USA; Lakhanr@berea.edu
2. Department of Social & Behavioral Health, School of Public Health, University of Nevada, Las Vegas, NV 89119, USA; manoj.sharma@unlv.edu
3. Office of Research, Kirk Kerkorian School of Medicine, University of Nevada, Las Vegas, NV 89102, USA
4. Graduate Department of Public Health, School of Health Sciences, Regis College, Weston, MA 02493, USA; frazier.beatty@regiscollege.edu
* Correspondence: kavita.batra@unlv.edu

Abstract: With the aging population, dementia emerges as a public health concern. In 2012, the Health and Retirement Study found that 8.8% of adults over 65 years suffered from dementia. The etiopathogenesis and treatment of dementia are not well understood. Antioxidant properties of Vitamin E and its major elements tocopherols and tocotrienols have been reported to be effective in slowing down the progression of dementia from its initial stage of Mild cognitive impairment (MCI). Therefore, the current review aims to explore the role of vitamin E on MCI. A literature search using the key words "Vitamin E, tocopherols, tocotrienols, and mild cognitive impairment" was conducted in MEDLINE (PubMed), CINAHL, and Google Scholar. The inclusion criteria were: (1) articles published in the past ten years; (2) published in English language; (3) published in peer-reviewed journals; and (4) descriptive and epidemiological or evaluation studies. Articles published prior to 2010, focused on other forms of dementia than MCI, grey literature and non-peer-reviewed articles were excluded. A total of 22 studies were included in the narrative synthesis. The results were equivocal. Eleven studies showed some level of the neuroprotective effect of Vitamin E, tocopherols and tocotrienols on the progression of MCI. The mixed results of this review suggest further exploration of the possible protective effects of Vitamin E on the development of dementia. Future studies can be conducted to decipher antioxidant properties of vitamin E and its association with slowing down the cognitive decline.

Keywords: dementia; mild cognitive impairment; vitamin E; amnesia

1. Introduction

Dementia is a serious public health concern with nearly 50 million people having some form of dementia globally [1]. Reportedly, about 60% of the dementia population live in low and middle-income countries (LMICs) [1]. Estimates suggest that about 10 million people get dementia every year and about 15–20% of elderly population reported having mild cognitive impairment (MCI) as the early stage of dementia [1–3]. MCI causes a slight but observable and measurable decline in the memory and thinking skills of an individual. In some individuals, MCI can be reversible (if physiological in origin), however, the likelihood of the reversal to the normal cognitive capability is less for majority of people if it is pathological [2,3]. With due course, MCI advances to the next stage with nearly 65% of people developing more severe forms [2,3].

According to the previous meta-analytical evidence presented by the American Academy of Neurology, the prevalence of MCI was nearly 7% among people with age 60–64 years, which increases with advancing age [3,4]. In the United States (U.S.), the highest prevalence was reported among elderly above 75 years of age [4]. These trends are not only limited to developed countries, low- and middle-income countries indicate

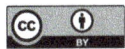

similar patterns [5]. However, due to lack of population-based studies, the true estimates are unavailable. According to the previous reports, the prevalence of MCI ranged from 4.5% to 15.4% among South Asian countries [6–9]. Differences in MCI by demographic characteristics (e.g., gender, race/ethnicity, education) were also noted with women being at greater lifetime risk for dementia compared to their male counterparts [10–12]. The occurrence of MCI is found delayed and lenient towards the end of life among whites and highly educated people while the onset of MCI is observed at younger age among blacks and those with lower education attainment [10–12]. The lifetime risk of dementia is 21% among men with an associate degree while it is 35% for those who have less than high school education [10–12]. White women have a shorter cognitively impaired life compared to black women (6 years vs. 12 to 13 years) [10–12]. The burden of dementia further translates into higher cost associated with its management [2]. According to the Alzheimer association, through identification of early stages of Alzheimer disease (AD) i.e., MCI, nearly $7 to $7.9 trillion in health and long-term care can be saved [2].

MCI has severe implications for the patients and their family members and challenges are multifactorial in origin [13]. Often time patients and their family members are unable to identify cognitive decline at earlier stages, particularly in older population groups, in whom cognitive decline is a normal physiological phenomenon. Moreover, cooccurrence of other age-associated diseases are likely to occur in this group with a limited ability to make a differential diagnosis [14,15]. Cognitive insufficiency impacts the quality of life, individual's functioning, their relationship with the family members, and their self-esteem [14,15]. Caregivers experience high level of caregiving burden for the larger population of MCI [16]. Given the unavailability of medication to treat, prevent, or slow the progression of MCI to dementia, preventive strategies take precedence for at-risk population groups to prevent progressive deficits [17]. Prevention of somatic diseases, promotion of physical and mental exercise, cognitive training, avoidance of toxins, reduction in stress, stopping smoking, and use of dietary compounds such as antioxidants and supplements are some of the suggested to address MCI [17,18]. Among antioxidants, vitamins play a critical role in reducing or delaying to the process of cognitive decline in people with MCI. Among all vitamins, vitamin E was found to be effective in reducing MCI [17–23]. Vitamin E is a fat-soluble vitamin and found in variety of foods [19]. Its usable form (i.e., alpha tocopherol) is considered a scavenger of free radicals in the body [19], which controls brain prostaglandin synthesis and regulates nucleic acid synthesis. While some studies have documented association of vitamin E intake in slowing down the progression of MCI, collective evidence to investigate its significance is still lacking [17–23]. Therefore, the purpose of this study was to review existing literature to decipher role of vitamin E in slowing down MCI progression.

2. Methods
2.1. Search Strategy

Bibliographical databases, including Medline (PubMed), CINAHL, and Google Scholar were quickly searched in January/February 2020. Pharmacological synonyms of vitamin E were used as related terms to locate potential evidence to be included in this review. Articles related to cognitive impairment were also sought using the Boolean operator "AND" to narrow down search results to include articles containing the specified terms. A detailed list of key words is shown in Table 1.

Table 1. List of keywords used for literature search.

Main Term	Related Terms Used
Vitamin E	Tocopherol * OR D1 alpha tocopherol OR Preventive therapy OR tocotrienols OR Aquasol E OR Antioxidant
	AND
Mild cognitive impairment	Dementia OR Alzheimer's disease OR Cognitive decline OR Amentia OR Mental disorder OR Paranoid Dementia OR Senile Paranoid

2.2. Inclusion Criteria and Data Abstraction

The inclusion criteria of this review were the following; (1) observational, randomized controlled trials, clinical and laboratory studies published over past ten years; (2) studies published in English language; (3) published in peer-reviewed journals; and (4) descriptive and epidemiological or evaluation-based studies. The exploration of preventive relationship of vitamin E with mild cognitive impairment is relatively new. Therefore, we selected to assign a broad range of criteria including human and animals-based studies published in the 10 years of timeframe. Articles published before 2010, focused on other forms of dementia than MCI, grey literature, abstracts—only studies, and non-peer-reviewed articles were excluded. We also conducted a post-hoc search in July 2021 to update our literature matrix used for this review. Details about the search results were saved in the spreadsheet by the lead author. Titles and abstracts were screened for relevancy and eligibility. If found relevant, full-texts were read thoroughly and data were extracted in a standardized data collection form. Variables such as year of publication, study type, outcomes, key findings, neuroprotective role of vitamin E, and conclusions were tabulated in the data collection form.

3. Results

Following keyword search, 53 articles in Medline/PubMed/Google Scholar and 5 in CINAHL database were found. Out of those, 48 studies met the inclusion criteria. Abstracts of all 48 studies were screened. Twenty-six studies were excluded for variety of reasons of being editorials, commentaries/letters, abstract-only study, combined vitamin E with other vitamins, focused on other form of dementia rather than MCI, reviews, narratives and opinion-based papers. Finally, 22 papers [19–41] were included in this review for the data summarization (Figure 1). Characteristics of finally included studies are provided in Table A1 in Appendix A.

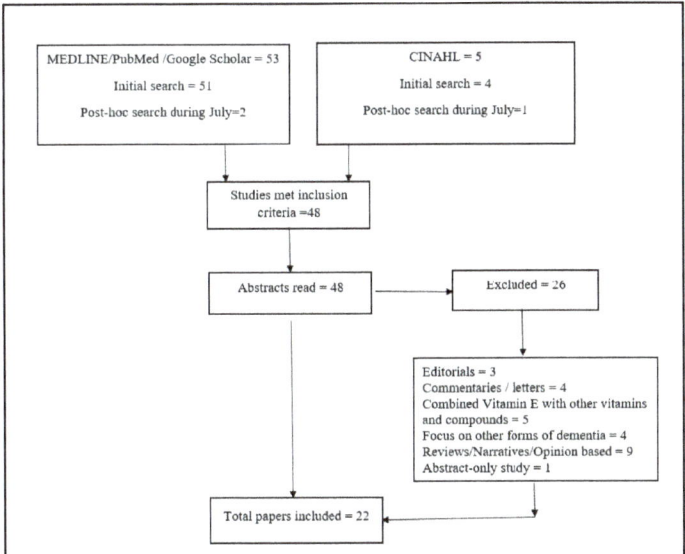

Figure 1. Flow diagram of the literature search and selection process.

Of 22 finally included studies, seven were conducted with animals. Out of seven, six studies conducted on rats, mice, and other animals exhibited some level of the neuroprotective effect of vitamin E by lowering the rate or delaying cognitive impairment progression. Similarly, out of 15 studies conducted on humans, eight studies reported

Vitamin E's role in lowering the risk or delaying cognitive impairment. Two studies, one cohort and a double-blind randomized placebo-controlled study, demonstrated Vitamin E's effect in improving learning and memory functions. Two studies of each experimental and double-blind randomized placebo-controlled did not find any effect of Vitamin E on cognitive impairment while a clinical study14 suggested a potentially favorable effect (Tables 2 and A1).

Table 2. Summary results of all studies in the review (n = 22).

	Categories	Delay or a Lower Rate of Cognitive Decline or Neuroprotective Effect	Improved Learning and Memory Functions	May Be Effective	Suggest Further Exploration	No Effect
Animals	Rats (n = 3)	3				
	Mice (n = 2)	1			1	
	Other animals (n = 2)	2				
Human	Cross-sectional (n = 1)	1				
	Case-control (n = 1)	1				
	Cohort (prospective) (n = 3)	2	1			
	Experimental (n = 4)	2				2
	Clinical (n = 2)	2		1		
	Double-blind, randomized, placebo-controlled (n = 4)	1	1			2
	Total (n = 22)	15	2	1	1	4

4. Discussion

The purpose of this review was to examine the effect of Vitamin E in slowing down cognitive decline in MCI. Some evidence from our literature synthesis points to the putative role of Vitamin E in slowing down MCI progression to dementia. Overall, the review collectively demonstrated through analysis of various experimental studies in rats, mice, and animals and cross-sectional, case-control, prospective cohort, experimental, clinical, and double-blind randomized in human that Vitamin E has some neuroprotective effect in slowing down progression to dementia. One clinical study carried out to lower the effect of cisplatin chemotherapy neurotoxicity, the supplementation with vitamin E (alpha tocopherol) has shown lower level of neurotoxicity, which indicates that vitamin E plays a neuroprotective role [42] even when the cause of neurotoxicity could be other than mild cognitive impairment. The findings of Gugliandolo et al. (2017) have reported similar physiological responses of Vitamin E on MCI [43–45]. Another study by Kaneai et al., indicated that vitamin E offers some neuroprotective benefits by improving neurotransmission [45]. Presently, no medication can treat, prevent, or slow the progression of MCI to dementia. However, it is important to explore the role of vitamins and antioxidants in reducing or delaying to the process of cognitive decline in people with MCI [17]. Studies show that high plasma Vitamin E levels have been associated with better cognitive performance in both ageing populations, dementia, and AD patients [42,43].

Consistent to previous studies it is understood that Vitamin E might have some therapeutic role when it comes to MCI and its progression to dementia. Since several studies in human as well as in rats and mice were MCI associated with lower level of tocopherol. Thus, it may be considered a good practice to maintain Vitamin E level through dietary sources. Vitamin E can also lead to toxicity that can be fatal in some cases which warrants careful monitoring of its levels in the aging population. The guidelines on the safe dose of vitamin E varies from 800–2000 IU/day as reported by previous studies [46,47]. Therefore, these findings should be considered rather carefully to prevent any toxic effects of vitamin E. In the meanwhile, more randomized controlled trials to further elucidate the role of Vitamin E on MCI must be conducted with larger sample sizes. Even though there are mixed results they favor a potential neuroprotective effect of Vitamin E in MCI. It would be recommended for clinical practice that the Vitamin E levels be checked annually in the elderly, and they should be provided Vitamin E supplementation in maintaining its adequate level.

Limitations

This review has certain limitations including that research articles focused on dementia, which have explored relationship of vitamin E on mild cognitive impairment but not necessarily mentioned MCI in the title or abstract, those articles might have left from inclusion. Authors utilized phrase searching, however, due to the lack of truncation rules for some terms of dementia, some articles might have been missed. Therefore, future studies using a systematic literature review with a well-defined and peer-reviewed search strategy can be conducted. Six animal studies are included in this review and comparison were made between findings in human and animals. Comparison of effect of an element between human and animal specially on cognitive function and process is extremely complex. In simpler terms, behavioral studies to investigate cognitive decline among humans offer higher inferential benefits than those being conducted among animals due to differences in their baseline intelligence levels and capabilities. Next, studies included in this review were heterogenous in terms of type of measures used to detect the cognitive decline and these measures had varied threshold criteria. These restricted our ability to generate pooled estimates, which otherwise might have helped us to quantify the association between vitamin E and neuroprotection in the form of appropriate effect sizes (such as odds ratios). In addition, understanding trajectories of change in cognitive function will be difficult with such a heterogeneity. On the other hand, the observation of physiological process relatively easier in animal population compared to human due to ethical consideration. The findings of animal studies showing favorable outcome of vitamin E on cognition process may not be rewarding when compared to human. The database such as LILACS were not explored. Few studies included in this review has a very small sample size or their results were mixed up with some other compound which might have impacted on the conclusion of this review.

Despite the limitations, the study has implications for practice. Vitamin E supplementation should be monitored closely when in combination with Vitamin E nutrients from food sources. Other than alpha tocopherol, no other component of vitamin was found helpful in slowing the process of cognitive decline. It is not known if the other form of vitamin E or its component has negative effect on cognitive process. Therefore, caution needs to be practiced in optimizing level of vitamin E that way the other components of vitamin E do not affect the properties of alpha tocopherol and its impact on MCI. In addition, this review indicates favorable physiological and neurochemical benefits of vitamin E in protecting or delaying cognitive decline process, however, effects may be different among animals and human-beings. These differences may be due to the varied vitamin E requirements and physiological mechanisms among these groups. Therefore, further research to understand associations between vitamin E requirements, consumption, and effects at organismal levels would be critical to unfold interactions of vitamin E with body mechanisms.

5. Conclusions

In conclusion, epidemiological, clinical, nor other studies have provided the conclusive answer to whether or not Vitamin E slows the progression of MCI. Further research with human subjects is needed to understand the safety and efficacy of Vitamin E as a nutritional supplement to promote health ageing. Future research to understand the physiological process of alpha tocopherol on cognitive process in human beings can be conducted.

Author Contributions: Conceptualization, R.L. and M.S.; methodology, R.L., M.S., K.B.; software, R.L., K.B.; validation, K.B., F.B.B., M.S.; data curation, R.L.; writing—original draft preparation, R.L., M.S., K.B., F.B.B.; writing—review and editing, K.B., F.B.B.; visualization, R.L., K.B.; project administration, R.L., M.S. All authors have read and agreed to the published version of the manuscript.

Funding: This research received no external funding.

Institutional Review Board Statement: Not applicable.

Informed Consent Statement: Not applicable.

Conflicts of Interest: The authors declare no conflict of interest.

Appendix A

Table A1. Reviewed studies and their salient findings (n = 22).

Authors	Year	Study Type	Sample Characteristics	Findings	Intrument Used to Screen Dementia	Conclusions
Wu et al.	2010	Experimental study in rats	Rats were fed 500 IU/Kg Vitamin E with their regular diets for four weeks before performing mild fluid percussion injury (FPI). The Vitamin E counter reacted against the effects of fluid percussion injury.	Vitamin E supplementation diet counteracts the molecular substrates underlying synaptic plasticity and cognitive function in the hippocampus.	Not Applicable	Vitamin E dietary supplementation can protect the brain against the effects of mild TBI on synaptic plasticity and cognition. Declines rate of cognitive impairment.
Huang et al.	2010	Experimental study in mice	The relationship between Vitamin E was observed with protein oxidation in mice.	Protein oxidation and nitration increased in MCI.	Not Applicable	The study suggested that the therapeutic role of vitamin E should be explored in MCI.
Alzoubi et al.	2013	Experimental, Animal study	The effect of Vitamin E against a high-fat high carbohydrate diet (HFCD) was observed. It is known that HFCD accelerates learning and cognitive impairment. In this study, the HFCD or Vitamin E was administered to animals for 6 weeks. Behavioral activities were conducted to test spatial learning and memory.	Vitamin E prevented memory impairment induced by HFCD and normalized the effect of HFCD on oxidative stress.	Not Applicable	Probably Vitamin E reduces the risk of MCI by reducing probably through normalizing antioxidant mechanisms in the hippocampus.
Giraldo et al.	2014	In vivo, mice study	The effect of Vitamin E was observed on the inhibition of p38 which prevents Aβ-induced tau phosphorylation that leads to cognitive impairment.	Vitamin E inhibited tau phosphorylation and reduced cognitive impairment.	Not Applicable	Vitamin E has a therapeutic role in protecting the decline of memory impairment.

Table A1. Cont.

Authors	Year	Study Type	Sample Characteristics	Findings	Intrument Used to Screen Dementia	Conclusions
McDougall et al.	2017	Animal experimental study	The study examined learning and memory impairment in zebrafish with vitamin E deficient and sufficient. Zebrafish fed with vitamin E for 45 days acquired sufficient vitamin E levels.	Learning ability was observed in association with vitamin E level by excluding the effect of avoidance conditioning and non-associative learning. Zebrafish with low vitamin E were found learning impaired.	Not Applicable	Study proves that vitamin E plays important role in protecting cognitive delay.
Nesari et al.	2019	Experimental study on rats	The effect of Alpha-tocopherol was evaluated in view of observing its protective effect on long-term memory impairment.	The Alpha-tocopherol reduced the passive avoidance memory performance, increased the level of malondialdehyde (MDE) and reactive oxygen specifies.	Not Applicable	Alpha-tocopherol was found to have a neuroprotective effect on memory impairment.
Mehrabadi & Sadr	2020	Experimental study on rats	The effect of vitamins D_3 and E, in a combination of both, was observed on learning and memory. 60 rats received different doses of vitamins.	Memory and learning were measured by the Novel Object Recognition (NOR) test found to improve in the rat group that received vitamin E.	Not Applicable	Vitamin E can improve learning and memory.
Iuliano et al.	2010	Case-control, experimental research	An enzymatic relationship between oxysterols (24S-hydroxycholesterol and 27 hydroxycholesterol, free radical related oxysterols of oxidative stress and Vitamin E were compared between 37 patients of Alzheimer's disease, 24 MCI, 29 multi-domains (md-MCI).	People with mild cognitive impairment with oxidative stress found to be lower in Vitamin E.	Mini Mental State Examination, Mental Deterioration Battery (MDB)	Vitamin E might have some role in reducing oxidative stress delay and cognitive delay.
Whitehair et al.	2010	Experimental research design	The relationship of Apolipoprotein E ε4 (APOE ε4) allele was observed for 36 months of the period in 516 MCI patients age between 55 to 90 years who were on Vitamin E in 516 MCI participants aged 55–90 years who received placebo.	Vitamin E did not find to be associated with the progression of Apolipoprotein E ε4.	Mini Mental State Examination, Alzheimer's Disease Assessment Scale-Cognitive subscale (ADAS-cog)	A direct connection between Vitamin E and the decline of cognitive function could not be found. However, the active status of APOE ε4 was found associated with a fast decline in cognitive function.

Table A1. Cont.

Authors	Year	Study Type	Sample Characteristics	Findings	Intrument Used to Screen Dementia	Conclusions
Mangialasche et al.	2012	Clinical study	This study examined the relationship between 8 natural compounds of Vitamin E with cognitive impairment. 166 MCI subjects were compared with cognitively normal people.	Low plasma tocopherols and tocotrienols levels of Vitamin E were found with increased odds of MCI in people with ID.	The Folstein Mini-Mental State Examination (MMSE), Clinical dementia rating scale and Hachinski ischemic scale	Vitamin E may have a role against the progression of MCI to AD.
Mangialasche et al.	2013	Cohort research design	140 non-cognitively impaired people were observed for 8 years. The baseline serum vitamin E and cognitive impairment were observed.	The risk of cognitive impairment was found lower among those who had a moderate level of tocopherol/cholesterol ratio than those who had the lowest level of tocopherols.	Mini-Mental State Examination (MMSE)	Vitamin E might play an important role in cognitive impairment in humans. Vitamin E's therapeutic role should be explored.
Shahar et al.	2013	Cross-sectional.	The relationship between MCI and Vitamin A and E was explored in a total of 333 participants age 60 years and above.	Vitamin E level was found lower in APOEe4 carriers that affect MCI.	The Folstein Mini-Mental State Examination (MMSE)	The role of vitamin E needs to be further explored in relation to MCI.
Dysken et al.	2014	Double-blind, placebo-controlled, parallel-group, randomized clinical trial	The effect of vitamin E on the progression of cognitive impairment was examined. 613 patients were recruited. They received either 2000 IU/d of alpha-tocopherol ($n = 152$), 20 mg/d of memantine ($n = 155$), the combination ($n = 154$), or placebo ($n = 152$).	Activities of Daily Living (ADCS-ADL) Inventory score declined in the group that was given vitamin E.	Activities of Daily Living (ADCS-ADL) Inventory score, Mini-Mental State Examination (MMSE)	Vitamin E can slow down the progression of cognitive impairment.
Zanotta, Puricelli & Bonoldi	2014	Prospective cohort	The effect of vitamin E in improving cognition in people diagnosed with MCI was assessed. 104 people about 70 years old were included in the research.	Vitamin E as a supplementary dietary found to be counteractive to cognitive impairment.	Alzheimer's Disease Assessment Scale-Cognitive subscale (ADAS-cog)	Vitamin E may have a role in lowering the risk of MCI.
Naeini et al.	2014	Double-blind randomized, placebo-controlled trial	256 elderly, ages between 65 to 75 were received 300 mg vitamin E with 400 mg of vitamin C or placebo for 1 year	Vitamin E reduced the malondialdehyde level and raised total antioxidant capacity and glutathione.	Mini-Mental State Examination (MMSE)	Vitamin E supplementation did not appear to be enhancing cognitive performance

Table A1. Cont.

Authors	Year	Study Type	Sample Characteristics	Findings	Intrument Used to Screen Dementia	Conclusions
Li et al.	2015	Prospective cohort	This study examined the effect of vitamin E and C together and both vitamins independently on cognitive functions in the elderly population. 276 elderly people received Vitamin E and C together and E independently.	Radioimmunoassay (RIA) results, MMSE, and HDS assessments indicated improvement in cognitive functions with vitamin E and also when vitamin E was given in combination with Vitamin C.	Mini-mental state examination and Hasegawa Dementia Scale	Vitamin E can improve cognitive functions in the elderly population.
De Beaumont et al.	2016	Experimental research	The relationship of apolipoprotein E4 (APOE-ε4) gene and butyryl cholinesterase (BCHE) was assessed on the effect of cognitive impairment.	The study did not mention vitamin E; however, it was designed on the premise of that lower levels of vitamin E increases apolipoprotein E4 (APOE-ε4) and butyryl cholinesterase (BCHE) activity that increases declines memory.	histopathological confirmation of AD according to NINCDS-ADRDA criteria	Vitamin E may have a role in lowering the rate of memory impairment.
Basambombo et al.	2017	Cohort research design	The effect of Vitamin E and also Vitamin C was observed in a cohort of 5269 individuals aged 65 years and above in the Canadian Study of Health and Aging (1991–2002).	The baseline memory and learning ability were compared on the same standardized tests. Vitamin E and C together and independently were found to be associated with a lower risk of memory decline.	Modified Mini-Mental State (3MS) Examination.	Vitamin E plays a role in reducing the risk of memory decline in individuals.
Liu et al.	2018	Randomized controlled study	A randomized controlled study in 7781 individuals of European descent.	No association was observed between dietary supplementation of vitamin E with cognitive impairment.	Not available, since this study utilized biomarkers	The study suggests no association between vitamin E supplementation and MCI in the general population.
Edmonds et al.	2018	Experimental research design	The effect of donepezil and Vitamin E was compared for 756 MCI participants.	The donepezil treatment group had a lower rate of progression from MCI to AD than the Vitamin E group.	The Wechsler Memory Scale–Revised Logical Memory II subtest, Mini-mental state examination.	Vitamin E may not have an effect on lowering the rate of MCI towards AD.

Table A1. Cont.

Authors	Year	Study Type	Sample Characteristics	Findings	Intrument Used to Screen Dementia	Conclusions
Kim et al.	2018	Cross-sectional	The effect of serum vitamin A, C, and E was evaluated for the risk of cognitive impairment in 230 participants aged 60 to 79 years.	Association between vitamin A and C serum was not observed while a negative relationship between vitamin E, beta-gamma tocopherol was observed with a lower risk of cognitive impairment.	Korean version of the Mini-Mental State Examination	Serum beta-gamma tocopherol levels tended to be inversely associated with the risk of cognitive impairment.
Casati et al.	2019	Experimental research design	The relationship between Vitamin E forms and leukocyte telomere length (LTL) in AD was explored for the purpose of knowing its effect on MCI. Vitamin E forms (α-, β-, γ- and δ-tocopherol, α-, β-, γ- and δ-tocotrienol), the ratio of α-tocopherylquinone/α-tocopherol and 5-nitro-γ-tocopherol/γ-tocopherol (markers of oxidative/nitrosative damage) and LTL were measured in 53 AD subjects and 40 cognitively healthy controls (CTs).	People suffering from AD found to have lower concentrations of α-, β-, γ- and δ-tocopherol, α- and δ-tocotrienol, total tocopherols, total tocotrienols, and total vitamin E compared to CTs.	Not available, since this study utilized telomere length as an indicator	The study suggests that Vitamin E deficiency may be playing a role in AD pathology in progressing MCI to AD.

References

1. World Health Organization (WHO). WHO Dementia. Available online: https://www.who.int/news-room/fact-sheets/detail/dementia (accessed on 20 November 2020).
2. Alzheimer Association. Mild Cognitive Impairment. 2020. Available online: https://www.alz.org/alzheimers-dementia/what-is-dementia/related_conditions/mild-cognitive-impairment (accessed on 21 September 2020).
3. Roberts, R.O.; Knopman, D.S.; Mielke, M.M.; Cha, R.H.; Pankratz, V.S.; Christianson, T.J.; Geda, Y.E.; Boeve, B.F.; Ivnik, R.J.; Tangalos, E.G.; et al. Higher risk of progression to dementia in mild cognitive impairment cases who revert to normal. *Neurology* **2014**, *82*, 317–325. [CrossRef]
4. American Academy of Neurology. Update, Mild Cognitive Impairment. Available online: https://www.aan.com/ (accessed on 19 May 2020).
5. Sosa, A.L.; Albanese, E.; Stephan, B.; Dewey, M.; Acosta, D.; Ferri, C.; Guerra, M.; Huang, Y.; Jacob, K.S.; Jiménez-Velázquez, I.Z.; et al. Prevalence, distribution, and impact of mild cognitive impairment in Latin America, China, and India: A 10/66 population-based study. *PLoS Med.* **2012**, *9*, e1001170. [CrossRef] [PubMed]
6. Das, S.K.; Bose, P.; Biswas, A.; Dutt, A.; Banerjee, T.K.; Hazra, A.; Raut, D.K.; Chaudhuri, A.; Roy, T. An epidemiologic study of mild cognitive impairment in Kolkata, India. *Neurology* **2007**, *68*, 2019–2026. [CrossRef] [PubMed]
7. Li, J.; Wang, Y.J.; Zhang, M.; Xu, Z.Q.; Gao, C.Y.; Fang, C.Q.; Yan, J.C.; Zhou, H.D. Vascular risk factors promote conversion from mild cognitive impairment to Alzheimer disease. *Neurology* **2011**, *76*, 1485–1491. [CrossRef] [PubMed]
8. Lee, L.K.; Shahar, S.; Chin, A.-V.; Yusoff, N.A.M.; Rajab, N.; Aziz, S.A. Prevalence of gender disparities and predictors affecting the occurrence of mild cognitive impairment (MCI). *Arch. Gerontol. Geriatr.* **2012**, *54*, 185–191. [CrossRef] [PubMed]
9. Kim, K.W.; Park, J.H.; Kim, M.-H.; Kim, M.D.; Kim, B.-J.; Kim, S.-K.; Kim, J.L.; Moon, S.W.; Bae, J.N.; Woo, J.I.; et al. A nationwide survey on the prevalence of dementia and mild cognitive impairment in South Korea. *J. Alzheimer's Dis.* **2011**, *23*, 281–291. [CrossRef]
10. Hale, J.M.; Schneider, D.C.; Mehta, N.K.; Myrskylä, M. Cognitive impairment in the U.S.: Lifetime risk, age at onset, and years impaired. *SSM—Popul. Healh* **2020**, *11*, 100577. [CrossRef]

11. Katz, M.J.; Lipton, R.B.; Hall, C.; Zimmerman, M.E.; Sanders, A.E.; Verghese, J.; Dickson, D.W.; Derby, C.A. Age-specific and sex-specific prevalence and incidence of mild cognitive impairment, dementia, and Alzheimer dementia in blacks and whites: A report from the einstein aging study. *Alzheimer Dis. Assoc. Disord.* **2012**, *26*, 335–343. [CrossRef]
12. McDougall, G.J., Jr.; Vaughan, P.W.; Acee, T.W.; Becker, H. Memory performance and mild cognitive impairment in Black and White community elders. *Ethn. Dis.* **2007**, *17*, 381–388.
13. Langa, K.M.; Levine, D.A. The diagnosis and management of mild cognitive impairment: A clinical review. *JAMA* **2014**, *312*, 2551–2561. [CrossRef]
14. Murman, D.L. The impact of age on cognition. *Semin. Hear.* **2015**, *36*, 111–121. [CrossRef] [PubMed]
15. Teng, E.; Tassniyom, K.; Lu, P.H. Reduced quality-of-life ratings in mild cognitive impairment: Analyses of subject and informant responses. *Am. J. Geriatr. Psychiatry* **2012**, *20*, 1016–1025. [CrossRef] [PubMed]
16. Connors, M.H.; Seeher, K.; Teixeira-Pinto, A.; Woodward, M.; Ames, D.; Brodaty, H. Mild cognitive impairment and caregiver burden: A 3-year-longitudinal study. *Am. J. Geriatr. Psychiatry* **2019**, *27*, 1206–1215. [CrossRef] [PubMed]
17. Eshkoor, S.A.; Mun, C.Y.; Ng, C.K.; Hamid, T.A. Mild cognitive impairment and its management in older people. *Clin. Interv. Aging* **2015**, *10*, 687–693. [CrossRef]
18. Vega, J.; Newhouse, P.A. Mild cognitive impairment: Diagnosis, longitudinal course, and emerging treatments. *Curr. Psychiatry Rep.* **2014**, *16*, 490. [CrossRef] [PubMed]
19. Farina, N.; Llewellyn, D.; Isaac, M.G.E.K.N.; Tabet, N. Vitamin E for Alzheimer's dementia and mild cognitive impairment. *Cochrane Database Syst. Rev.* **2017**, *4*, CD002854. [CrossRef]
20. Wu, A.; Ying, Z.; Gomez-Pinilla, F. Vitamin E protects against oxidative damage and learning disability after mild traumatic brain injury in rats. *Neurorehabilit. Neural Repair* **2009**, *24*, 290–298. [CrossRef]
21. Huang, Q.; Aluise, C.D.; Joshi, G.; Sultana, R.; Clair, D.K.S.; Markesbery, W.R.; Butterfield, D.A. Potential in vivo amelioration by N-acetyl-L-cysteine of oxidative stress in brain in human double mutant APP/PS-1 knock-in mice: Toward therapeutic modulation of mild cognitive impairment. *J. Neurosci. Res.* **2010**, *88*, 2618–2629. [CrossRef]
22. Alzoubi, K.H.; Khabour, O.F.; Salah, H.A.; Hasan, Z. Vitamin E prevents high-fat high-carbohydrates diet-induced memory impairment: The role of oxidative stress. *Physiol. Behav.* **2013**, *119*, 72–78. [CrossRef]
23. Giraldo, E.; Lloret, A.; Fuchsberger, T.; Vina, J. Aβ and tau toxicities in Alzheimer's are linked via oxidative stress-induced p38 activation: Protective role of vitamin E. *Redox Biol.* **2014**, *2*, 873–877. [CrossRef]
24. Nesari, A.; Mansouri, M.T.; Khodayar, M.J.; Rezaei, M. Preadministration of high-dose alpha-tocopherol improved memory impairment and mitochondrial dysfunction induced by proteasome inhibition in rat hippocampus. *Nutr. Neurosci.* **2021**, *24*, 119–129. [CrossRef]
25. Mehrabadi, S.; Sadr, S.S. Administration of Vitamin D3 and E supplements reduces neuronal loss and oxidative stress in a model of rats with Alzheimer's disease. *Neurol. Res.* **2020**, *42*, 862–868. [CrossRef]
26. Iuliano, L.; Monticolo, R.; Straface, G.; Spoletini, I.; Gianni, W.; Caltagirone, C.; Bossu, P.; Spalletta, G. Vitamin E and enzymatic/oxidative stress-driven oxysterols in amnestic mild cognitive impairment subtypes and Alzheimer's disease. *J. Alzheimer's Dis.* **2010**, *21*, 1383–1392. [CrossRef]
27. Whitehair, D.C.; Sherzai, A.; Emond, J.; Raman, R.; Aisen, P.S.; Petersen, R.C.; Fleisher, A.S. Alzheimer's disease cooperative study influence of apolipoprotein E ε4 on rates of cognitive and functional decline in mild cognitive impairment. *Alzheimer's Dement.* **2010**, *6*, 412–419. [CrossRef] [PubMed]
28. Mangialasche, F.; Xu, W.; Kivipelto, M.; Costanzi, E.; Ercolani, S.; Pigliautile, M.; Cecchetti, R.; Baglioni, M.; Simmons, A.; Soininen, H.; et al. Tocopherols and tocotrienols plasma levels are associated with cognitive impairment. *Neurobiol. Aging* **2012**, *33*, 2282–2290. [CrossRef] [PubMed]
29. Mangialasche, F.; Solomon, A.; Kåreholt, I.; Hooshmand, B.; Cecchetti, R.; Fratiglioni, L.; Soininen, H.; Laatikainen, T.; Mecocci, P.; Kivipelto, M. Serum levels of vitamin E forms and risk of cognitive impairment in a Finnish cohort of older adults. *Exp. Gerontol.* **2013**, *48*, 1428–1435. [CrossRef] [PubMed]
30. Shahar, S.; Lee, L.K.; Rajab, N.; Lim, C.L.; Harun, N.A.; Noh, M.F.N.M.; Mian-Then, S.; Jamal, R. Association between vitamin A, vitamin E and apolipoprotein E status with mild cognitive impairment among elderly people in low-cost residential areas. *Nutr. Neurosci.* **2013**, *16*, 6–12. [CrossRef]
31. Dysken, M.W.; Sano, M.; Asthana, S.; Vertrees, J.E.; Pallaki, M.; Llorente, M.; Love, S.; Schellenberg, G.D.; McCarten, J.R.; Malphurs, J.; et al. Effect of vitamin E and memantine on functional decline in Alzheimer disease: The TEAM-AD VA cooperative randomized trial. *JAMA* **2014**, *311*, 33–44. [CrossRef]
32. Zanotta, D.; Puricelli, S.; Bonoldi, G. Cognitive effects of a dietary supplement made from extract of *Bacopa monnieri*, astaxanthin, phosphatidylserine, and vitamin E in subjects with mild cognitive impairment: A noncomparative, exploratory clinical study. *Neuropsychiatr. Dis. Treat.* **2014**, *10*, 225–230. [CrossRef]
33. Naeini, A.M.A.; Elmadfa, I.; Djazayery, A.; Barekatain, M.; Ghazvini, M.R.A.; Djalali, M.; Feizi, A. The effect of antioxidant vitamins E and C on cognitive performance of the elderly with mild cognitive impairment in Isfahan, Iran: A double-blind, randomized, placebo-controlled trial. *Eur. J. Nutr.* **2013**, *53*, 1255–1262. [CrossRef]
34. De Beaumont, L.; Pelleieux, S.; Lamarre-Theroux, L.; Dea, D.; Poirier, J. Butyrylcholinesterase K and apolipoprotein E-ε4 reduce the age of onset of Alzheimer's disease, accelerate cognitive decline, and modulate donepezil response in mild cognitively impaired subjects. *J. Alzheimer's Dis.* **2016**, *54*, 913–922. [CrossRef] [PubMed]

35. Basambombo, L.L.; Carmichael, P.-H.; Côté, S.; Laurin, D. Use of vitamin E and C supplements for the prevention of cognitive decline. *Ann. Pharmacother.* **2016**, *51*, 118–124. [CrossRef] [PubMed]
36. Liu, G.; Zhao, Y.; Jin, S.; Hu, Y.; Wang, T.; Tian, R.; Han, Z.; Xu, D.; Jiang, Q. Circulating vitamin E levels and Alzheimer's disease: A mendelian randomization study. *Neurobiol. Aging* **2018**, *72*, 189-e1. [CrossRef] [PubMed]
37. Li, Y.; Liu, S.; Man, Y.; Li, N.; Zhou, Y.U. Effects of vitamins E and C combined with β-carotene on cognitive function in the elderly. *Exp. Ther. Med.* **2015**, *9*, 1489–1493. [CrossRef]
38. Edmonds, E.C.; Ard, M.C.; Edland, S.D.; Galasko, D.R.; Salmon, D.P.; Bondi, M.W. Unmasking the benefits of donepezil via psychometrically precise identification of mild cognitive impairment: A secondary analysis of the ADCS vitamin E and donepezil in MCI study. *Alzheimer's Dement.* **2018**, *4*, 11–18. [CrossRef] [PubMed]
39. Casati, M.; Boccardi, V.; Ferri, E.; Bertagnoli, L.; Bastiani, P.; Ciccone, S.; Mansi, M.; Scamosci, M.; Rossi, P.D.; Mecocci, P.; et al. Vitamin E and Alzheimer's disease: The mediating role of cellular aging. *Aging Clin. Exp. Res.* **2019**, *32*, 459–464. [CrossRef]
40. Kim, S.H.; Park, Y.M.; Choi, B.Y.; Kim, M.K.; Roh, S.; Kim, K.; Yang, Y.J. Associations of serum levels of vitamins A, C, and E with the risk of cognitive impairment among elderly Koreans. *Nutr. Res. Pract.* **2018**, *12*, 160–165. [CrossRef]
41. McDougall, M.; Choi, J.; Magnusson, K.; Truong, L.; Tanguay, R.; Traber, M.G. Chronic vitamin E deficiency impairs cognitive function in adult zebrafish via dysregulation of brain lipids and energy metabolism. *Free Radic. Biol. Med.* **2017**, *112*, 308–317. [CrossRef]
42. Pace, A.; Savarese, A.; Picardo, M.; Maresca, V.; Pacetti, U.; Del Monte, G.; Biroccio, A.; Leonetti, C.; Jandolo, B.; Cognetti, F.; et al. Neuroprotective effect of vitamin E supplementation in patients teated with cisplatin chemotherapy. *J. Clin. Oncol.* **2003**, *21*, 927–931. [CrossRef]
43. Gugliandolo, A.; Bramanti, P.; Mazzon, E. Role of vitamin E in the treatment of Alzheimer's disease: Evidence from animal models. *Int. J. Mol. Sci.* **2017**, *18*, 2504. [CrossRef] [PubMed]
44. La Torre, M.E.; Villano, I.; Monda, M.; Messina, A.; Cibelli, G.; Valenzano, A.; Pisanelli, D.; Panaro, M.A.; Tartaglia, N.; Ambrosi, A.; et al. Role of vitamin E and the orexin system in neuroprotection. *Brain Sci.* **2021**, *11*, 1098. [CrossRef] [PubMed]
45. Kaneai, N.; Arai, M.; Takatsu, H.; Fukui, K.; Urano, S. Vitamin E inhibits oxidative stress-induced denaturation of nerve terminal proteins involved in neurotransmission. *J. Alzheimer's Dis.* **2012**, *28*, 183–189. [CrossRef] [PubMed]
46. La Fata, G.; Weber, P.; Mohajeri, M.H. Effects of vitamin E on cognitive performance during ageing and in Alzheimer's disease. *Nutrients* **2014**, *6*, 5453–5472. [CrossRef] [PubMed]
47. Lloret, A.; Badía, M.-C.; Mora, N.J.; Pallardó, F.V.; Alonso, M.-D.; Viña, J. Vitamin E paradox in Alzheimer's disease: It does not prevent loss of cognition and may even be detrimental. *J. Alzheimer's Dis.* **2009**, *17*, 143–149. [CrossRef]

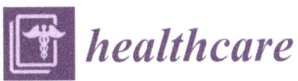

Systematic Review

Correction of Breech Presentation with Moxibustion and Acupuncture: A Systematic Review and Meta-Analysis

Jian-An Liao [1], Shih-Chieh Shao [2,3,4], Chian-Ting Chang [2], Pony Yee-Chee Chai [2], Kok-Loon Owang [2], Tse-Hung Huang [1], Chung-Han Yang [4,5], Tsai-Jen Lee [1] and Yung-Chih Chen [4,6,*]

[1] Department of Traditional Chinese Medicine, Keelung Chang Gung Memorial Hospital, Keelung 204, Taiwan; frank771124@cgmh.org.tw (J.-A.L.); kchuang@cgmh.org.tw (T.-H.H.); cs8336@gmail.com (T.-J.L.)

[2] Department of Pharmacy, Keelung Chang Gung Memorial Hospital, Keelung 204, Taiwan; s.c.shao@hotmail.com (S.-C.S.); rrrctc@cgmh.org.tw (C.-T.C.); ponychai@cgmh.org.tw (P.Y.-C.C.); thenight_eve@hotmail.com (K.-L.O.)

[3] School of Pharmacy, Institute of Clinical Pharmacy and Pharmaceutical Sciences, College of Medicine, National Cheng Kung University, Tainan 701, Taiwan

[4] Center of Evidence-Based Medicine, Keelung Chang Gung Memorial Hospital, Keelung 204, Taiwan; dr3939@gmail.com

[5] Division of Rheumatology, Allergy, and Immunology, Department of Internal Medicine, Linkou Chang Gung Memorial Hospital, Taoyuan 333, Taiwan

[6] Division of General Internal Medicine, Department of Internal Medicine, Keelung Chang Gung Memorial Hospital, Keelung 204, Taiwan

* Correspondence: yungchihc@gmail.com; Tel.: +886-2-24329292

Abstract: Acupuncture-type interventions (such as moxibustion and acupuncture) at Bladder 67 (BL67, Zhiyin point) have been proposed to have positive effects on breech presentation. The aim of this systematic review and meta-analysis was to evaluate the effectiveness and safety of moxibustion and acupuncture in correcting breech presentation. We searched PubMed, MEDLINE, Embase, the Cochrane Central Register of Controlled Trials (CENTRAL), the Chinese Electronic Periodical Services (CEPS), and databases at ClinicalTrials.gov to identify relevant randomized controlled trials (RCTs). In this study, sixteen RCTs involving 2555 participants were included. Compared to control, moxibustion significantly increased cephalic presentation at birth (RR = 1.39; 95% CI = 1.21–1.58). Moxibustion also seemed to elicit better clinical outcomes in the Asian population (RR = 1.42; 95% CI = 1.21–1.67) than in the non-Asian population (RR = 1.20; 95% CI = 1.01–1.43). The effects of acupuncture on correcting breech presentation after sensitivity analysis were inconsistent relative to control. The effect of moxibustion plus acupuncture was synergistic for correcting breech presentation (RR = 1.53; 95% CI = 1.26–1.86) in one RCT. Our findings suggest that moxibustion therapy has positive effects on correcting breech presentation, especially in the Asian population.

Keywords: breech; pregnancy; maternal and prenatal health; moxibustion; acupuncture; systematic review; meta-analysis

1. Introduction

Breech presentation is a common malposition in the third trimester of pregnancy. The frequency of breech presentation in term pregnancies is 3%–4% in America and approximately 2% in China [1,2]. Risk factors for breech presentation include preterm labor, uterine anomaly, multiparity, placenta previa, and polyhydramnios [3]. Serious complications, such as traumatic injuries or asphyxia, can occur during vaginal delivery [4]. Therefore, a planned Caesarean section is recommended for pregnant women with breech presentation at childbirth [3]. However, Caesarean section is not free from complications, including wound infection, adhesions, hemorrhage, or scar rupture during subsequent labor [5]. Some non-invasive therapies are available, including knee-chest position management and external cephalic version (ECV). However, there is insufficient evidence to support knee-chest position management, and ECV is a painful procedure for pregnant women [6,7].

Moxibustion and acupuncture have a long history in the treatment of various problems, including fetal malposition. The interventions are similar because they both stimulate acupoints to achieve a therapeutic effect. Moxibustion is a traditional Chinese procedure that utilizes the heat generated from a burning moxa stick (made from herbal preparations containing *Artemisia vulgaris*) to stimulate acupuncture points [8,9]. Several clinical trials have shown that moxibustion at Bladder 67 (BL67), also known as the Zhiyin point, elicits positive effects on breech presentation without serious adverse events [10,11]. However, systematic reviews and meta-analysis have reported conflicting results regarding the effects of moxibustion on breech presentation. For example, Vas et al. [12] and Li et al. [13] reported that moxibustion has positive effects on non-vertex presentation. However, Coyle et al. [14] suggested that moxibustion treatment may not improve non-cephalic presentations at birth relative to no treatment. To determine the efficacy of moxibustion on breech presentation, additional clinical trials since 2012 have investigated the effects of moxibustion [15,16]. Acupuncture has also been reported to correct fetal malposition, although evidence from systematic reviews and meta-analysis is lacking [17]. To fill this research gap, we conducted an updated systematic review and meta-analysis to evaluate the effects and safety of these acupuncture-type interventions in correcting breech presentation.

2. Materials and Methods

This systematic review and meta-analysis study are reported in accordance with the statement of preferred reporting items for systematic reviews and meta-analysis (PRISMA). The protocol was registered on PROSPERO with a registration number: CRD42020192572.

2.1. Search Strategy

In this systematic review, we included all RCTs on the use of acupuncture-type interventions (i.e., moxibustion and acupuncture) in the management of breech presentation, regardless of whether the RCTs were blinded. We performed literature searches in PubMed, MEDLINE, Embase, the Cochrane Central Register of Controlled Trials (CENTRAL), the Chinese Electronic Periodical Services (CEPS), and databases at ClinicalTrials.gov from the inception of the source to 31 January 2021. Keywords for literature search included "breech," "labor presentation," "acupuncture," "electroacupuncture," "acupressure," and "moxibustion." We explored our literature search with MeSH headings without restrictions of language, publication type, or date. We applied a filter to narrow the number of articles which fit the specific study type (e.g., RCTs) and study question (e.g., intervention). The details of the search strategy are presented in Supplementary Materials (Table S1). We also searched the reference lists of included studies and related articles in PubMed and clinical trial databases to identify relevant RCTs.

2.2. Study Selection and Data Extraction

We selected eligible studies based on the following inclusion criteria: (1) the study was an RCT; (2) pregnant women in the 28th–35th week of gestation with a normal pregnancy and an ultrasound diagnosis of breech (non-vertex) presentation were included; (3) the interventions consisted of moxibustion alone, traditional acupuncture or electro-acupuncture alone, or moxibustion and acupuncture; (4) comparisons between interventions and control measures (e.g., observation, usual care, or knee-chest position) were conducted; and (5) outcome measures (e.g., fetal presentation at birth and adverse events) were reported. Studies were excluded based on the following criteria: (1) the study was non-randomized, quasi-experimental, observational, qualitative, or did not involve human subjects; (2) had wrong or no comparators; or (3) had incomplete outcome data. Two authors independently selected articles according to the inclusion and exclusion criteria by screening the titles, abstracts, and full texts of included studies. We extracted the following information from studies that met the inclusion criteria: study characteristics (e.g., author, publication year, study design and settings, inclusion/exclusion criteria, methods of randomization), participant characteristics (age, gender, co-morbidities), interventions (types, duration), comparisons (types of control groups) and outcomes (types of outcome measures, adverse events). We retrieved data from individual studies having an intention-to-treat principle. Any disagreements about whether to include a study were resolved by a third reviewer.

2.3. Assessment of the Risk of Bias in Included Studies

Two authors independently assessed the methodological quality of each included clinical trial, according to the Cochrane risk of bias tool for randomized controlled trials (RoB 2.0) [18]. RoB 2.0 is composed of five domains, including bias arising from the randomization process (allocation), bias due to deviations from the intended interventions (performance), bias due to missing outcome data (follow-up), bias in the outcome measurement (measurement), and bias in the selection of the reported results (reporting). The authors rated each domain as either low risk, some concerns (uncertain risk of bias), or high risk. Discrepancies were resolved by the third reviewer.

2.4. Data Synthesis and Statistical Analysis

We compared moxibustion with control, acupuncture with control, and moxibustion plus acupuncture with control. The primary outcome was the fetal presentation at birth, and the secondary outcome was adverse events.

Data were analyzed using Review Manager Software (version 5.3.5). Dichotomous outcomes were extracted from each study to compute the RR with a 95% CI. The pooled RR and the associated 95% CI were estimated by the Mantel-Haenszel method. Numbers needed to treat (NNT) were calculated from the formula (NNT = 1/absolute risk reduction). We assessed clinical heterogeneity by comparing the methodologies and study designs of the included studies. Statistical heterogeneity of effect sizes between studies was assessed using the I^2 statistic and Q statistic with an X^2 test. We defined statistical heterogeneity using $p \leq 0.1$ for the X^2 test or $I^2 \geq 50\%$. In the meta-analysis, a fixed-effect model was performed when there was no significant heterogeneity, and a random-effects model was performed when the heterogeneity was significant. A funnel plot was produced to detect possible publication bias. Sensitivity analysis was performed to test the robustness of results by excluding trials that used low-quality methodologies. To assess between-group differences and explain heterogeneity, we carried out a subgroup analysis. Because regional differences may exist, we reported treatment effects on breech presentation separately.

3. Results
3.1. Study Selection and Characteristics

We identified 198 studies using our search strategy and included 16 studies based on our inclusion and exclusion criteria. We summarize the process of study identification and selection in Figure 1, and present the characteristics of each of the included studies in Table 1. All included studies were randomized controlled trials. The size of the study populations ranged from 20 to 406 persons. The 16 studies included a total of 2555 participants; eight studies included participants from China [10,11,19–24], two studies included participants from Italy [25,26], and the others included participants from France [27], Australia [28], Switzerland [29], Croatia [17], Denmark [16], and Spain [15]. Most studies were published in English (56.3%); others were published in Chinese (37.5%) and French (6.2%).

Regarding study interventions, 13 RCTs compared moxibustion with control [10,11,15,16,19,21–25,27–29]; two RCTs compared acupuncture with control [17,22]; two RCTs compared moxibustion plus acupuncture with control [20,26]. Treatment was applied to BL67 in all included studies. The duration of each intervention was distinct from study to study. The typical application time of moxibustion or acupuncture was 15–20 min. The treatment sessions were typically conducted over 7–14 days. The gestational age was different among studies, ranging from 28 to 37 weeks, when acupuncture or/and moxibustion was performed.

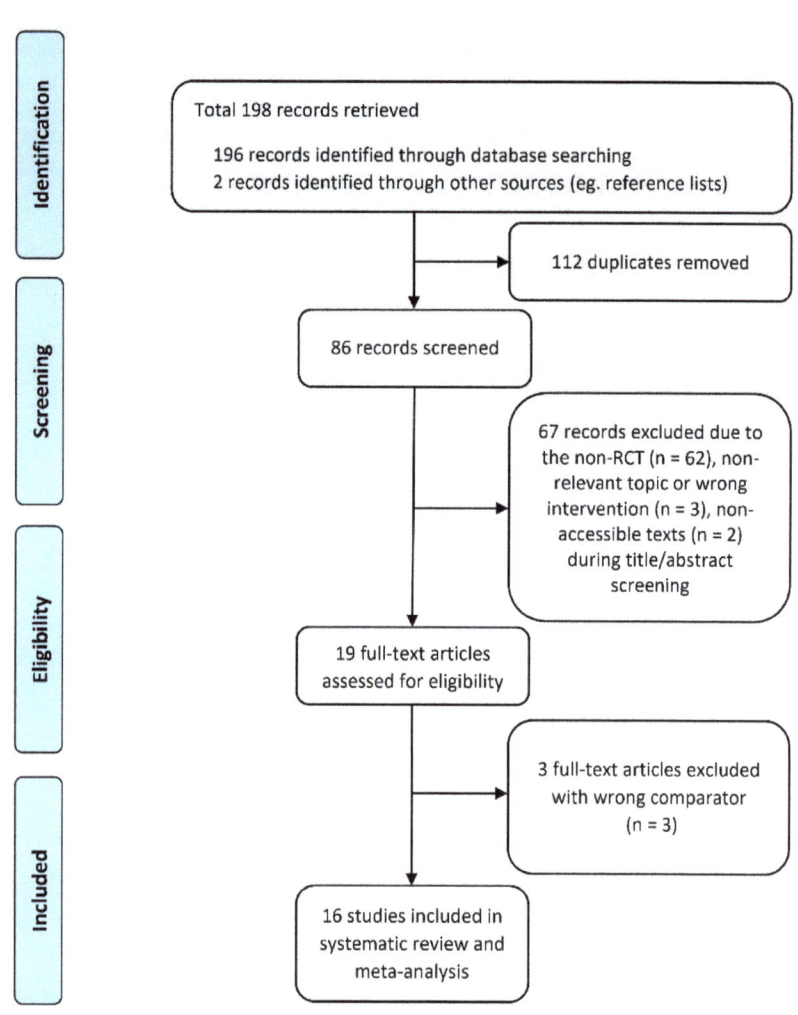

Figure 1. Flow chart of the identification and selection of studies for inclusion.

Table 1. Characteristics of the included studies.

Study	Study Design	Patient Population	Intervention	Control	Outcomes
Bue 2016 [16]	RCT	200	Moxibustion at BL67; daily for 15–20 mins, preferably in the evening; 14 days	Observation	Cephalic presentation; rate of ECV and Cesarean delivery
Cardini 1998 [10]	RCT	260	Moxibustion at bilateral BL67; 15 mins on each side; 7 days	Observation	Cephalic presentation; Cesarean delivery rate
Cardini 2005 [25]	RCT	123	Moxibustion at BL67; 15 mins; twice daily; 7 days	Observation	Cephalic presentation

Table 1. Cont.

Study	Study Design	Patient Population	Intervention	Control	Outcomes
Chen 2004 [23]	RCT	142	Moxibustion at BL67; twice daily, 10–15 mins each time; up to 14 days	Observation and knee-chest position	Cephalic presentation
Chen 2007 [21]	RCT	150	Moxibustion at bilateral BL67; 20 mins a day; up to 15 days	Knee-chest position	Cephalic presentation
Do 2011 [28]	RCT	20	Moxibustion at bilateral BL67; 10 mins on each side; 10 days	Observation	Cephalic presentation
Guittier 2009 [29]	RCT	212	Moxibustion at bilateral BL67; 10 mins on each side; 14 days	Observation	Cephalic presentation
Habek 2003 [17]	RCT	67	Acupuncture at BL67; 30 mins; twice a week	Observation	Cephalic presentation; Cesarean delivery rate
Li 1996 [22]	RCT	111	Electro-acupuncture at bilateral BL67; 30 mins; 6 days Moxibustion at bilateral BL67; 20 mins; 6 days	Observation	Cephalic presentation
Lin 2002 [24]	RCT	122	Moxibustion at bilateral BL67; twice daily for 20 mins	Knee-chest position	Cephalic presentation
Millereau 2009 [27]	RCT	68	Moxibustion at BL67; 15–20 mins; 7 days	Observation	Cephalic presentation
Neri 2004 [26]	RCT	240	Moxibustion plus acupuncture at bilateral BL 67; total 40 mins; twice a week; 14 days	Observation	Cephalic presentation; Cesarean section rate
Vas 2013 [15]	RCT	406	Moxibustion at bilateral BL67; 20 mins; 14 days	Observation	Cephalic presentation; Cesarean delivery rate
Yang 2006 [11]	RCT	206	Moxibustion at BL67; 15–20 mins; 7 days	Knee-chest position	Cephalic presentation
Yang 2008 [19]	RCT	226	Moxibustion at bilateral BL67; 15 mins; up to 14 days	Knee-chest position	Cephalic presentation
Yang 2010 [20]	RCT	120	Moxibustion plus acupuncture at bilateral BL67; once daily; 14 days	Knee-chest position	Cephalic presentation

BL67: Bladder67 (Zhiyin point), ECV: external cephalic version, RCT: randomized controlled trials.

3.2. Methodological Quality of Included Studies

The risk of bias for included studies is shown in Figures 2 and 3. All studies were assessed as having low or uncertain levels of risk of bias, except in the domains of allocation and follow-up. We present the details of the risk of bias assessment in Supplementary Materials (Table S2). In general, the quality was moderate in all included studies, except for four studies [20,22,23,25] that were assessed as having a high risk of bias in the domain of either allocation or follow-up.

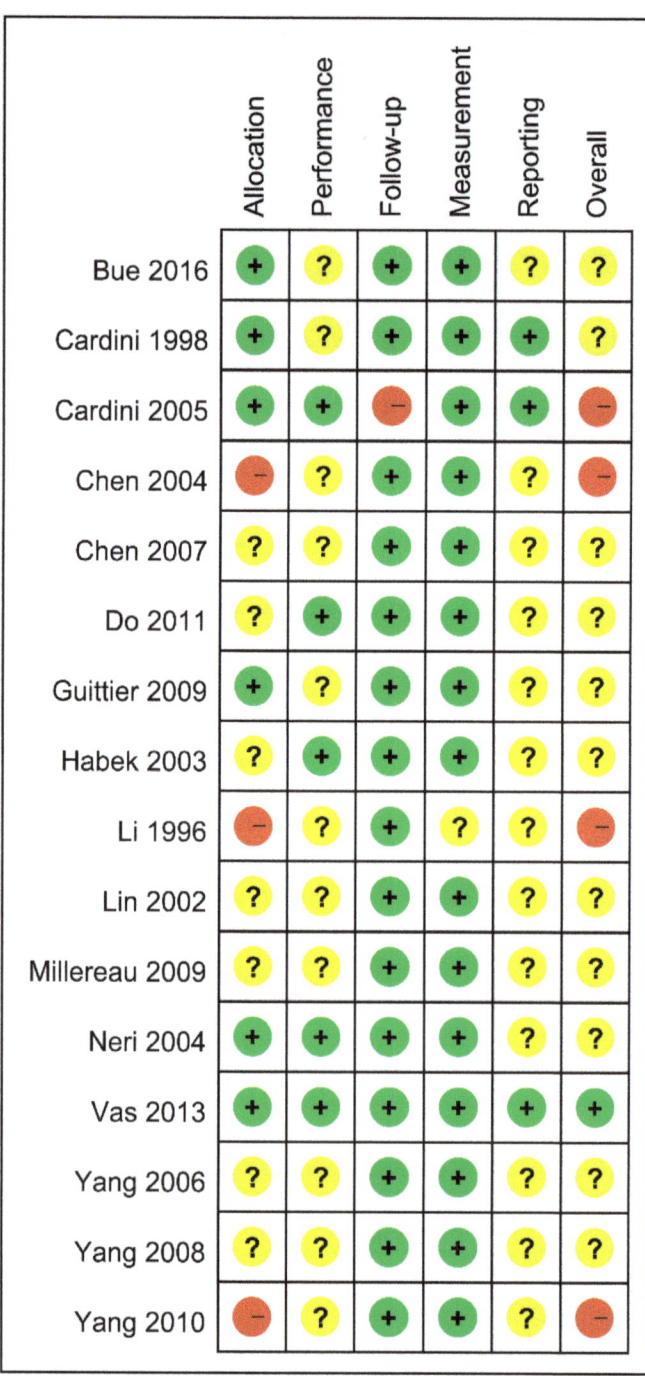

Figure 2. Methodological quality summary: reviews authors' judgement on each methodological quality item for each included study.

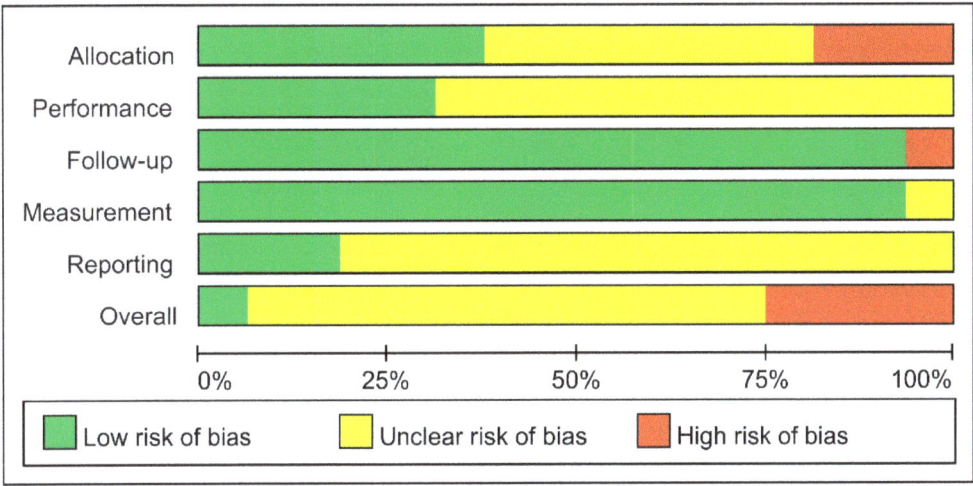

Figure 3. Methodological quality graph: reviews authors' judgement on each methodological quality item presented as percentage for each included study.

3.3. Efficacy of Interventions

The meta-analysis of the included studies revealed a beneficial effect of acupuncture-type interventions on correcting breech presentation at delivery (average RR = 1.45; 95% CI = 1.28–1.65; random effect model, $I^2 = 66\%$) (Figure 4). The forest plot was divided into three subgroups: (1) moxibustion, (2) acupuncture, and (3) moxibustion plus acupuncture.

Fetal presentation was investigated in the results of 13 studies with 2063 participants comparing moxibustion with control [10,11,15,16,19,21–25,27–29]. The pooled data show a significant increase in cephalic presentation at birth (RR = 1.39; 95% CI = 1.21–1.58; random effect model, I2 = 64%). The NNT is 6 (95% CI = 4–11).

Two clinical trials involving 146 patients compared acupuncture with control [17,22]. The meta-analysis reveals no differences between treatment and control groups (RR = 2.78; 95% CI = 0.84–9.19; random effect model, I2 = 85%).

Pooled data from two trials with 346 participants reveals significant difference between moxibustion plus acupuncture and control groups in the meta-analysis [20,26] (RR = 1.53; 95% CI = 1.26–1.86; random effect model, I2 = 0%). The NNT is 5 (95% CI = 3–9).

3.4. Sensitivity Analysis: Excluding Four Trials with a High Risk of Bias

Limiting the meta-analysis to the 12 trials with moderate to low risk of bias [10,11,15–17,19,21,24,26–29] which investigated the effects of acupuncture-type interventions including moxibustion, acupuncture, and moxibustion plus acupuncture reveal significant effects on correcting fetal malposition (RR = 1.36; 95% CI = 1.23–1.51; random effect model, $I^2 = 41\%$) (Figure 5). The sensitivity analysis for the moxibustion subgroup reveals a result like that of the previous analysis (RR = 1.34; 95% CI = 1.19–1.51; random effect model, $I^2 = 47\%$). The NNT is 7 (95% CI = 5–12). Only one trial that evaluated acupuncture versus control shows more cephalic presentation in the acupuncture group (RR = 1.68; 95% CI = 1.11–2.55). The NNT is 4 (95% CI = 2–20). Only one trial reports that moxibustion plus acupuncture had more cephalic presentation relative to control (RR = 1.42; 95% CI = 1.06–1.90). The NNT is 7 (95% CI = 3–45).

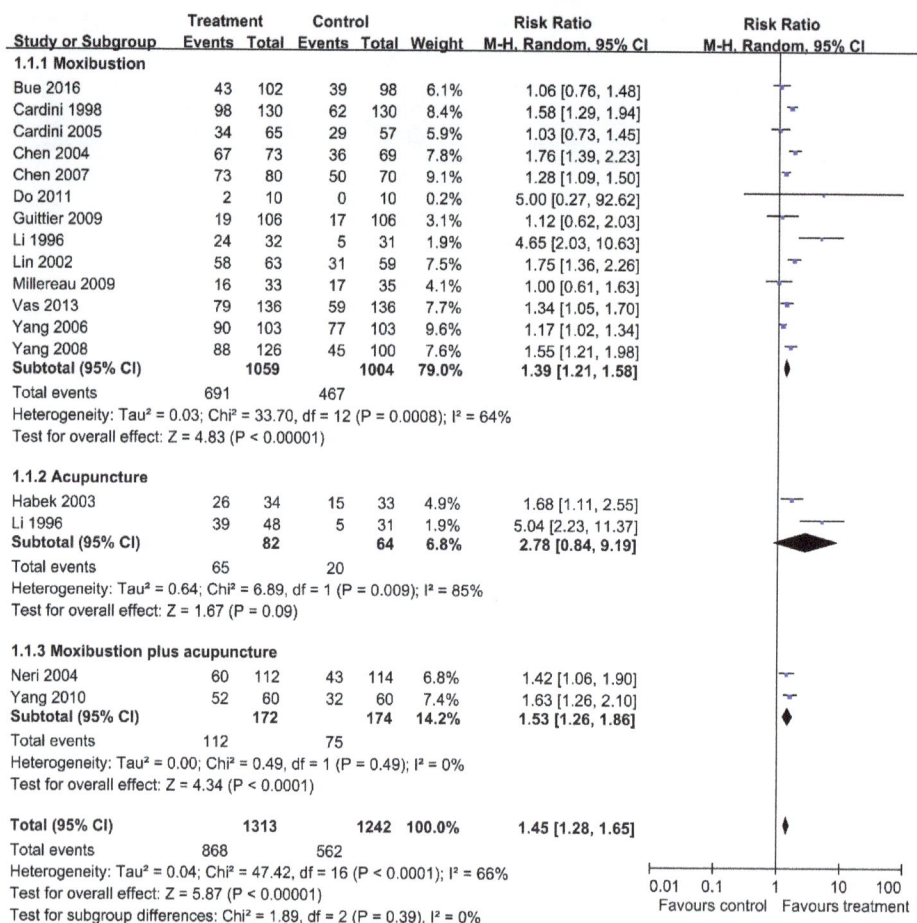

Figure 4. Forest plot of each comparison: Acupuncture-type interventions versus Control; Outcome: Cephalic presentation.

3.5. Subgroup Analysis of Moxibustion

Moxibustion is effective in the Asian population (RR = 1.42; 95% CI = 1.21–1.67; random effect model, I^2 = 71%) and in the non-Asian population (RR = 1.20; 95% CI = 1.01–1.43; random effect model, I^2 = 0%) (Figure 6).

3.6. Adverse Events

Information on adverse events was presented in four trials. Because of the clinical heterogeneity between the included studies, we did not perform a meta-analysis of adverse events. Cardini et al. in 2005 reported adverse events (41.5%) related to moxibustion [25]. Patients had abdominal pain, throat problems, and unpleasant odor with or without nausea. Cardini et al. in 1998 and Vas et al. reported that no adverse events occurred in the moxibustion or control groups [10,15]. Neri et al. observed no adverse effects on participants who received moxibustion plus acupuncture or usual care [26].

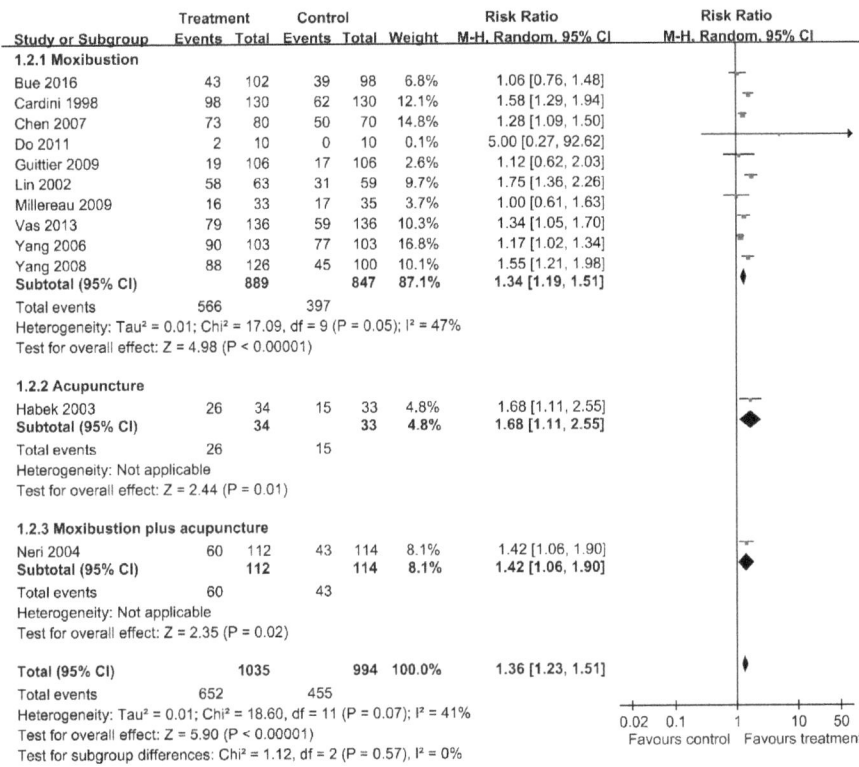

Figure 5. Sensitivity analysis: Acupuncture-type interventions versus Control; Outcome: Cephalic presentation.

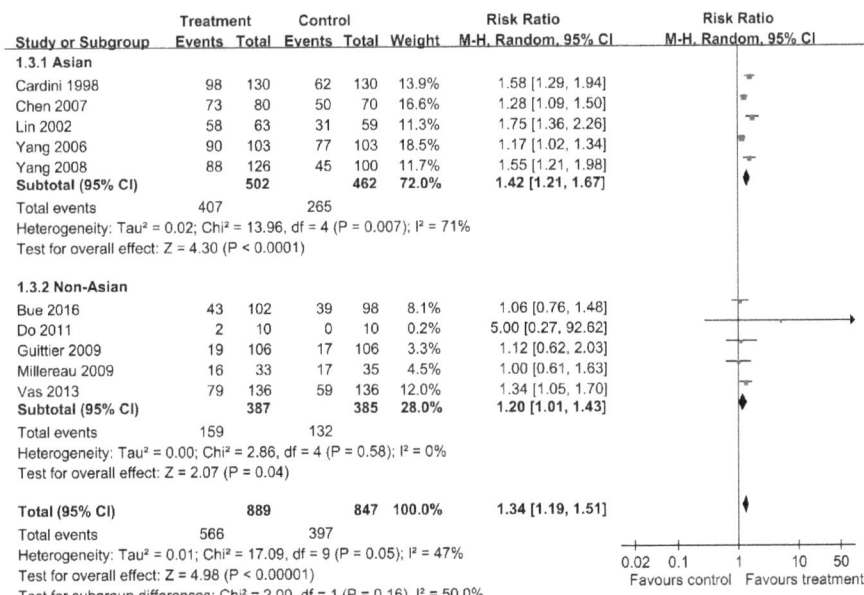

Figure 6. Subgroup analysis: Moxibustion versus Control; Outcome: Cephalic presentation.

3.7. Publication Bias

We used Review Manager Software (Version 5.3.5) to evaluate the publication bias. The sample size of most studies was >100 participants with two comparison arms except for Do 2011 [28], Li 1996 [22], and Millereau 2009 [27]. Funnel plots are typically symmetrical for studies with large sample sizes (Figure 7). However, for studies with small sample sizes, no study reported a negative result, which suggests that publication bias is probable in the literature reporting correction of breech presentation with moxibustion and acupuncture.

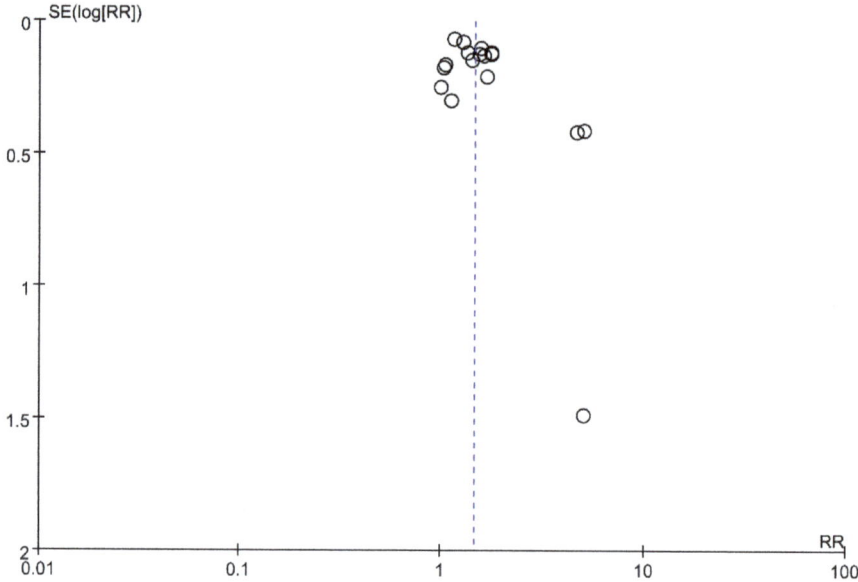

Figure 7. Funnel plot of the studies included in the meta-analysis.

4. Discussion

Our study found that acupuncture-type interventions (including moxibustion, acupuncture, and moxibustion plus acupuncture) at BL67 increase the frequency of cephalic presentation at birth. Moxibustion seemed to be more effective in correcting non-vertex presentation in the Asian population than in the non-Asian population.

Previously, Vas et al. found that moxibustion had positive effects on correcting non-vertex presentation, although they noted that there was considerable heterogeneity among studies [12]. Li et al. demonstrated that moxibustion was effective in correcting breech presentation, but non-randomized controlled trials were included in this study [13]. The results of these two studies differed from those of Coyle et al. [14], who found that moxibustion did not reduce the frequency of non-cephalic presentation relative to no treatment [14]. This discrepancy could be attributed to emerging clinical trials in recent years. In addition, Coyle et al. did not include all relevant trials, such as Chen, 2007 [21], Do, 2011 [28], Li, 1996 [22], Millereau, 2009 [27], and Yang, 2008 [19]. Our study included only RCTs that were eligible and up-to-date.

To minimize the impact of potential bias, a sensitivity analysis was performed; such an analysis was not reported as being conducted in most previous studies. After comparing the net effects of different acupuncture-type interventions before and after sensitivity analysis, a positive effect on correcting breech presentation, particularly with moxibustion alone or in combination with acupuncture, is consistent. Our findings provide robust support of the effectiveness of moxibustion on correcting breech presentation.

The mechanism of moxibustion is not fully understood. Moxibustion at BL67 is thought to stimulate the production of prostaglandin and estrogen, which increases uterus contractions that lead to fetal movements [30,31]. Traditional Chinese medicine (TCM) theory teaches that disharmony of qi and blood may cause fetal malposition. It is thought that moxibustion at BL67 tonifies Yang qi and dredges channels to correct fetal position [19,21].

Some studies suggest that the effects of treatment might be related to ethnicity [32,33]. We performed a subgroup analysis to assess differences between ethnic groups and found that moxibustion seemed to be more effective in correcting non-vertex presentation in Asians than in non-Asian populations. To the authors' best knowledge, this is the first article that investigates the effect of moxibustion on breech presentation in different races. However, the mechanism of this phenomenon is unclear.

During pregnancy, acupuncture has been hypothesized to have beneficial effects on pelvic pain or labor pain [34,35]. In TCM theory, moxibustion or acupuncture applied at BL67 is thought to activate blood circulation and dredge channels to correct fetal malposition [20]. However, there have been few studies on the use of acupuncture to treat breech presentation, and there has been no systematic review or meta-analysis in the literature to date. In our study, only two clinical trials were retrieved and included in the meta-analysis, but the risk of bias in one of those trials [22] was rated as "high." The result of the subsequent sensitivity analysis revealed that the effect of acupuncture was inconsistent. Therefore, reports on the effects of acupuncture should be interpreted with caution.

According to Coyle et al., there was a positive effect on breech presentation using moxibustion combined with acupuncture [14]. Nevertheless, only one trial was included in the meta-analysis. Our study included a new trial [20], and the result was similar. The pooled RR of moxibustion versus moxibustion plus acupuncture was 1.39 vs. 1.53 without analysis and 1.34 vs. 1.42 with sensitivity analysis. The combination of moxibustion and acupuncture appears to exert a synergistic effect on correcting breech presentation.

Previous systematic reviews included RCTs with different controls, including knee-chest position or observation [12,13]. However, one systematic review by Hofmeyr et al. found that there was no difference in cephalic presentation between knee-chest position and observation [7]. Therefore, we included clinical trials with no-effect controls, including knee-chest position and observation.

Moxibustion and acupuncture are generally safe when administrated by experienced clinicians, and both are less expensive than Caesarean section in general practice. In a study by Ineke et al., moxibustion reduced the number of Caesarean sections performed in pregnant woman with breech presentation and was cost-effective when compared to expectant management [36]. A previous study pointed out that there were no significant differences in the comparison of moxibustion with usual care, with respect to premature births or premature rupture of the membranes [12]. We performed meta-analysis of these two outcomes, and had similar results (see Supplementary Materials Figure S1). Because the use of TCM theories is increasing in many countries, the modality of using moxibustion might be more widely deemed as being beneficial in obstetric patients.

This study was limited in several aspects. First, there might be publication bias in the meta-analysis. Second, the sample sizes of some included studies were too small for RCT design. Finally, the application time of treatment (15–20 min) and treatment duration (7–14 days) differed between studies

5. Conclusions

Our updated systematic review and meta-analysis suggested that moxibustion has a positive effect on correcting breech presentation. However, more randomized, controlled clinical trials are needed to evaluate whether our estimate of the magnitude of the effect of moxibustion remains constant.

Supplementary Materials: The following are available online at https://www.mdpi.com/article/10.3390/healthcare9060619/s1, Table S1: Literature search strategy, Table S2: Summary of risk of bias assessment, Figure S1: Forest plot of comparison: Moxibustion versus Control; Outcome: Preterm delivery & Premature rupture of membranes.

Author Contributions: J.-A.L., S.-C.S. and Y.-C.C. designed this study; C.-T.C., P.Y.-C.C., K.-L.O., T.-H.H., C.-H.Y., T.-J.L. analyzed and interpreted study results. J.-A.L. and S.-C.S. were major contributors in writing the manuscript. All authors have read and agreed to the published version of the manuscript.

Funding: This research received no external funding.

Institutional Review Board Statement: Not applicable.

Informed Consent Statement: Not applicable.

Data Availability Statement: Not applicable.

Acknowledgments: We thank all researchers involved in the individual trials.

Conflicts of Interest: The authors declare no conflict of interest.

References

1. Hickok, D.E.; Gordon, D.C.; Milberg, J.A.; Williams, M.A.; Daling, J.R. The frequency of breech presentation by gestational age at birth: A large population-based study. *Am. J. Obstet. Gynecol.* **1992**, *166*, 851–852. [CrossRef]
2. Cui, H.; Chen, Y.; Li, Q.; Chen, J.; Liu, C.; Zhang, W. Cesarean Rate and Risk Factors for Singleton Breech Presentation in China. *J. Reprod. Med.* **2016**, *61*, 270–274.
3. Sharshiner, R.; Silver, R.M. Management of fetal malpresentation. *Clin. Obstet. Gynecol.* **2015**, *58*, 246–255. [CrossRef] [PubMed]
4. Kotaska, A.; Menticoglou, S.; Gagnon, R. Vaginal delivery of breech presentation. *J. Obstet. Gynaecol. Can.* **2009**, *31*, 557–566. [CrossRef]
5. Hofmeyr, G.J.; Hannah, M.; Lawrie, T.A. Planned caesarean section for term breech delivery. *Cochrane Database Syst. Rev.* **2015**, *7*, 18–20. [CrossRef] [PubMed]
6. *External Cephalic Version and Reducing the Incidence of Term Breech Presentation: Green-top Guideline No. 20a*; Royal College of Obstetricians and Gynaecologists: London, UK, 2017; Volume 124, pp. e178–e192.
7. Hofmeyr, G.J.; Kulier, R. Cephalic version by postural management for breech presentation. *Cochrane Database Syst Rev.* **2012**, *10*, 5–6. [CrossRef]
8. Deng, H.; Shen, X. The mechanism of moxibustion: Ancient theory and modern research. *Evidence Based Complementary Altern. Med.* **2013**, *2013*, 379291. [CrossRef]
9. Park, J.W.; Lee, B.H.; Lee, H. Moxibustion in the management of irritable bowel syndrome: Systematic review and meta-analysis. *BMC Complement Altern. Med.* **2013**, *13*, 247. [CrossRef]
10. Cardini, F.; Weixin, H. Moxibustion for correction of breech presentation: A randomized controlled trial. *JAMA* **1998**, *280*, 1580–1584. [CrossRef] [PubMed]
11. Yang, F.Q. Comparison of knee-chest position plus moxibustion on Zhiyin with knee-chest position for breech presentation. *J. Sichuan Tradit. Chin. Med.* **2006**, *2006*, 106–107.
12. Vas, J.; Aranda, J.M.; Nishishinya, B.; Mendez, C.; Martin, M.A.; Pons, J.; Liu, P.J.; Wang, C.Y.; Milla, P.E. Correction of nonvertex presentation with moxibustion: A systematic review and metaanalysis. *Am. J. Obstet. Gynecol.* **2009**, *201*, 241–259. [CrossRef] [PubMed]
13. Li, X.; Hu, J.; Wang, X.; Zhang, H.; Liu, J. Moxibustion and other acupuncture point stimulation methods to treat breech presentation: A systematic review of clinical trials. *Chin. Med.* **2009**, *4*, 4. [CrossRef] [PubMed]
14. Coyle, M.E.; Smith, C.A.; Peat, B. Cephalic version by moxibustion for breech presentation. *Cochrane Database Syst. Rev.* **2012**, *5*, 7–10. [CrossRef] [PubMed]
15. Vas, J.; Aranda, J.R.; Modesto, M.; Monserrat, M.; Baron, M.; Aguilar, I.; Parejo, N.; Ramirez, C.; Rivas, F. Using moxibustion in primary healthcare to correct non-vertex presentation: A multicentre randomised controlled trial. *Acupunct. Med.* **2013**, *31*, 31–38. [CrossRef]
16. Bue, L.; Lauszus, F.F. Moxibustion did not have an effect in a randomised clinical trial for version of breech position. *Dan. Med. J.* **2016**, *63*, 2–4.
17. Habek, D.; Cerkez Habek, J.; Jagust, M. Acupuncture conversion of fetal breech presentation. *Fetal. Diagn. Ther.* **2003**, *18*, 418–421. [CrossRef]
18. A Revised Tool for Assessing Risk of Bias in Randomized Trials. Available online: https://methods.cochrane.org/bias/resources/rob-2-revised-cochrane-risk-bias-tool-randomized-trials (accessed on 20 March 2021).
19. Yang, W.-W.; Zheng, W. Warm Argy Moxibustion Correct Abnormal Fetal Position 126 Cases. *J. Zhe Jiang Coll. Tradit. Chin. Med.* **2008**, *32*, 386.

20. Yang, Y.; Yin, S.C.; Syu, S.Y. Integration Treatment of Traditional Chinese Medicine and Western Medicine in Breech Presentation: A Clinical Observation of 60 Cases. *J. Shanhai Med Coll. Contin. Educ.* **2010**, *20*, 54–55.
21. Chen, Y. Moxibustion of zhiyin in breech presentation: 80 cases. *Shaanxi Zhongyi* **2007**, *28*, 334–335.
22. Li, Q.; Wang, L. Clinical observation on correcting malposition of fetus by electro-acupuncture. *J. Tradit. Chin. Med.* **1996**, *16*, 260–262. [PubMed]
23. Chen, Y.; Yang, L.W. Moxibustion on Zhiyin plus raising buttocks in a lateral position for correction fetal presentation in 73 cases. *Clin. J. Tradit. Chin. Med.* **2004**, *333*, 1.
24. Lin, Y.P.; Deqing, Z.; Yongqing, H. Combination of moxibustion at point Zhiyin and knee-chest position for correction of breech pregnancy in 63 cases. *Chin. Acupunct. Moxibustion* **2002**, *2002*, 811–812.
25. Cardini, F.; Lombardo, P.; Regalia, A.L.; Regaldo, G.; Zanini, A.; Negri, M.G.; Panepuccia, L.; Todroc, T. A randomised controlled trial of moxibustion for breech presentation. *BJOB* **2005**, *112*, 743–747. [CrossRef] [PubMed]
26. Neri, I.; Airola, G.; Contu, G.; Allais, G.; Facchinetti, F.; Bnedetto, C. Acupuncture plus moxibustion to resolve breech presentation: A randomized controlled study. *J. Matern. Fetal. Neonatal. Med.* **2004**, *15*, 247–252. [CrossRef]
27. Millereau, M.; Branger, B.; Darcel, F. Fetal version by acupuncture (moxibustion) versus control group. *J. Gynecol. Obstet. Biol. Reprod.* **2009**, *38*, 481–487. [CrossRef] [PubMed]
28. Do, C.K.; Smith, C.A.; Dahlen, H.; Bisists, A.; Schimied, V. Moxibustion for cephalic version: A feasibility randomised controlled trial. *BMC Complement. Altern Med.* **2011**, *11*, 81. [CrossRef]
29. Guittier, M.J.; Pichon, M.; Dong, H.; Irion, O.; Boulvain, M. Moxibustion for breech version: A randomized controlled trial. *Obstet. Gynecol.* **2009**, *114*, 1034–1040. [CrossRef]
30. West, Z. *Acupuncture in Pregnancy and Childbirth*; Elsevier Health Sciences: New York, NY, USA, 2008.
31. Schlaeger, J.M.; Stoffel, C.L.; Bussell, J.L.; Cai, H.Y.; Takayama, M.; Yajima, H.; Takakura, N. Moxibustion for Cephalic Version of Breech Presentation. *J. Midwifery Womens Health* **2018**, *63*, 309–322. [CrossRef]
32. O'Donnell, P.H.; Dolan, M.E. E. Cancer pharmacoethnicity: Ethnic differences in susceptibility to the effects of chemotherapy. *Clin. Cancer Res.* **2009**, *15*, 4806–4814. [CrossRef]
33. Campbell, C.M.; Edwards, R.R. Ethnic differences in pain and pain management. *Pain Manag.* **2012**, *2*, 219–230. [CrossRef]
34. Pennick, V.E.; Young, G. Interventions for preventing and treating pelvic and back pain in pregnancy. *Cochrane Database Syst. Rev.* **2007**, *2*, CD001139.
35. Smith, C.A.; Collins, C.T.; Crowther, C.A.; Levett, K.M. Acupuncture or acupressure for pain management in labour. *Cochrane Database Syst Rev.* **2011**, *7*, CD009232. [CrossRef] [PubMed]
36. Van den Berg, I.; Kaandorp, G.C.; Bosch, L.J.; Duvekot, J.J.; Arends, L.R.; Huning, M.G.M. Cost-effectiveness of breech version by acupuncture-type interventions on BL 67, including moxibustion, for women with a breech foetus at 33 weeks gestation: A modelling approach. *Complement. Ther Med.* **2010**, *18*, 67–77. [CrossRef] [PubMed]

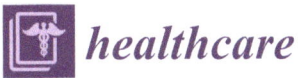

Review

Comparative Effectiveness of Western and Eastern Manual Therapies for Chronic Obstructive Pulmonary Disease: A Systematic Review and Network Meta-Analysis

Chan-Young Kwon [1,†], Boram Lee [2,†], Beom-Joon Lee [3,4], Kwan-Il Kim [3,4,*] and Hee-Jae Jung [3,4,*]

1. Department of Oriental Neuropsychiatry, Dong-eui University College of Korean Medicine, Busan 47227, Korea; beanalogue@naver.com
2. Department of Clinical Korean Medicine, Kyung Hee University, Seoul 02447, Korea; qhfka9357@naver.com
3. Department of Internal Korean Medicine, Kyung Hee University Korean Medicine Hospital, Seoul 02453, Korea; franchisjun@naver.com
4. Division of Allergy, Immune and Respiratory System, Department of Internal Medicine, College of Korean Medicine, Kyung Hee University, Seoul 02447, Korea
* Correspondence: myhappy78@naver.com (K.-I.K.); hanfish@khmc.or.kr (H.-J.J.); Tel.: +82-2-958-9124 (K.-I.K.); +82-2-958-9147 (H.-J.J.)
† These authors are co-first authors.

Citation: Kwon, C.-Y.; Lee, B.; Lee, B.-J.; Kim, K.-I.; Jung, H.-J. Comparative Effectiveness of Western and Eastern Manual Therapies for Chronic Obstructive Pulmonary Disease: A Systematic Review and Network Meta-Analysis. *Healthcare* 2021, 9, 1127. https://doi.org/10.3390/healthcare9091127

Academic Editors: Manoj Sharma and Kavita Batra

Received: 13 July 2021
Accepted: 25 August 2021
Published: 30 August 2021

Publisher's Note: MDPI stays neutral with regard to jurisdictional claims in published maps and institutional affiliations.

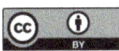

Copyright: © 2021 by the authors. Licensee MDPI, Basel, Switzerland. This article is an open access article distributed under the terms and conditions of the Creative Commons Attribution (CC BY) license (https://creativecommons.org/licenses/by/4.0/).

Abstract: Background: Manual therapy (MT) is considered a promising adjuvant therapy for chronic obstructive pulmonary disease (COPD). Comparing the effectiveness among different Western and Eastern MTs being used for the management of COPD could potentially facilitate individualized management of COPD. This systematic review attempted to estimate the comparative effectiveness of Western and Eastern MTs for COPD patients using a network meta-analysis (NMA) methodology. Methods: Nine electronic databases were comprehensively searched for relevant randomized controlled trials (RCTs) published up to February 2021. Pair-wise meta-analysis and NMA were conducted on the outcomes of COPD, which included lung function and exercise capacity. Results: The NMA results from 30 included RCTs indicated that the optimal treatment for each outcome according to the surface under the cumulative ranking curve was massage, acupressure, massage, and tuina for forced expiratory volume in 1 s (FEV1), forced vital capacity (FVC), FEV1/FVC, and 6 min walking distance, respectively. Conclusions: MTs such as massage, acupressure, and tuina have shown comparative benefits for lung function and exercise capacity in COPD. However, the methodological quality of the included studies was poor, and the head-to-head trial comparing the effects of different types of MTs for COPD patients was insufficient. Therefore, further high-quality RCTs are essential.

Keywords: chronic obstructive pulmonary disease; manual therapy; systematic review; meta-analysis; network meta-analysis

1. Introduction

Chronic obstructive pulmonary disease (COPD) is a common pulmonary disease characterized by persistent airflow limitation, which is usually associated with an enhanced chronic inflammatory response [1]. In addition, the harmful effects of toxic chemical particles or gases on the lungs often cause COPD; therefore, smoking is an important risk factor [1]. Epidemiological studies indicate that the prevalence of COPD is very common, ranging from 8% to 10% [2], and it causes significant economic and social burden worldwide [3].

The main therapeutic approaches for COPD include pharmacological treatment and lifestyle management such as cessation of smoking [4]. In pharmacological treatment for COPD, long-acting β2-agonist, long-acting muscarinic antagonists, inhaled corticosteroids, and bronchodilators, among others, may be used alone or in combination, depending on the patient's condition or comorbidity [4].

COPD is a pathological condition associated with altered chest wall mechanics and musculoskeletal changes, and various manual therapies have been used as adjuvant therapy in combination with conventional medicine [5]. Although manual therapy is frequently used in clinical practice, some systematic reviews have pointed out that there is not enough evidence to support its therapeutic effect [6,7]. According to its theoretical basis, manual therapy can be classified as either based on Western medicine or on Eastern medicine. In the former case, it is applied based on the anatomical knowledge of the human body, such as manual therapy currently used in COPD, but in the latter case, manual therapy from a holistic perspective is applied within the body-mind-spirit model [8,9]. Previous studies that pointed out the lack of evidence for manual therapy for COPD have the limitation that they did not consider manual therapy based on Eastern medicine [6,7].

Various manual therapies take a common approach when the practitioner's body comes in contact with the patient's body; therefore, they will have a common expected effect along with the unique effect of each therapy, which leads to unique results for multiple outcomes of COPD. For example, advocators of Western manual therapy may explain that by improving musculoskeletal changes of altered chest wall mechanics, manual therapy can affect chest wall compliance of patients with COPD [5]. On the other hand, Eastern manual therapies are regarded as manual therapy combined with the traditional concept of meridian massage, and in this medical system, there is a view that both function and structure are systematically correlated [10]. Therefore, several Western and Eastern manual therapies can each have their own effectiveness for COPD, and comparative analysis of them can promote important individualized therapy in COPD management [11]. In addition, comparative analysis of Western and Eastern manual therapies for COPD could potentially help establish an integrative medical perspective for patients with COPD by combining the advantages of each.

Network meta-analysis (NMA) is a methodology that enables simultaneous comparison of various interventions at the same time [12]. By creating indirect evidence, it enables comparisons between interventions that are not directly compared by the existing clinical trials [12]. Therefore, this methodology can suggest the best intervention for each outcome to obtain optimal results for patients; further, it can be used to deduce clinical practice guidelines [13]. Until now, the effect of various manual therapies from the East and West on the outcome of COPD has not been comprehensively reviewed, and no attempts have been made to investigate the comparative effect of NMA. Therefore, this review aimed to compare the effectiveness and safety of several Western and Eastern manual therapies in COPD management. The results of this study will help to understand not only the clinical evidence of manual therapy for COPD more comprehensively but also understand the comparative effects of the presence or absence of a holistic approach (Western vs. Eastern).

2. Materials and Methods

The pre-registered protocol of this review can be found in OSF registries (doi:10.17605/OSF.IO/T2WM4). This systematic review complied with the Preferred Reporting Items for Systematic Reviews and Meta-Analyses (PRISMA) 2020 statement [14].

2.1. Data Sources and Search Strategy

To find relevant studies, a total of nine electronic databases, including Medline via PubMed, Excerpta Medica dataBASE (EMBASE) via Elsevier, the Cochrane Central Register of Controlled Trials, Allied and Complementary Medicine, Korean Studies Information Service System, Korea Citation Index, China National Knowledge Database, Wanfang Database, and Chinese Scientific Journals Database (CSJD-VIP), were comprehensively searched by one researcher (BL), without any limitations on language and publication status. The search date was 12 February 2021, and all published studies up to the search date were considered. In addition, we reviewed the reference list of included or related literature to find gray literature and requested advice from systematic review experts (Supplement S1).

2.2. Eligibility Criteria

The inclusion criteria for this review were as follows: (1) Study type: Only randomized controlled trials (RCTs) were included in this review, while quasi-RCTs were excluded. (2) Types of participants: Adult patients (over 18 years of age) diagnosed with COPD were included in this study regardless of sex, COPD stage, and history of exacerbations. Patients with COPD having other significant diseases affecting the respiratory system, such as lung or other cancers, were excluded. Studies including people with COPD as well as other respiratory diseases (such as asthma or asthma COPD overlap syndrome) were also excluded. (3) Types of interventions: Western and Eastern manual therapies were included as interventions of interest, including manipulative therapy, joint mobilization, chiropractic, massage, reflexology, soft tissue therapy, muscle stretching, tuina, and acupressure passively applied using the practitioners' hands. In this review, Western manual therapy was defined as manual therapy based on conventional Western anatomy. Specifically, manual therapy that mainly targets musculoskeletal changes of altered chest wall mechanics was considered Western manual therapy, which may include spinal manipulation, osteopathic manipulative treatment, manual diaphragm release technique, and soft tissue massage [5]. On the other hand, Eastern manual therapy was defined as manual therapy based on East Asian traditional medicine (EATM) theory such as meridian theory as well as conventional anatomy. Specifically, manual therapy targeting the meridian, a unique energy flow that connects the whole body in EATM, or based on a holistic perspective, was considered Eastern manual therapy, which may include tuina, reflexology, and acupressure [10]. Exercise therapy, self-treatment, active stretching, and therapies not performed by a practitioner were excluded. Additionally, acupressure with needles, seeds, or magnetic pieces on acupoints was also excluded. Although eligible treatments could be employed with or without other conventional interventions, it was imperative that the primary tested intervention applied manual therapy techniques. Oral or external herbal medicine, pharmacopuncture, acupuncture, moxibustion, qigong, taichi, and psychotherapy, which could not be considered conventional interventions, were excluded. (4) Types of controls: Comparators included no treatment, wait-list, sham treatment, routine pulmonary rehabilitation, medication, and other active controls. (5) Types of outcomes: The primary outcome was lung function parameters, such as forced expiratory volume in 1 s (FEV1), forced vital capacity (FVC), or FEV1/FVC, and exercise capacity, such as the 6 min walking distance (6MWD). Secondary outcomes were clinical symptoms such as the severity of dyspnea assessed using the Medical Research Council (MRC) dyspnea scale developed in England. Alternatively, other assessment tools such as patient-reported measures, self-assessment, and/or questionnaires could be used. In addition, quality of life measured using the COPD assessment test (CAT) was included as a secondary outcome. When CAT was not used, an alternate assessment tool, such as the St. George Respiratory Questionnaire (SGRQ), was allowed. Finally, the incidence of adverse events (AEs) or safety measurements was included as a secondary outcome. The outcome for the respiratory function was included in the analysis, but other outcomes such as constipation, anxiety, depression, and sleep disorder were not analyzed because they were not of interest to us. However, symptoms of sputum were considered, as they were indirectly related to respiratory function.

2.3. Study Selection

Two independent reviewers (CYK and BL) screened the titles and abstracts of the searched studies to determine their eligibility. Then, the full text of the screened studies was reviewed by two independent reviewers (CYK and BL) for inclusion. Discrepancies were resolved by discussion with a third researcher (KIK). EndNote X7 (Clarivate, Philadelphia, PA, USA), a reference management tool, was used in the study selection process.

2.4. Data Extraction

The data that were extracted from the eligible studies by two independent researchers (CYK and BL) were entered into a Microsoft Excel file. The following data were extracted: first author, country, information related to the risk of bias assessment, sample size, mean age and sex ratio of participants, the condition of COPD (acute exacerbations of COPD (AECOPD) and stable COPD), diagnostic criteria for COPD, pattern identification, details of intervention, methods of manual therapy, treatment duration, timing of assessment, outcomes, and results. Discrepancies were resolved by discussion with a third researcher (KIK).

2.5. Risk of Bias Assessment

The risk of bias of the included studies was assessed according to the Cochrane Handbook version 5.1.0. assessment tool by two independent researchers (CYK and BL) [15]. In the Cochrane's risk of bias tool, domains for random sequence generation, allocation concealment, blinding of participants and personnel, blinding of outcome assessment, incomplete outcome data, selective reporting, and other sources of bias are evaluated as "low," "high," or "unclear" [15]. The risk of bias summary figure was produced using the RevMan Software version 5.4 (The Cochrane Collaboration, London, England). Discrepancies were resolved by discussion with a third researcher (KIK).

2.6. Data Analysis and Synthesis

The baseline characteristics and outcomes of all the included studies were analyzed descriptively.

2.6.1. Conventional Pair-Wise Meta-Analysis

When there was adequate homogeneous data, quantitative synthesis was performed using RevMan 5.4 (The Cochrane Collaboration, London, England). Dichotomous data were presented as risk ratio (RR) with 95% confidence interval (CI), and continuous data were reported as mean difference (MD) with 95% CI. Heterogeneity between the studies in terms of effect measures was assessed using both the χ^2 test and the I^2 statistic. I^2 values of $\geq 50\%$ and $\geq 75\%$ were considered indicative of substantial and considerable heterogeneity, respectively. Due to the nature of non-pharmacological therapies, which are the interventions of interest in this review, it was difficult to guarantee the homogeneity of the implementation of the interventions, so we applied the random-effects model to meta-analyses [16]. When a sufficient number of studies (≥ 10) were included in each meta-analysis, publication bias was evaluated using a funnel plot.

2.6.2. Network Meta-Analysis

NMA was performed on primary outcomes to provide both direct and indirect evidence. Routine care (ROC) was used as the reference treatment. NMA based on the frequent framework was carried out using mvmeta and network packages in Stata software version 16 (StataCorp, College Station, TX, USA). Inconsistency was assessed using the node-splitting method and the design-by-treatment interaction model, and a random-effects NMA model was selected. Potential publication bias was assessed using a net funnel plot, provided a sufficient number of studies (≥ 10) were included. In addition, we examined the surface under the cumulative ranking curve (SUCRA) statistic to identify the best treatment. The overall NMA method in this review followed that of Shim et al. (2017) [17].

2.7. Dealing with Missing Data

The authors contacted the corresponding author via email regarding any unclear information in the concerned study. If the data were still insufficient after contacting the corresponding author or if contact was not possible, it was analyzed using the available data.

3. Results

3.1. Study Selection

Through database searching, a total of 2623 articles were searched, and no studies were identified through other sources. After removing 843 duplicates, the titles and abstracts of 1780 articles were screened for first inclusion, and 1714 studies were excluded. After assessing full-text of the remaining 66 articles, 36 studies including eight only abstract available with no details, one case series, four quasi-RCTs, two review articles, 10 not meeting intervention criteria, five without outcomes of interest, four using duplicated data, and two unavailable full-text were excluded (Supplement S2). Finally, total 30 RCTs [18–47] were included in qualitative synthesis, and 21 RCTs [19,20,22–24,27–31,33,35,36,38,41–47] were included in meta-analysis (Figure 1).

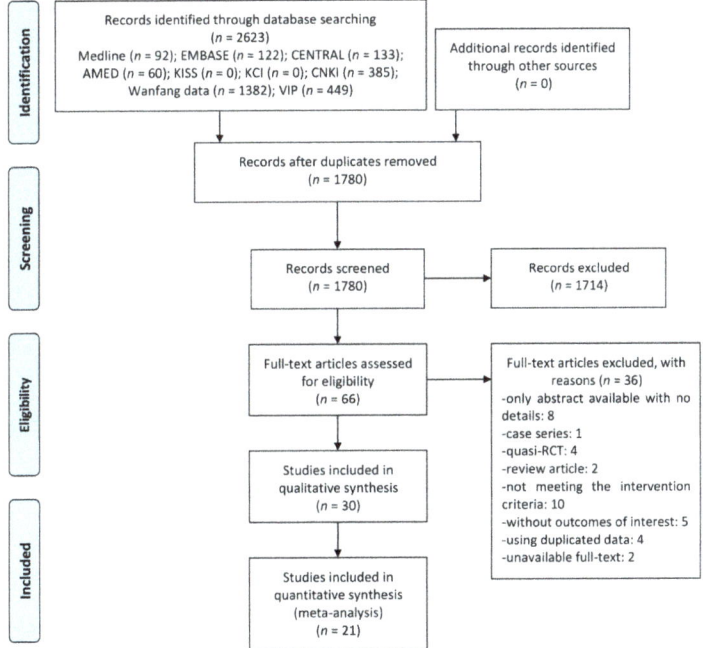

Figure 1. A PRISMA flow diagram of the literature screening and selection process. AMED—Allied and Complementary Medicine Database; CENTRAL—Cochrane Central Register of Controlled Trials; CNKI—China National Knowledge Infrastructure; KCI—Korea Citation Index; KISS—Korean Studies Information Service System; RCT—randomized controlled trial.

3.2. Study Characteristics

In total, 19 studies [19,22–30,33,35,38,41,43–47] were published in China, two were published in Italy [18,42], Poland [31,34], and the United Kingdom [20,39], and one was published in the USA [36], Brazil [37], Australia [21], Turkey [32], and Taiwan [40]. There were 11 studies [18,20,21,31,32,34,36–38,42,47] using Western manual therapy, of which four [18,34,36,42] were related to manipulation, four [21,31,32,47] were regarding massage, and one study each was related to release technique [37], manual chest technique [20], and manual percussion [38]. Nineteen studies [19,22–30,33,35,39–41,43–46] used Eastern manual therapy, of which 10 [22–24,28,30,33,40,41,45,46] were related to acupressure, five [25–27,29,39] pertained to foot reflexology, and four [19,35,43,44] were regarding tuina. As for the COPD stage, 16 studies [18,19,25–30,34–37,39,42,43,45] targeted stable COPD participants, eight studies [20,22–24,31,33,38,46] were on AECOPD, and six studies [21,32,40,41,44,47] did not specify the stage. Nine studies [22–24,28–30,35,41,45] targeted participants with specific pattern identification, of which four focused on participants with phlegm-heat [22], phlegm turbidity [23,41], or phlegm-blood stasis [24] obstructing the lung, and five [28–30,35,45] targeted dual deficiency of lung–spleen or lung–kidney. Twelve studies [18,20–24,32,34,36,37,42,45] were approved by the Institutional Review Board prior to study commencement, and 19 studies [18,20–26,29,32,34–37,40–42,45,47] received consent forms from the participants (Tables 1 and 2).

3.3. Risk of Bias Assessment

Thirteen studies [22–29,34,37,40,42,43] that used an appropriate random sequence generation method such as random number tables were evaluated as having a low risk of selection bias, and three studies [21,32,37] that properly concealed allocation using an opaque sealed envelope were also evaluated as having a low risk of selection bias. Three studies [34,36,37] that reported that the practitioners who were not blinded were at high risk of performance bias, and one study [42] that reported that both participants and personnel were blinded was evaluated as having a low risk of performance bias. Five studies [20,21,36,37,42] reporting blindness of outcome assessors were evaluated as having a low risk of detection bias. Three studies [32,39,43] that performed per-protocol analysis without specifying the reason for dropout were evaluated as having a high risk of attrition bias. Three studies [18,39,43] did not report raw data, and four studies [23,24,41,46] that did not report pulmonary function-related outcomes were evaluated as having a high risk of reporting bias. One study [28] without baseline characteristic data and one study [34] with cross-over design was evaluated as having a high risk of other potential biases (Figure 2).

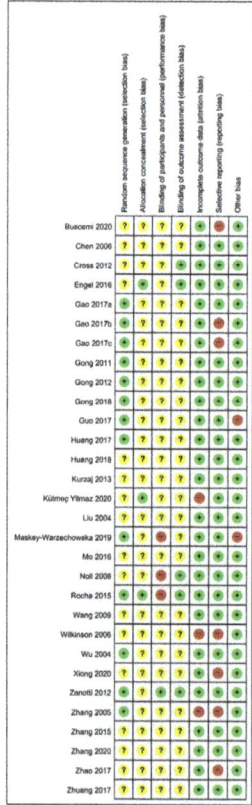

Figure 2. Risk of bias for all included studies. Low, unclear, and high risk, respectively, are represented with the following symbols: "+", "?", and "−".

Table 1. Characteristics of included studies using Western manual therapy.

First Author (Year), Country	Sample Size (Included →Analyzed)	Mean Age (Year)	Diagnosis	(A) Treatment Intervention	(B) Control Intervention	Duration of Treatment/Follow-Up	Outcome of Interest
Stable COPD							
Noll (2008), USA	35(18:17)→35(18:17)	(A) 69.6 ± 6.6 (B) 72.2 ± 7.1	Known COPD history, FEV1/FVC < 70%	Osteopathic manipulative treatment	Sham (light touch)	20 min one session/none	1. FEV1 (L); 2. FVC (L); 3. FEV1/FVC (%); 4. Adverse events
Zanotti (2012), Italy	20(10:10)→20(10:10)	(A) 63.5 ± 4.7 (B) 64.2 ± 5.5	GOLD	Osteopathic manipulative treatment	Sham (light touch)	45 min once a week for 4 weeks/none	1. VC (L); 2. FEV1 (L); 3. FVC (L); 4. 6MWD (m); 5. Adverse events
Maskey-Warzechowska (2019), Poland	38(19:19)→38(19:19)	68	Severe-very severe (FEV1 < 50%), GOLD 2016	Osteopathic manipulative treatment	Sham	25 min one session/none	Note. Only median (IQR) value was reported. 1. FEV1 (L, %pv); 2. FVC (L, %pv); 3. FEV1/FVC (%); 4. VAS (dyspnea); 5. Adverse events
Buscemi (2020), Italy	32→32	71	Moderate-severe COPD	Osteopathic manipulative treatment + (B)	Conventional pharmacotherapy	once a week for 8 weeks/15 days	Note. Raw data were not reported except adverse events. 1. FVC (L); 2. FEV1 (L); 3. CAT; 4. 6MWD (m); 5. Adverse events
Rocha (2015), Brazil	20(11:9)→19(10:9)	(A) 71 ± 5 (B) 71 ± 6	GOLD 2011	Manual diaphragm release technique	Sham (light touch)	6 times on non-consecutive days within 2 weeks/none	Note. Only change value was reported. 1. 6MWD (m)
AECOPD							
Kurzaj (2013), Poland	30(20:10)→30(20:10)	(A) 57 (B) 55	NR	Massage + (B)	Basic physiotherapy (Respirometric training)	30 min daily for 6 days/none	1. FEV1 (L, %pv); 2. 6MWD (m); 3. MRC; 4. BODE index

Table 1. Cont.

First Author (Year), Country	Sample Size (Included →Analyzed)	Mean Age (Year)	Diagnosis	(A) Treatment Intervention	(B) Control Intervention	Duration of Treatment/Follow-Up	Outcome of Interest
Cross (2012), UK	522(258:264)→372(186:186)	(A) 69.08 ± 9.85 (B) 69.58 ± 9.51	NR	Manual chest technique + (B)	Breathing technique	1–41 min, total 1–21 sessions/6 mon	Note. Raw data of sputum volume and SpO2 were not reported. 1. SGRQ; 2. Breathlessness Cough and Sputum Scale; 3. EQ-5D; 4. EQ-VAS; 5. Sputum volume (mL); 6. SpO2; 7. Hospitalization period; 8. Adverse events
Wang (2009), China	120(60:60)→120(60:60)	NR	NR	Manual percussion	Mechanical percussion	twice a day for 7 days/none	1. Sputum excretion (mL); 2. SpO2; 3. Hospitalization period; 4. Time to improvement/disappearance of cough, dyspnea, and sputum sound in lungs; 5. FVC (L); 6. FEV1 (L)
Unclear COPD							
Engel (2016), Australia	33(9:9:15)→31(8:8:15)	(A1) 67.6 ± 3.5 (A2) 65.0 ± 4.1 (B) 64.5 ± 4.1	NR	(A1) Massage + (B) (A2) Massage + Spinal manipulation + (B)	Pulmonary rehabilitation	twice a week for 8 weeks/none	Note. Only change value was reported. 1. FEV1 (L); 2. FVC (L); 3. SGRQ; 4. 6MWD (m); 5. Adverse events
Zhuang (2017), China	70(35:35)→70(35:35)	(A) 64.98 ± 4.98 (B) 65.23 ± 5.25	NR	Massage + (B)	Routine care (medication, exercise education, diet education, etc.)	NR/none	1. FEV1 (L); 2. FEV1/FVC (%); 3. TER (respiratory symptom)
Kütmeç Yılmaz (2020), Turkey	91(49:42)→58(28:30)	70.6	NR	Back massage + (B)	Routine care	15 min, daily for 4 days/none	Note. Only median (IQR) value was reported. 1. SpO2

Abbreviations: AECOPD—acute exacerbations of chronic obstructive pulmonary disease; BODE—body-mass index, obstruction of airways, dyspnea, exercise capacity; CAT—chronic obstructive pulmonary disease assessment test; COPD—chronic obstructive pulmonary disease; EQ-VAS—EuroQol-visual analogue scale; EQ-5D—EuroQol-5 dimension; FEV1—forced expiratory volume in one second; FVC—forced vital capacity; GOLD—global initiative for chronic obstructive lung disease; IQR—interquartile range; MRC—medical research council dyspnea scale; NR—not recorded; pv—predicted value; SGRQ—St. George respiratory questionnaire; TER—total effective rate; VAS—visual analogue scale; VC—vital capacity; 6MWD—6 min walking distance.

Table 2. Characteristics of included studies using Eastern manual therapy.

First Author (Year), Country	Sample Size (Included→Analyzed)	Mean Age (Year)	Diagnosis	(A) Treatment Intervention	(B) Control Intervention	Duration of Treatment/Follow-Up	Outcome of Interest
Stable COPD							
Guo (2017), China	200(100:100)→200(100:100)	NR	Criteria used by associations or guidelines in China	Acupressure + (B)	Basic physiotherapy (Respirometric training)	2–3 min per acupoint, once a day for 6 mon/none	1. FEV1 (L); 2. FEV1/FVC (%); 3. SGRQ
Huang (2018), China	68(34:34)→68(34:34)	(A) 52.43 ± 3.96 (B) 54.43 ± 1.27	COPD	Acupressure + (B)	Basic physiotherapy (Respirometric training)	2 min per acupoint twice a day for 3 mon/none	1. FEV1 (L, %pv); 2. FEV1/FVC (%); 3. 6MWD (m); 4. CAT
Zhang (2020), China	90(45:45)→90(45:45)	(A) 67.46 ± 5.23 (B) 67.85 ± 5.62	Criteria used by associations or guidelines in China	Acupressure + (B)	Basic physiotherapy (Respirometric training)	2–3 min per acupoint once a day for 6 mon/none	1. FVC (L); 2. FEV1 (L); 3. FEV1/FVC (%)
Wilkinson (2006), UK	14(7:7)→14(7:7)	(A) 77 (B) 75	Moderate–severe COPD	Foot reflexology	No intervention	50 min once a week for 4 weeks/none	Note. Raw data were not reported. 1. Quality of life (questionnaire); 2. SpO2
Gong (2011), China	60(30:30)→60(30:30)	(A) 67.03 ± 9.48 (B) 69.93 ± 8.18	Criteria used by associations or guidelines in China	Foot reflexology + (B)	Health education	30 min once a day for 3 mon/none	Note. Only change value was reported. 1. SGRQ; 2. FEV1 (L, %pv); 3. FEV1/FVC (%)
Gong (2012), China	60(30:30)→60(30:30)	(A) 67.03 ± 9.48 (B) 69.93 ± 8.18	Criteria used by associations or guidelines in China	Foot reflexology + (B)	Health education	30 min once a day for 3 mon/none	Note. On 6MWD and MRC, only change values were reported. 1. 6MWD (m); 2. MRC; 3. TER (respiratory symptom)
Huang (2017), China	60(30:30)→59(29:30)	(A) 69.52 ± 4.31 (B) 69.37 ± 4.56	Criteria used by associations or guidelines in China	Foot reflexology + (B)	Health education	30 min once a day for 6 mon/none	1. 6MWD (m)

Table 2. Cont.

First Author (Year), Country	Sample Size (Included→Analyzed)	Mean Age (Year)	Diagnosis	(A) Treatment Intervention	(B) Control Intervention	Duration of Treatment/Follow-Up	Outcome of Interest
Gong (2018), China	60(30:30)→59(29:30)	(A) 69.52 ± 4.31 (B) 69.37 ± 4.56	Criteria used by associations or guidelines in China	Foot reflexology + (B)	Health education	30 min once a day for 6 mon/none	Note. Only change value was reported. 1. BODE index; 2. 6MWD (m); 3. modified MRC; 4. FEV1 (%)
Zhang (2005), China	66(33:33)→63(31:32)	(A) 68.3 ± 6.79 (B) 67.7 ± 7.92	Criteria used by associations or guidelines in China	Tuina	Basic physiotherapy (Respirometric training)	20 min 3 times a week for 3 mon/none	1. FVC (%); 2. FEV1 (L); 3. FEV1/FVC (%); 4. 6MWD (m); 5. TER (SGRQ); 6. Quality of life (questionnaire)
Chen (2006), China	30(15:15)→30(15:15)	(A) 69.12 ± 6.21 (B) 67.63 ± 7.01	Criteria used by associations or guidelines in China	Tuina + (B)	Conventional pharmacotherapy	20 min 5 times a week for 8 weeks/none	1. TER (dyspnea); 2. FEV1/FVC (%); 3. FEV1 (L); 4. FVC (L); 5. 6MWD (m)
Mo (2016), China	60(30:30)→57(29:28)	(A) 56.5 ± 6.2 (B) 58.4 ± 5.6	Criteria used by associations or guidelines in China	Tuina + (B)	Conventional pharmacotherapy	6 times a week for 4 weeks/none	1. CAT; 2. 6MWD (m); 3. Adverse events
AECOPD							
Liu (2004), China	127(64:63)	(A) 65.33 ± 4.44 (B) 64.49 ± 5.63	Criteria used by associations or guidelines in China	Acupressure + (B)	Routine care	1hr once a day for 7 days/none	1. TER (respiratory symptom); 2. Time to improve cough, sputum, and dyspnea; 3. PaO2; 4. PaCO2
Gao (2017a), China	60(30:30)→60(30:30)	(A) 66.65 ± 3.70 (B) 68.77 ± 4.28	Criteria used by associations or guidelines in China	Acupressure + (B)	Routine care	1 min per acupoint for 10 min twice a day for 7 days/none	1. TER (respiratory symptom); 2. Symptom score (cough, sputum, wheezing, shortness of breath); 3. PaO2; 4. PaCO2; 5. SaO2
Gao (2017b), China	60(30:30)→60(30:30)	(A) 70.5 ± 4. (B) 68.5 ± 4.7	Criteria used by associations or guidelines in China	Acupressure + (B)	Routine care	20 min twice a day for 7 days/none	1. Sputum excretion (mL); 2. SpO2; 3. PaO2; 4. PaCO2

Table 2. Cont.

First Author (Year), Country	Sample Size (Included→Analyzed)	Mean Age (Year)	Diagnosis	(A) Treatment Intervention	(B) Control Intervention	Duration of Treatment/Follow-Up	Outcome of Interest
Gao (2017c), China	60(30:30)→60(30:30)	(A) 69.36 ± 5.65 (B) 70.84 ± 4.76	Criteria used by associations or guidelines in China	Acupressure + (B)	Routine care	15 min twice a day for 7 days/none	1. Symptom score (cough, sputum, dyspnea); 2. PaCO2; 3. PaO2; 4. SaO2; 5. TER (respiratory symptom); 6. Hospitalization period
Zhao (2017), China	58(29:29)→58(29:29)	(A) 67.5 ± 3.6 (B) 68.5 ± 4.1	NR	Acupressure + (B)	Routine care	10 min twice a day for 7 days/none	1. Sputum excretion (mL); 2. SpO2; 3. PaO2; 4. PaCO2
Unclear COPD							
Wu (2004), Taiwan	44(22:22)→44(22:22)	73 ± 9.7	NR	Acupressure	Sham (unrelated acupoint)	16 min five times a week for 4 weeks/none	Note. Only change value was reported. 1. 6MWD (m); 2. SpO2
Xiong (2020), China	120(60:60)→120(60:60)	(A) 50.89 ± 4.58 (B) 55.72 ± 4.54	NR	Acupressure + (B)	Routine care	30 min twice a day for 1 mon/none	1. TER (respiratory symptom); 2. Sputum excretion (mL)
Zhang (2015), China	80(40:40)→80(40:40)	(A) 45 ± 2.5 (B) 43 ± 3.4	Criteria used by associations or guidelines in China	Tuina + (B)	Routine care (medication)	~25 min five times a week for 7 weeks/none	1. TER (respiratory symptom); 2. FEV1/FVC (%); 3. FEV1 (L); 4. FVC (L)

Abbreviations: AECOPD—acute exacerbations of chronic obstructive pulmonary disease; BODE—body-mass index, obstruction of airways, dyspnea, exercise capacity; CAT—chronic obstructive pulmonary disease assessment test; COPD—chronic obstructive pulmonary disease; FEV1—forced expiratory volume in one second; FVC—forced vital capacity; MRC—medical research council dyspnea scale; NR—not recorded; pv—predicted value; SGRQ—St. George respiratory questionnaire; TER—total effective rate; 6MWD—6 min walking distance.

3.4. Effectiveness and Safety of Manual Therapies Using Pair-Wise Meta-Analysis

Manipulation showed no differences compared with sham in lung functions (FEV1: MD 0.23 L, 95% CI from −0.12 to 0.58; FVC: MD −0.02 L, 95% CI from −0.57 to 0.53; FEV1/FVC: MD 3.01%, 95% CI from −6.90 to 12.92), exercise capacity (6MWD: MD 64.80 m, 95% CI from −12.94 to 142.54), and incidence of AE (RR 0.50, 95% CI: from 0.11 to 2.38). Additional massage significantly improved FEV1/FVC (MD 20.00%, 95% CI from 15.46 to 24.54) and total effective rate (TER) calculated using the severity of respiratory symptoms (RR 1.17, 95% CI from 1.00 to 1.38), compared with ROC alone. However, there were no differences between them in the FEV1 (MD 0.68 L, 95% CI from −0.62 to 1.99), 6MWD (MD 56.20 m, 95% CI from −8.18 to 120.58), and incidence of AE (RR 8.89, 95% CI from 0.48 to 165.55). When comparing additional acupressure with ROC alone, although there was no difference in FEV1 (MD 0.05 L, 95% CI from −0.24 to 0.34) and FEV1/FVC (MD 0.84%, 95% CI from −4.60 to 2.27), other outcomes including FVC (MD 0.33 L, 95% CI from 0.17 to 0.49), 6MWD (MD 14.38 m, 95% CI from 3.71 to 25.05), TER based on the respiratory symptom (RR 1.14, 95% CI from 1.06 to 1.23), sputum secretion (MD −5.31 mL, 95% CI from −6.00 to −4.62), SpO2 (MD 3.44%, 95% CI from 1.64 to 5.23), PaO2 (MD 13.38 mmHg, 95% CI from 9.16 to 17.60), PaCO2 (MD −8.91 mmHg, 95% CI from −12.09 to −5.72), and SaO2 (MD 9.10%, 95% CI from 5.29 to 12.91) significantly improved. Additional tuina significantly improved FEV1/FVC (MD 2.65%, 95% CI from 0.10 to 5.20), and 6MWD (MD 49.53 m, 95% CI from 27.05 to 72.00) compared with ROC alone, although there were no differences in FEV1 (MD 0.10 L, 95% CI from −0.05 to 0.25), FVC (MD 0.26 L, 95% CI from −0.05 to 0.58), and TER based on the respiratory symptom (RR 1.10, 95% CI from 0.94 to 1.28). When conducting foot reflexology in addition to ROC, 6MWD (MD 36.08 m, 95% CI from 8.45 to 63.71), and TER based on the respiratory symptom (RR 2.13, 95% CI from 1.09 to 4.16) significantly improved compared with ROC alone (Supplement S3).

3.5. Comparative Effectiveness of Manual Therapies Using NMA

NMA was possible only for the outcomes of FEV1, FVC, FEV1/FVC, and 6MWD. Therefore, pair-wise meta-analysis was performed for other outcomes because the network had no degrees of freedom for heterogeneity due to the small number of studies included. Figure 3 shows the network map of the interventions belonging to each NMA.

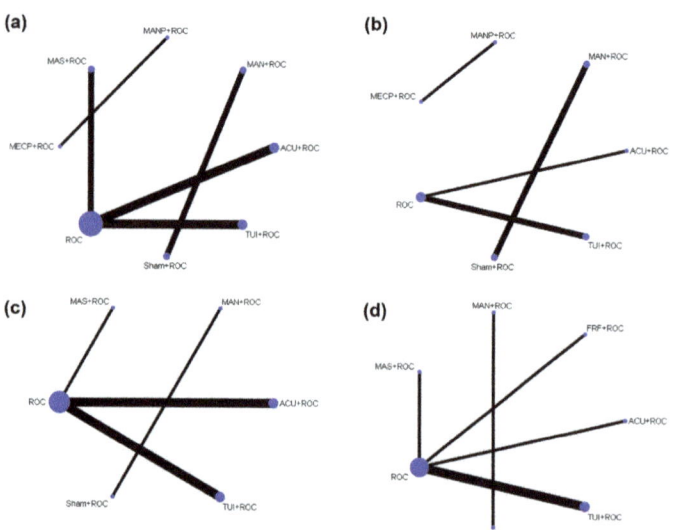

Figure 3. Network map of (**a**) FEV1 (L), (**b**) FVC (L), (**c**) FEV1/FVC (%), and (**d**) 6 min walking distance. ACU—acupuncture; FRF—foot reflexology; MAN—manipulation; MANP—manual percussion; MAS—massage; MECP—mechanical percussion; ROC—routine care; TUI—tuina.

3.5.1. Lung Function

In FEV1, only additional massage showed significantly better results compared to ROC alone (MD 0.74 L, 95% CI 0.08 to 1.40). In FVC, additional acupressure resulted in significant improvement while tuina showed borderline better results compared to ROC alone (MD 0.33 L, 95% CI from 0.17 to 0.47; MD 0.26 L, 95% CI from −0.05 to 0.58) (Table 3). In FEV1/FVC, additional massage showed significantly better results not only compared to ROC alone (MD 20.00%, 95% CI from 12.16 to 27.84) but also compared to additional acupressure (MD 19.18%, 95% CI from 10.23 to 28.13) and additional tuina (MD 16.99%, 95% CI from 7.86 to 26.13). No statistically significant differences between the interventions were observed (Table 4). The most optimal treatment based on SUCRA in FEV1 and FEV1/FVC was additional massage, followed by additional tuina and acupuncture, and ROC. Furthermore, the most optimal treatment in FVC was additional acupressure, followed by additional tuina and ROC (Table 5).

Table 3. Network league table of FEV1 (L) (right upper part) and FVC (L) (left lower part).

ROC	0.04 (−0.48, 0.55)	0.74 (0.08, 1.40)	0.09 (−0.46, 0.65)
0.33 (0.17, 0.49)	ACU + ROC	0.70 (−0.13, 1.54)	0.05 (−0.70, 0.81)
		MAS + ROC	−0.65 (−1.51, 0.21)
0.26 (−0.05, 0.58)	−0.07 (−0.42, 0.28)		TUI + ROC

Note: Data are presented in mean difference (95% confidence interval). The result underlined meant it had statistical significance. Abbreviations. ACU—acupuncture; FEV1—forced expiratory volume in one second; FVC—forced vital capacity; MAS—massage; ROC—routine care; TUI—tuina.

Table 4. Network league table of FEV1/FVC (%) (right upper part) and 6 min walking distance (m) (left lower part).

ROC	0.82 (−3.50, 5.14)		20.00 (12.16, 27.84)	3.01 (−1.68, 7.69)
14.38 (−12.74, 41.50)	ACU + ROC		19.18 (10.23, 28.13)	2.19 (−4.18, 8.56)
36.08 (−1.14, 73.30)	21.70 (−24.35, 67.75)	FRF + ROC		
56.20 (−12.84, 125.24)	41.82 (−32.36, 116.00)	20.12 (−58.31, 98.55)	MAS + ROC	−16.99 (−26.13, −7.86)
49.49 (25.60, 73.38)	35.11 (−1.03, 71.26)	13.41 (−30.81, 57.64)	−6.71 (−79.77, 66.35)	TUI + ROC

Note: Data are presented in mean difference (95% confidence interval). The result underlined meant it had statistical significance. Abbreviations. ACU—acupuncture; FEV1—forced expiratory volume in one second; FRF—foot reflexology; FVC—forced vital capacity; MAS—massage; ROC—routine care; TUI—tuina.

Table 5. SUCRA for interventions on each outcome.

Interventions	FEV1 (L)	FVC (L)	FEV1/FVC (%)	6MWD (m)
ROC	27.9	2.5	15.4	6
ACU + ROC	35.1	82.4	29.9	30
FRF + ROC				59.5
MAS + ROC	95.6		100	76.5
TUI + ROC	41.4	65.1	54.7	78

Abbreviations. ACU—acupuncture; FEV1—forced expiratory volume in one second; FRF—foot reflexology; FVC—forced vital capacity; MAS—massage; ROC—routine care; TUI—tuina; 6MWD—6 min walking distance.

3.5.2. Exercise Capacity

In 6MWD, additional tuina showed significantly better results compared to ROC alone (MD 49.49 m, 95% CI from 25.60 to 73.38) and borderline better results compared to additional acupressure (MD 35.11 m, 95% CI from −1.03 to 71.26). Furthermore, additional foot reflexology showed borderline significant results compared to ROC alone (MD 36.08 m, 95% CI from −1.14 to 73.30) (Table 4). The most optimal treatment based on SUCRA in 6MWD was additional tuina, followed by additional massage, foot reflexology, acupressure, and ROC (Table 5).

4. Discussion

4.1. Summary of Evidence

This systematic review attempted to estimate the comparative effectiveness of Western and Eastern manual therapies for COPD patients based on a total of 30 RCTs [18–47]. Data for five interventions, including manipulation, massage, acupressure, tuina, and foot reflexology, were obtained from the pair-wise meta-analysis results. Additional massage (FEV/FVC), acupressure (FVC, 6MWD), tuina (FEV1/FVC, 6MWD), and foot reflexology (6MWD) showed significantly improved results compared to ROC alone in one or more outcomes of lung functions and/or exercise capacity. However, manipulation did not show significantly better results (FEV1, FVC, FEV1/FVC, 6MWD) compared to sham treatment. In addition, there was evidence that additional acupressure and tuina could significantly improve the quality of life of COPD patients (CAT and SGRQ), although meta-analysis could not be carried out because there was only one study that evaluated this outcome. Additional acupressure could significantly improve some objective outcomes of COPD patients, including sputum secretion, SpO2, PaO2, PaCO2, and SaO2. There were no interventions that significantly differed in the incidence of AEs compared to the controls. The number of interventions included in the NMA for FEV1, FVC, FEV1/FVC, and 6MWD was four, three, four and five, respectively. According to the results, only additional massage for FEV1 and only additional acupressure for FVC showed significantly better results than ROC. On the other hand, additional massage for FEV1/FVC showed significantly better results than ROC, acupressure, and tuina. Only additional tuina showed significantly better results for 6MWD than ROC. However, the comparative effect of foot reflexology was not significant for any outcome. The optimal treatment for each outcome according to SUCRA was massage, acupressure, massage, and tuina for FEV1, FVC, FEV1/FVC, and 6MWD, respectively.

The methodological quality of the included studies was generally poor. Limitations of methodological quality were found throughout the evaluated domains in the Cochrane's risk of bias tool, and more than half of the studies were evaluated as having an unclear or high risk of bias in relation to random sequence generation, allocation concealment, and blinding procedures. This suggests that the study results derived from the included studies may have been influenced by the placebo effect or overestimated.

4.2. Clinical Implications

Although the main therapeutic approaches for COPD are pharmacological approaches and lifestyle management [4], manual therapy is considered a promising adjuvant therapy [5]. In this review, various types of manual therapies were categorized as therapies derived from the East or West according to their origins, and the most effective manual therapy for individual outcomes related to COPD was explored through the NMA methodology. Although with limited certainty, some clinical evidence indicated that massage was the most effective treatment for FEV1 and FEV1/FVC, acupressure for FVC, and tuina for 6MWD. Since manual therapies are generally used as a complement to conventional treatment for COPD in clinical settings, the findings of this review suggest that it may be helpful to select a specific manual therapy method according to the individual patient's characteristics and target symptoms.

COPD is a long-standing problem, and the development of non-pharmacological therapies to improve the quality of life of COPD patients is important [48]. In this review, manual therapies that showed significant improvement in some outcomes of the quality of life in COPD patients were acupressure and tuina belonging to Eastern manual therapy. These therapies may not only affect lung function or exercise capacity in COPD patients but may also help improve other disturbing symptoms, including pain [49], insomnia [50,51], and fatigue [50], as seen in previously published studies, thereby contributing to the improvement in the quality of life of COPD patients.

4.3. Limitations

This systematic review attempted to conduct a comprehensive review of the various types of manual therapies utilized for COPD and to investigate its comparative effectiveness on lung function and exercise capacity of COPD patients using the NMA methodology. However, the results of this review should be interpreted considering the following limitations.

First, given the heterogeneity of interventions investigated, the number of studies that were included in this review (30 in total) was not sufficient to provide strong evidence through quantitative synthesis. In addition, given that most of the included studies had small sample sizes, there is a possibility that the findings of this review were greatly influenced by small-study effects [52]. Second, the quality of the included studies was poor overall. In particular, as aforementioned, the results from these studies may have been influenced by placebo effects or could have been overestimated, as random sequence generation, allocation concealment, and blinding procedures were described unclearly or with a high risk of bias. Third, in our prior protocol, evaluation of publication bias of the included studies was planned using funnel plots and net funnel plots. However, the lack of included studies consequently made it impossible to visually evaluate publication bias using funnel plots. This implies that we cannot rule out the possibility that the results reported in the studies included in this review may be biased. Finally, comparisons between manual therapies performed in this review primarily came from NMA, and the data are lacking in conventional pair-wise meta-analysis. That is, the head-to-head trial comparing the comparative effects of different types of manual therapies for COPD patients in conventional RCTs was insufficient. In particular, head-to-head trials between Western manual therapy and Eastern manual therapy, one of the rationales of this systematic review, did not exist. Although the NMA methodology enables indirect comparison between interventions that have not previously been directly compared with each other [12], the overall poor methodological quality of the included studies suggests that large-scale, high-quality head-to-head trials can provide more reliable results. Given that various manual therapies are being used and studied for COPD patients in both East and West, robust clinical trials evaluating the comparative effectiveness of these treatments may be of interest to future researchers.

5. Conclusions

This systematic review estimated the comparative effectiveness of Western and Eastern manual therapies for patients with COPD using the NMA methodology. The optimal treatment for each outcome according to SUCRA was massage, acupressure, massage, and tuina for FEV1, FVC, FEV1/FVC, and 6MWD, respectively. However, the methodological quality of the included studies was generally poor, and the head-to-head trial comparing different types of manual therapies for COPD patients was inadequate. Given the complementary role and promise of manual therapies in the treatment of patients with COPD, high-quality RCTs in this area should be implemented in the future.

Supplementary Materials: The following are available online at https://www.mdpi.com/article/10.3390/healthcare9091127/s1, Supplement S1. Search strategy used in each database; Supplement S2. List of excluded studies after full-text review; Supplement S3. Results of pair-wise meta-analysis; Supplement S4. PRISMA 2020 Checklist.

Author Contributions: Conceptualization, C.-Y.K. and K.-I.K.; Methodology, C.-Y.K. and B.L.; Writing—original draft, C.-Y.K. and B.L.; Writing—review and editing, K.-I.K., B.-J.L., and H.-J.J.; Funding, H.-J.J.; Supervision, K.-I.K. and H.-J.J. All authors have read and agreed to the published version of the manuscript.

Funding: This research was supported by a grant of the Korea Health Technology R&D Project through the Korea Health Industry Development Institute (KHIDI), funded by the Ministry of Health & Welfare, Republic of Korea (grant number: HF20C0030).

Institutional Review Board Statement: Ethical review and approval were waived for this study, as this study is a systematic review of previously published studies.

Informed Consent Statement: Patient consent was waived, as this study is a systematic review of previously published studies.

Data Availability Statement: The data presented in this study are available in the article and supplementary materials.

Conflicts of Interest: The authors have no conflict of interest to declare.

References

1. Vestbo, J. COPD: Definition and phenotypes. *Clin. Chest Med.* **2014**, *35*, 1–6. [CrossRef]
2. Diaz-Guzman, E.; Mannino, D.M. Epidemiology and prevalence of chronic obstructive pulmonary disease. *Clin. Chest Med.* **2014**, *35*, 7–16. [CrossRef]
3. Iheanacho, I.; Zhang, S.; King, D.; Rizzo, M.; Ismaila, A.S. Economic burden of chronic obstructive pulmonary disease (COPD): A systematic literature review. *Int. J. Chronic Obstr. Pulm. Dis.* **2020**, *15*, 439–460. [CrossRef]
4. Nici, L.; Mammen, M.J.; Charbek, E.; Alexander, P.E.; Au, D.H.; Boyd, C.M.; Criner, G.J.; Donaldson, G.C.; Dreher, M.; Fan, V.S.; et al. Pharmacologic management of chronic obstructive pulmonary disease. An official American thoracic society clinical practice guideline. *Am. J. Respir. Crit. Care Med.* **2020**, *201*, e56–e69. [CrossRef]
5. Clarke, S.; Munro, P.E.; Lee, A.L. The role of manual therapy in patients with COPD. *Healthcare* **2019**, *7*, 21. [CrossRef]
6. Simonelli, C.; Vitacca, M.; Vignoni, M.; Ambrosino, N.; Paneroni, M. Effectiveness of manual therapy in COPD: A systematic review of randomised controlled trials. *Pulmonology* **2019**, *25*, 236–247. [CrossRef]
7. Wearing, J.; Beaumont, S.; Forbes, D.; Brown, B.; Engel, R. The use of spinal manipulative therapy in the management of chronic obstructive pulmonary disease: A systematic review. *J. Altern. Complement. Med.* **2016**, *22*, 108–114. [CrossRef]
8. Chan, C.; Ho, P.S.; Chow, E. A body-mind-spirit model in health: An Eastern approach. *Soc. Work. Health Care* **2001**, *34*, 261–282. [CrossRef]
9. Shim, J.M.; Kim, J. Cross-national differences in the holistic use of traditional East Asian medicine in East Asia. *Health Promot. Int.* **2018**, *33*, 536–544. [CrossRef]
10. Park, T.Y.; Moon, T.W.; Cho, D.C.; Lee, J.H.; Ko, Y.S.; Hwang, E.H.; Heo, K.H.; Choi, T.Y.; Shin, B.C. An introduction to Chuna manual medicine in Korea: History, insurance coverage, education, and clinical research in Korean literature. *Integr. Med. Res.* **2014**, *3*, 49–59. [CrossRef]
11. Singh, D.; Miravitlles, M.; Vogelmeier, C. Chronic Obstructive Pulmonary Disease Individualized Therapy: Tailored Approach to Symptom Management. *Adv. Ther.* **2017**, *34*, 281–299. [CrossRef] [PubMed]
12. Tonin, F.S.; Rotta, I.; Mendes, A.M.; Pontarolo, R. Network meta-analysis: A technique to gather evidence from direct and indirect comparisons. *Pharm. Pract.* **2017**, *15*, 943. [CrossRef]
13. Rouse, B.; Cipriani, A.; Shi, Q.; Coleman, A.L.; Dickersin, K.; Li, T. Network meta-analysis for clinical practice guidelines: A case study on first-line medical therapies for primary open-angle glaucoma. *Ann. Intern. Med.* **2016**, *164*, 674–682. [CrossRef] [PubMed]
14. Page, M.J.; Moher, D.; Bossuyt, P.M.; Boutron, I.; Hoffmann, T.C.; Mulrow, C.D.; Shamseer, L.; Tetzlaff, J.M.; Akl, E.A.; Brennan, S.E.; et al. PRISMA 2020 explanation and elaboration: Updated guidance and exemplars for reporting systematic reviews. *BMJ (Clin. Res. Ed.)* **2021**, *372*, n160. [CrossRef]
15. Higgins, J. Cochrane Handbook for Systematic Reviews of Interventions. Version 5.1.0 [Updated March 2011]. The Cochrane Collaboration. Available online: https://handbook-5-1.cochrane.org/ (accessed on 11 March 2021).
16. Spineli, L.M.; Pandis, N. The importance of careful selection between fixed-effect and random-effects models. *Am. J. Orthod. Dentofac. Orthop.* **2020**, *157*, 432–433. [CrossRef]
17. Shim, S.; Yoon, B.H.; Shin, I.S.; Bae, J.M. Network meta-analysis: Application and practice using Stata. *Epidemiol. Health* **2017**, *39*, e2017047. [CrossRef]
18. Buscemi, A.; Pennisi, V.; Rapisarda, A.; Pennisi, A.; Coco, M. Efficacy of osteopathic treatment in patients with stable moderate-to-severe chronic obstructive pulmonary disease: A randomized controlled pilot study. *J. Complement. Integr. Med.* **2020**, *17*, 20180128. [CrossRef] [PubMed]
19. Chen, Q.; Zhong, L.W.; Liu, H.B.; Zhang, J.F.; Xie, G.G.; Jin, X.Q.; Zhou, X. Massage therapy for chronic obstructive pulmonary disease. *Chin. J. Clin. Rehabil.* **2006**, *10*, 10–12.
20. Cross, J.L.; Elender, F.; Barton, G.; Clark, A.; Shepstone, L.; Blyth, A.; Bachmann, M.O.; Harvey, I. Evaluation of the effectiveness of manual chest physiotherapy techniques on quality of life at six months post exacerbation of COPD (MATREX): A randomised controlled equivalence trial. *BMC Pulm. Med.* **2012**, *12*, 33. [CrossRef] [PubMed]
21. Engel, R.M.; Gonski, P.; Beath, K.; Vemulpad, S. Medium term effects of including manual therapy in a pulmonary rehabilitation program for chronic obstructive pulmonary disease (COPD): A randomized controlled pilot trial. *J. Man. Manip. Ther.* **2016**, *24*, 80–89. [CrossRef]

22. Gao, L. Application effect of midnight-noon ebb-flow of acupoint massage timing in COPD patients with accumulation of phlegm-heat in lung. *J. Nurs. Sci.* **2017**, *32*, 41–43.
23. Gao, L.; Sheng, H.; Zhu, Y. Application of mechanical-assisted expectoration combined with acupoint massage in nursing care of phlegm obstructing lung type of chronic obstructive pulmonary disease patients. *Chin. Nurs. Res.* **2017**, *31*, 182–185.
24. Gao, L.; Tang, Y. Observation of effect of treating acute exacerbation of chronic obstructive pulmonary disease by applying midnight-midday ebb-flow acupoint massage. *Chin. J. Pract. Nurs.* **2017**, *33*, 689–692.
25. Gong, H.; Chen, J. Effects of foot's reflection area therapy on quality of life and pulmonary function of patients with stable COPD. *J. Fujian Univ. TCM* **2011**, *21*, 10–12.
26. Gong, H.; Huang, M. The intervention effect of foot reflex zone massage for patients with stable COPD. *J. Shenyang Med. Coll.* **2018**, *20*, 407–409.
27. Gong, H.R.; Zhuang, H.L.; Liu, Z.H. The impact of foot reflex zone therapy on exercise tolerance and dyspnea of stable COPD patients. *J. Clin. Exp. Med.* **2012**, *11*, 12–13, 15. [CrossRef]
28. Guo, X.T.; Zhan, X.P.; Jin, X.Z.; Huang, Q.H.; Jin, C.C.; Hu, L.D.; Yu, N.N.; Qi, X. Effect of acupoint massage and respiratory function exercise on pulmonary function and quality of life of patients with chronic obstructive pulmonary disease in stable stage. *Chin. Gen. Pract.* **2017**, *20*, 345–347.
29. Huang, M.C.; Gong, H.R.; Deng, Y.C. Rehabilitation effect of foot reflex zone massage on 60 patients with stable COPD with lung and spleen qi deficiency. *Fujian Med. J.* **2017**, *39*, 43–45.
30. Huang, Y.L.; Feng, L.Y.; Lin, D.Y. Clinical observation on the effect of acupoint massage on pulmonary rehabilitation of COPD patients with lung-spleen-qi deficiency in the stable period. *J. Front. Med.* **2018**, *8*, 344–345. [CrossRef]
31. Kurzaj, M.; Wierzejski, W.; Dor, A.; Stawska, J.; Rozek, K. The impact of specialized physiotherapy methods on BODE index in COPD patients during hospitalization. *Adv. Clin. Exp. Med.* **2013**, *22*, 721–730.
32. Kütmeç Yilmaz, C.; Duru Aşiret, G.; Çetinkaya, F. The effect of back massage on physiological parameters, dyspnoea, and anxiety in patients with chronic obstructive pulmonary disease in the intensive care unit: A randomised clinical trial. *Intensive Crit. Care Nurs.* **2021**, *63*, 102962. [CrossRef] [PubMed]
33. Liu, S.; Zhou, Y.; Chen, Y.F. Study on effect of point massage on promoting sputum exclude in treatment of chronic obstructive pulmonary disease (COPD) during acute episode. *Mod. Prev. Med.* **2004**, *31*, 588–589.
34. Maskey-Warzechowska, M.; Mierzejewski, M.; Gorska, K.; Golowicz, R.; Jesien, L.; Krenke, R. Effects of osteopathic manual therapy on hyperinflation in patients with chronic obstructive pulmonary disease: A randomized cross-over study. *Adv. Exp. Med. Biol.* **2019**, *1222*, 17–25. [CrossRef]
35. Mo, F. Observation of Clinical Efficacy on Stable COPD (Lung and Kidney Qi Deficiency) by Replenishing Kidney Holding Qi Down. Master's Thesis, Changchun University of Chinese Medicine, Changchun, China, 2016.
36. Noll, D.R.; Degenhardt, B.F.; Johnson, J.C.; Burt, S.A. Immediate effects of osteopathic manipulative treatment in elderly patients with chronic obstructive pulmonary disease. *J. Am. Osteopath. Assoc.* **2008**, *108*, 251–259.
37. Rocha, T.; Souza, H.; Brandão, D.C.; Rattes, C.; Ribeiro, J.; Campos, S.L.; Aliverti, A.; de Andrade, A.D. The manual diaphragm release technique improves diaphragmatic mobility, inspiratory capacity and exercise capacity in people with chronic obstructive pulmonary disease: A randomised trial. *J. Physiother.* **2015**, *61*, 182–189. [CrossRef]
38. Wang, X.Y.; Wu, X.H.; Cao, C.F.; Liu, X.H. A comparative study on the effect of different sputum excretion methods on patients with COPD and pulmonary infection. *World Health Dig. Med. Period.* **2009**, *6*, 39–40. [CrossRef]
39. Wilkinson, I.S.A.; Prigmore, S.; Rayner, C.F. A randomised-controlled trail examining the effects of reflexology of patients with chronic obstructive pulmonary disease (COPD). *Complement. Ther. Clin. Pract.* **2006**, *12*, 141–147. [CrossRef]
40. Wu, H.S.; Wu, S.C.; Lin, J.G.; Lin, L.C. Effectiveness of acupressure in improving dyspnoea in chronic obstructive pulmonary disease. *J. Adv. Nurs.* **2004**, *45*, 252–259. [CrossRef]
41. Xiong, Y.; Yang, F. Study on the application of mechanical sputum drainage combined with acupoint massage in the nursing of patients with phlegm turbid and dammed lung type chronic obstructive pulmonary disease. *Chin. Foreign Med. Res.* **2020**, *18*, 90–92.
42. Zanotti, E.; Berardinelli, P.; Bizzarri, C.; Civardi, A.; Manstretta, A.; Rossetti, S.; Fracchia, C. Osteopathic manipulative treatment effectiveness in severe chronic obstructive pulmonary disease: A pilot study. *Complement. Ther. Med.* **2012**, *20*, 16–22. [CrossRef]
43. Zhang, J.F.; Zong, L.W.; Liu, H.B.; Chen, Q. Treatment of chronic obstructive pulmonary disease in remission stage by tuina. *J. Acupunct. Tuina Sci.* **2005**, *3*, 44–47.
44. Zhang, W. Study on the effect of massage therapy on chronic obstructive pulmonary disease. *Guide China Med.* **2015**, *13*, 195.
45. Zhang, X.; Huang, Y.; Zhang, D. The application of acupoint massage combined with respiratory function exercise in patients with stable chronic obstructive pulmonary disease. *Guangming J. Chin. Med.* **2020**, *35*, 557–559.
46. Zhao, L. Application of mechanical assisted expectoration combined with acupoint massage in the nursing of patients with chronic obstructive pulmonary disease. *J. Aerosp. Med.* **2017**, *28*, 1410–1411.
47. Zhuang, Y. Observation on the effect of comprehensive rehabilitation nursing in improving lung function of elderly patients with chronic obstructive pulmonary disease. *J. Contemp. Clin. Med.* **2017**, *30*, 2788–2790. [CrossRef]
48. Vu, G.V.; Ha, G.H.; Nguyen, C.T.; Vu, G.T.; Pham, H.Q.; Latkin, C.A.; Tran, B.X.; Ho, R.C.M.; Ho, C.S.H. Interventions to Improve the Quality of Life of Patients with Chronic Obstructive Pulmonary Disease: A Global Mapping During 1990–2018. *Int. J. Environ. Res. Public Health* **2020**, *17*, 3089. [CrossRef]

49. Li, T.; Li, X.; Huang, F.; Tian, Q.; Fan, Z.Y.; Wu, S. Clinical Efficacy and Safety of Acupressure on Low Back Pain: A Systematic Review and Meta-Analysis. *Evidence-Based Complement. Altern. Med. eCAM* **2021**, *2021*, 8862399. [CrossRef]
50. Lee, E.J.; Frazier, S.K. The efficacy of acupressure for symptom management: A systematic review. *J. Pain Symptom Manag.* **2011**, *42*, 589–603. [CrossRef]
51. Feng, G.; Han, M.; Li, X.; Geng, L.; Miao, Y. Clinical effectiveness of Tui Na for insomnia compared with estazolam: A systematic review and meta-analysis of randomized controlled trials. *Complement. Ther. Med.* **2019**, *47*, 102186. [CrossRef]
52. Sterne, J.A.; Gavaghan, D.; Egger, M. Publication and related bias in meta-analysis: Power of statistical tests and prevalence in the literature. *J. Clin. Epidemiol.* **2000**, *53*, 1119–1129. [CrossRef]

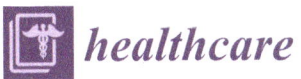

Article

Testing Multi-Theory Model (MTM) in Explaining Sunscreen Use among Florida Residents: An Integrative Approach for Sun Protection

Manoj Sharma [1], Matthew Asare [2], Erin Largo-Wight [3,4], Julie Merten [3], Mike Binder [5], Ram Lakhan [6] and Kavita Batra [7,*]

[1] Department of Social and Behavioral Health, School of Public Health, University of Nevada, Las Vegas, NV 89119, USA; manoj.sharma@unlv.edu
[2] Department of Public Health, Baylor University, Waco, TX 76798, USA; matt_asare@baylor.edu
[3] Department of Public Health, University of North Florida, Jacksonville, FL 32224, USA; largo.wight@unf.edu (E.L.-W.); jmerten@unf.edu (J.M.)
[4] Institute of Environmental Research and Education, University of North Florida, Jacksonville, FL 32224, USA
[5] Department of Political Science and Public Administration, University of North Florida, Jacksonville, FL 32224, USA; m.binder@unf.edu
[6] Department of Health and Human Performance, Berea College, Berea, KY 40404, USA; Lakhanr@berea.edu
[7] Office of Research, Kirk Kerkorian School of Medicine, University of Nevada, Las Vegas, NV 89102, USA
* Correspondence: kavita.batra@unlv.edu

Abstract: Florida residents have the second highest incidence of skin cancer in the nation. Sunscreen usage was found to be the one of the most effective integrative health approaches for reducing risk of skin cancer. Given the limited information on the likelihood of adopting and continuing sunscreen usage behavior, this cross-sectional study aimed to examine the correlates of initiating and sustaining sunscreen usage behavior among Florida dwellers, using the fourth-generation, multi-theory model (MTM) of behavior change. A web-based survey containing 51 questions was emailed to Florida residents aged 18 years or above, who were randomly selected from the state voter file. Psychometric validity of the survey instrument was established using structural equation modeling, and Cronbach's alpha values were calculated for assessing the internal consistency. An independent-samples-t-test and hierarchical multiple regression tests were used to analyze the data. The results indicated that participants who engaged in sunscreen usage behavior, participatory dialogue (β = 0.062, $p < 0.05$), behavioral confidence (β = 0.636, $p < 0.001$), and changes in the physical environment (β = 0.210, $p < 0.001$) were statistically significant and accounted for 73.6% of the variance in initiating sunscreen usage behavior. In addition, the constructs of emotional transformation (β = 0.486, $p < 0.001$) and practice for change (β = 0.211, $p < 0.001$), as well as changes in the social environment (β = 0.148, $p < 0.001$) were significant predictors of maintaining sunscreen usage behavior and contributed to 59% of variance in sustenance. These findings offer a valuable insight regarding the applicability of MTM models to guiding public health interventions promoting sunscreen usage and preventing UV radiation risk and related skin cancer.

Keywords: multi-theory model; skin cancer; sunscreen; Florida; integrative medicine

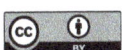

1. Introduction

Sunscreen offers an integrative health approach to sun protection, to prevent skin cancers. Skin cancer is among the most common forms of cancers in the United States (U.S.), affecting nearly 10,000 people every day [1]. Over three million cases of non-melanoma skin cancers (NMSC), including basal cell carcinoma (BCC) and squamous cell carcinoma (SCC), are diagnosed annually, with one in five Americans projected to develop the cancer during their lifetime [2]. The incidence rates may vary across states and regions, depending upon sociodemographic and environmental factors, and rates of cancer screening [1,3].

Florida has the second highest incidence rate of skin cancers in the U.S., which can be partly explained by its high ultraviolet (UV) index [3–5]. Over 600 Floridians die of skin cancer each year, and this mortality rate has doubled over the past few decades [3]. These rates are also underestimated, due to lack of NMSC reporting in cancer registries [1,6]. However, a report of the Medical Expenditure Panel Survey indicated that nearly 4.3 million people were treated for NMSC in 2015 in the U.S. [6]. Collective evidence suggests an increase in the national, as well as global, incidence of NMSC compared to other forms of non-preventable cancers combined [1,7–10].

Given the continued increase in incidence, the healthcare cost associated with skin cancer is substantial, making it the fifth most expensive disease in the U.S. [1,11]. Nearly five million people have been treated for some form of skin cancer, which cost the nation over eight billion dollars [4]. This underscores the need for adopting and reinforcing cost-effective yet simple preventive strategies, especially sunscreen use, which is the single most modifiable risk factor of skin cancer, other than avoiding ultraviolet (UV) exposure [2,12].

Other risk factors for skin cancer include old age, race, family history, male gender, long-term skin inflammation, and immunocompromised status [7,13,14]. NMSC occurs more often in white people than people of color, due to lower melanin (photo-protective pigment) production in the former group [14]. However, the worst prognosis was noted among people of color [15,16]. According to the previous reports, incidence and mortality associated with NMSC among people of color may be underestimated, given the scarcity of data [14]. UV radiation from the sun or indoor tanning machines has been directly associated with the development of skin cancer [12]. The risk of skin cancer can be significantly reduced by limiting sun exposure [12]. The American Cancer Society (ACS) recommends avoiding the sun during peak hours (10 am–4 pm), seeking shade when outdoors, wearing sun protective clothing, including sunglasses and a wide-brimmed hat, and frequently applying sunscreen (SPF > 30) with both UVA and UVB (broadband) protection [17].

Proper sunscreen use has been linked to a reduction in squamous cell and malignant melanoma skin cancer development, by 40% and 50%, respectively [18,19]. The best method of preventing skin cancer in the population is to increase sunscreen usage in the community, to protect skin from harmful UV radiation exposure. Regrettably, the utilization of sunscreen is low despite the well-established protective benefits of sunscreen in preventing skin cancers [18,19]. Personal barriers (dislike of the appearance or feel of sunscreen), time constraints, and economic barriers were commonly cited contributing factors to sunscreen underuse [20]. According to the 2015 National Health Interview Survey-Cancer Control Supplement analysis, sunscreen use in U.S adults was only 31.5% [21]. Only 10% of Americans reported using sunscreen daily with nearly half (47%) indicating that they have never used sunscreen. This highlights the importance of behavior change community-based interventions to address the underutilization of sunscreen [21].

Previous studies utilized a range of theoretical frameworks, including a transtheoretical model, health belief model, precaution adoption model, social cognitive theory, protection motivation theory, inoculation theory, and theory of planned behaviors in guiding public health interventions targeted at reducing the risk of skin cancer by promoting sunscreen usage, and thereby decreasing sun exposure [22–26]. Such theoretical interventions have received some success in identifying gaps in knowledge, attitudes, and practices, but overall, their impact has been limited in promoting sunscreen usage behaviors. Additionally, public health experts and behavior change theorists have been cognizant of the limitations of public health theories, as many of these do not provide robust estimations of the likelihood of initiation and sustenance. Behavioral change is a long-term process, and if a behavior is not sustained long enough then a relapse is more likely. Therefore, it is vital to obtain a better understanding of the initiation and sustenance of sunscreen usage in the community, to reduce the increasing incidence risk of skin cancer. Sharma (2015) attempted to address these gaps by combining constructs of popular theories and models in a way that predicted the initiation and sustenance of a behavior [27]. Therefore, this study aims to investigate the predictability of adopting and continuing sunscreen usage behavior among a high UV index risk population: Florida residents.

2. Materials and Methods

2.1. Setting, Study Design, and Sample

This study is a cross-sectional study of the general population of Florida, which is the third largest state in the U.S., with a diverse demography [28]. The data for this study were collected through a web-based survey; launched on 11 June 2021 and closed on 27 June 2021. All participants were required to be 18 years or above, current residents of Florida, and able to read and write in English. No other exclusion criteria were applied.

2.2. Sample Recruitment

Invitations to participate in this study were sent through emails, which were randomly selected from the Florida vote file. Initial emails were sent to all potential respondents (~100 k) and a follow-up reminder email was sent after 4 days to the non-respondents. We oversampled (~41 k) to reach underrepresented populations to yield a representative sample comparable to the census distribution according to the latest American Community Survey population estimates.

2.3. Study Approval and Data Protection Compliance

The study (protocol #1015079-8) received an exempt status by the Institutional Review Board (IRB), University of North Florida. All participants received a detailed participant information sheet outlining the purpose of the study, exact details related to participation (associated risks and benefits), and how information would be stored and disseminated as one or another form of scholarly product. Participants were also informed about their voluntary participation and that they could withdraw from the study at any time. Detailed contact information of the principal investigator was provided if participants had any questions about the study. Data integrity was ensured in accordance with all data privacy laws and regulations. Principal investigators shared deidentified password protected data files with the analyst of this study. The data were stored in a locked computer and analysis results were shared in an aggregate form with the rest of the research team members.

2.4. Quality Control and Authenticity of Responses

Several quality control measures were applied to ensure authenticity of the responses. The "Prevent Ballot Box Stuffing" option was selected in the Qualtrics to limit only one response from each participant to collect unique responses. Invalid or incomplete entries were removed.

2.5. Survey Instrument

The initial draft of the survey was sent to seven panelists (including three authors). All were experts in instrumentation in social and behavioral health sciences, five were experts on MTM, two were experts in sun protection research, and three were chosen from the target population. The instrument was validated for face and content validity, along with readability, in two rounds. A total of 16 changes were made during two rounds. Consensus was reached between the experts after two rounds, to finalize the survey instrument. To minimize observer bias, all reviewers were blinded. A 51-item survey MTM based questionnaire was created to examine determinants of sunscreen use among Florida residents. The Flesch reading ease of the entire scale was 66.9 and the Flesch–Kincaid grade level was 5.7 (or less than sixth grade). The survey was composed of 20 questions related to demography, outdoor activities, sunscreen use, and medical history. In addition, 31 items were related to two primary MTM theoretical constructs (initiation and sustenance). The initiation component comprised three constructs which included participatory dialogue, behavioral confidence, and changes in physical environments. "Participatory dialogue" between interventionist and subject evaluates the advantages and disadvantages of initiating an action [28–30]. "Behavioral confidence" is like self-efficacy but with subtle differences, it focuses on the self-confidence of the individual in acting. "Changes in physical environment" emphasizes the need for the subject to modify available resources and settings for a behavior to occur. The other component, sustenance (a continuation of behavior) comprises another three constructs: emotional transformation, practice for change, and changes in social environment. "Emotional transformation" involves changes in feelings and attitude and in this process, an individual prepares mentally to sustain the action [28–30]. "Practice for change" is a reflective process that continues while person is in action phase. The individual monitors behavioral progress and brings needed changes to sustain the behavior. "Changes in social environment" captures the available support around the individual that is conducive to sustaining the behavior [28–30]. A visual representation of MTM constructs is provided in Figure 1.

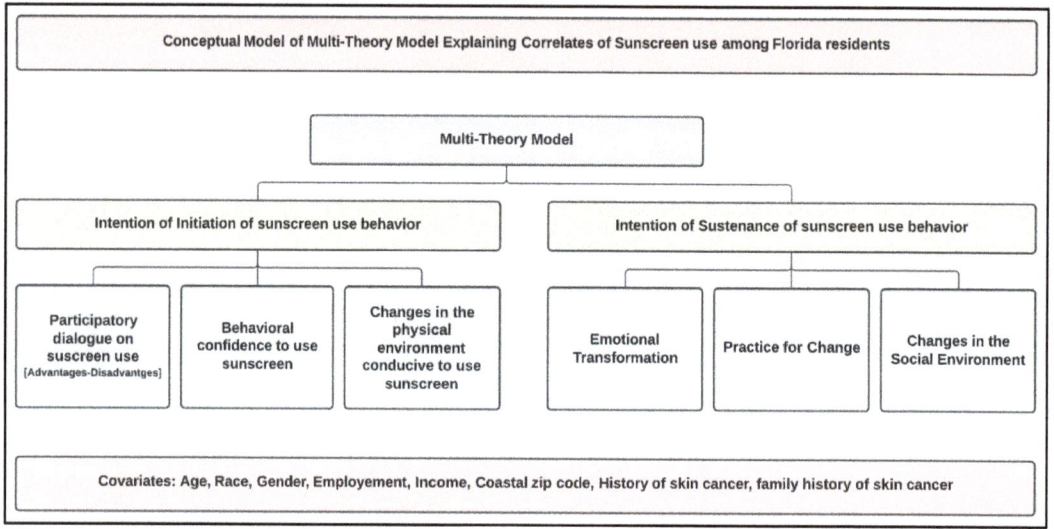

Figure 1. Multi-theory model framework.

2.6. Statistical Analysis

Participants' responses were first preprocessed and then exported to IBM SPSS version 27.0 (IBM Corp. Armonk, NY, USA) for statistical analyses. Incomplete responses and those with invalid data entries were excluded. Mean and standard deviation were used to represent continuous variables. Counts and proportions were used to express categorical variables. Inferential statistics were conducted through independent samples-t-tests to perform group-wise comparisons. Cronbach's alpha values were computed for the entire scale and subscales to assess the internal consistency. Two hierarchical regression models (HRM) were fit to explain the variance in the likelihood of initiation and sustenance of sunscreen use behavior by MTM individual constructs, besides the demographic variables. Structural equation modeling (SEM) was utilized for the construct validation. The Analysis of Moment Structure, AMOS (Chicago, IL, USA) was used for SEM [27]. We used indices such as chi-square (χ^2), root mean square error of approximation (RMSEA), comparative fit index (CFI), and Tucker–Lewis (TLI) to assess how well our models fit the data [31–33]. Models were considered to have adequate fit if they met the less stringent, but traditionally accepted, values of 0.90 or greater for CFI and TLI, and values less than 0.08 for RMSEA. P-values less than 0.05 were considered statistically significant.

2.7. Sample Size Justification

Sample size estimation of independent-samples-test was conducted using G * Power software packages, using a Cohen's small effect size of 0.2 at the power of 95% [34,35]. After factoring a 15% attrition rate ($n = 163$), the minimum sample required was 1247 participants. For the purpose of structural equation analyses, a minimum sample size of 300 was determined to be acceptable, as indicated by previous studies [36].

3. Results

A total of 1284 valid responses were included in the analysis. The mean age of the sample was 50.2 ± 18.1 years. Nearly 86% participants reported living in zip codes not touching an ocean or gulf area (Table 1). About 75 percent of the sample population reported having no college level education or degree. White respondents represented nearly half of the sample population. Six out of 10 respondents reported being employed and having an annual income under USD 100,000 (Table 1). About 13 percent of respondents had a history of skin cancer. Noticeably, 4 in 10 respondents had a family history of skin cancer (Table 1). Sunscreen users had a statistically significant higher mean scores for initiation (2.10 ± 1.49 vs 0.41 ± 1.2) and sustenance (1.82 ± 1.46 vs 0.36 ± 0.74) compared to sunscreen non-users (Table 2).

Table 1. Demographic characteristics of the sample population of Floridians ($N = 1284$).

Characteristics or Variables	n	Percentage
Age (in years)		
18–24	146	11.34
25–34	204	15.91
35–44	194	15.09
45–54	203	15.81
55–64	214	16.63
65 and over	324	25.23
Gender		
Male	619	48.24
Female	664	51.76
Coastal Zip Code		
Not Touching Ocean or Gulf	1104	86.02
Touches Ocean or Gulf	180	13.98
Race		
White	689	53.69
Black	194	15.15
Hispanic	333	25.91
Other	67	5.25
Education		
No College Degree	900	70.08
College Degree	371	28.90
Employed		
Yes	777	60.55
No	487	37.91
Annual Income		
Less than $ 50,000	434	33.81
$ 50,001 to $ 100,000	402	31.28
$ 100,001 to $ 150,000	185	14.39
$ 150,001 to $ 200,000	71	5.56
More than $ 200,000	89	6.95
Skin cancer history		
Yes	171	13.35
No	1107	86.21
Family history of skin cancer		
Yes	318	24.75
No	960	74.74

Note: Percentage may not add to 100%, due to some missing data.

Table 2. Possible and observed range and mean scores of multi-theory model constructs of behavior change across participants who engaged in sunscreen usage behavior and those who did not engage in sunscreen usage behavior (n = 1284).

Groups Constructs	Participants Who Engaged in Sunscreen Usage Behavior (n = 523)			Participants Who Did Not Engage in Sunscreen Usage Behavior (n = 761)			p-Value
	Possible Score Range	Observed Score Range	Mean ± SD	Possible Score Range	Observed Score Range	Mean ± SD	
Initiation	0–4	0–4	2.10 ± 1.49	0–4	0–4	0.41 ± 0.80	<0.001
Participatory dialogue: advantages	0–24	0–24	15.91 ± 5.00	0–24	0–24	10.76 ± 6.30	<0.001
Participatory dialogue: disadvantages	0–24	0–22	5.75 ± 4.07	0–24	0–24	8.26 ± 5.25	<0.001
Participatory dialogue	−24 to (+24)	−16 to (+24)	10.17 ± 7.07	−24 to (+24)	−24 to (+24)	2.52 ± 8.48	<0.001
Behavior confidence	0–20	0–20	9.35 ± 6.73	0–20	0–20	1.61 ± 3.12	<0.001
Changes in the physical environment	0–12	0–12	7.43 ± 3.63	0–12	0–12	4.19 ± 3.65	<0.001
Sustenance	0–4	0–4	1.82 ± 1.46	0–4	0–4	0.36 ± 0.74	<0.001
Emotional transformation	0–12	0–12	6.73 ± 3.93	0–12	0–12	2.50 ± 3.18	<0.001
Practice for change	0–12	0–12	4.65 ± 3.30	0–12	0–12	1.98 ± 2.78	<0.001
Changes in the social environment	0–12	0–12	4.48 ± 3.73	0–12	0–12	2.76 ± 3.36	<0.001

Among participants who were engaged in sunscreen usage behaviors, the final model containing the demographic variables and all three constructs to predict initiation was statistically significant (adjusted R^2 = 0.736, F = 113.572, $p < 0.001$; Table 3). In the same group, constructs of emotional transformation, practice for change, and changes in social environment (besides family history of skin cancer) were significant predictors of the sustenance of sunscreen usage behavior (adjusted R^2 = 0.590, F = 59.565, $p < 0.001$; Table 3). Among participants who were not engaged in sunscreen usage behaviors, the model containing all constructs of initiation that were significant predictors of initiation was statistically significant; adjusted R^2 = 0.500, F = 61.305, $p < 0.001$; Table 4. In the sustenance model, emotional transformation, practice for change, and changes in the social environment explained 23.9% of variance in sustaining sunscreen usage behaviors among those who did not engage in sunscreen usage behavior (adjusted R^2 = 0.239, F = 19.80, $p < 0.001$; Table 4).

Table 3. Hierarchical multiple regression (HRM) predicting likelihood of initiation and sustenance among respondents who used sunscreen (n = 523).

Variables	Model 1		Model 2		Model 3		Model 4	
	B	β	B	β	B	β	B	β
The likelihood of initiation as a dependent variable								
(Constant)	1.927		0.640		−0.224		−0.553	
Age	0.001	0.001	0.004	0.047	0.007 *	0.084	0.007 **	0.088
Gender (Female Ref.)	−0.445 **	−0.147	−0.376 **	−0.124	−0.243 **	−0.081	−0.205 *	−0.068
Race (White Ref.)	0.696 **	0.232	0.531 **	0.177	0.480 **	0.160	0.602 **	0.201
Employment (Not working Ref.)	−0.065	−0.021	−0.014	−0.005	−0.001	0.000	−0.007	−0.002
Annual Income (<$100,000 Ref.)	−0.016	−0.005	−0.008	−0.003	−0.128	−0.042	−0.152	−0.050
Education (No college degree Ref.)	−0.006	−0.002	−0.107	−0.034	0.079	0.025	0.017	0.005
Coastal Zip Code (Not touch ocean Ref.)	0.185	0.042	0.088	0.020	0.100	0.023	0.092	0.021
Skin Cancer (No Ref.)	0.052	0.013	−0.045	−0.011	−0.184	−0.045	−0.195	−0.048
Family History of Skin Cancer (No Ref.)	0.364 *	0.109	0.269 **	0.081	0.288 **	0.087	0.278 **	0.083
Participatory dialogue	-	-	0.117 **	0.552	0.026 **	0.123	0.013 *	0.062
Behavioral confidence	-	-	-	-	0.166 **	0.746	0.141 **	0.636
Changes in the physical environment	-	-	-	-	-	-	0.086 **	0.210
R^2	0.062	-	0.360	-	0.724	-	0.742	-
F	3.517 **	-	26.758 **	-	112.985 **	-	113.572 **	-
Δ R^2	0.062	-	0.298	-	0.364	-	0.018	-
Δ F	3.517 **	-	221.294 **	-	624.447 **	-	33.888 **	-

Table 3. Cont.

Variables	Model 1 B	β	Model 2 B	β	Model 3 B	β	Model 4 B	β
The likelihood of sustenance as a dependent variable								
Constant	1.924	-	−0.165	-	−0.274	-	−0.392	-
Age	−0.008	−0.094	−0.002	−0.023	−0.001	−0.014	0.000	−0.004
Gender (Female Referent)	−0.382 *	−0.128	−0.115	−0.039	−0.101	−0.034	−0.114	−0.038
Race (White Ref.)	0.539 **	0.182	0.486 **	0.165	0.508 **	0.172	0.493	0.167
Employment (Not working Ref.)	0.124	0.041	0.099	0.033	0.042	0.014	0.088	0.029
Annual Income (<$100,000 Ref.)	0.013	0.004	−0.074	−0.025	−0.048	−0.016	−0.054	−0.018
Education (No college degree Ref.)	−0.060	−0.019	−0.041	−0.013	−0.061	−0.019	0.006	0.002
Coastal Zip Code (Not touching ocean Ref.)	0.224	0.051	0.034	0.008	0.052	0.012	0.029	0.007
Skin Cancer (No Ref.)	0.125	0.031	0.045	0.011	0.047	0.012	0.036	0.009
Family History of Skin Cancer (No Ref.)	0.286	0.087	0.223 *	0.068	0.246 **	0.075	0.216 *	0.066
Emotional transformation	-	-	0.265 **	0.709	0.201 **	0.538	0.181 **	0.486
Practice for change	-	-	-	-	0.110 **	0.249	0.094 **	0.211
Changes in the social environment	-	-	-	-	-	-	0.058 **	0.148
R^2	0.068	-	0.554	-	0.586	-	0.600	-
F	3.902 **	-	59.502 **	-	61.344 **	-	59.565 **	-
ΔR^2	0.068	-	0.486	-	0.031	-	0.014	-
ΔF	3.902 **	-	521.764 **	-	36.102 **	-	17.157 **	-

B (Unstandardized coefficient); β (Standardized coefficient), * p-value < 0.05; ** p-value < 0.001; Adjusted R^2 of initiation = 0.736; Adjusted R^2 of sustenance = 0.590.

Table 4. Hierarchical Multiple Regression (HRM) predicting likelihood of initiation and sustenance among respondents who did not use sunscreen (n = 761).

Variables	Model 1 B	β	Model 2 B	β	Model 3 B	β	Model 4 B	β
The likelihood of initiation as a dependent variable								
(Constant)	0.474	-	0.429	-	0.115	-	0.019	-
Age	−0.001	−0.023	−0.001	−0.020	0.000	−0.009	0.000	−0.008
Gender (Female Referent)	−0.256 **	−0.158	−0.238 **	−0.147	−0.113 *	−0.070	−0.117 *	−0.072
Race (White Ref.)	0.130	0.081	0.102	0.063	0.091	0.056	0.112 *	0.069
Employment (Not working Ref.)	0.030	0.018	0.009	0.005	0.057	0.034	0.052	0.031
Annual Income (<$100,000 Ref.)	0.070	0.040	0.044	0.025	0.008	0.004	−0.009	−0.005
Education (No college degree Ref.)	0.080	0.044	0.041	0.023	0.012	0.007	−0.018	−0.010
Coastal Zip Code (Not touching ocean Ref.)	−0.036	−0.016	−0.089	−0.038	−0.014	−0.006	−0.011	−0.005
Skin Cancer (No Ref.)	−0.084	−0.033	−0.104	−0.041	−0.117	−0.046	−0.138	−0.054
Family History of Skin Cancer (No Ref.)	0.091	0.047	0.040	0.021	0.082	0.043	0.084	0.044
Participatory dialogue	-	-	0.037 **	0.394	0.016 **	0.174	0.013 **	0.143
Behavioral confidence	-	-	-	-	0.154 **	0.601	0.146 **	0.568
Changes in the physical environment	-	-	-	-	-	-	0.029 **	0.133
R^2	0.038	-	0.190	-	0.494	-	0.508	-
F	3.129 **	-	16.768 **	-	63.323 **	-	61.305 **	-
ΔR^2	0.038	-	0.152	-	0.304	-	0.014	-
ΔF	3.129 **	-	134.267 **	-	428.455 **	-	20.275 **	-
The likelihood of sustenance as a dependent variable								
Constant	0.218	-	−0.091	-	−0.087	-	−0.139	-
Age	0.001	0.034	0.002	0.054	0.002	0.052	0.003	0.065
Gender (Female Referent)	−0.190 **	−0.127	−0.123 *	−0.082	−0.135 *	−0.090	−0.147 **	−0.098
Race (White Ref.)	0.192 **	0.129	0.143 *	0.096	0.132 *	0.088	0.137 *	0.092
Employment (Not working Ref.)	0.072	0.047	0.081	0.052	0.065	0.042	0.073	0.048
Annual Income (< $100,000 Ref.)	−9.921	0.000	−0.040	−0.025	−0.013	−0.008	−0.029	−0.018
Education (No college degree Ref.)	0.058	0.035	0.033	0.020	0.039	0.023	0.042	0.025
Coastal Zip Code (Not touching ocean Ref.)	0.064	0.030	0.086	0.040	0.089	0.042	0.087	0.041
Skin cancer (No Ref.)	−0.084	−0.036	−0.106	−0.045	−0.117	−0.050	−0.111	−0.047
Family History of skin Cancer (No Ref.)	0.132	0.074	0.129 *	0.072	0.129 *	0.072	0.129 *	0.072
Emotional transformation	-	-	0.107 **	0.455	0.084 **	0.358	0.080 **	0.340
Practice for change	-	-	-	-	0.036 *	0.135	0.028 *	0.107
Changes in the social environment	-	-	-	-	-	-	0.019 *	0.085
R^2	0.036	-	0.239	-	0.247	-	0.252	-
F	2.927 **	-	22.143 **	-	21.028 **	-	19.800 **	-
ΔR^2	0.036	-	0.0203	-	0.008	-	0.005	-
ΔF	2.927 **	-	188.128 **	-	7.758 *	-	4.980 *	-

B (Unstandardized coefficient); β (Standardized coefficient), * p-value < 0.05; ** p-value < 0.001; Adjusted R^2 of initiation = 0.500; Adjusted R^2 of sustenance = 0.239.

Construct Validation through Structural Equation Modeling

The structural equation modeling results (e.g., χ^2 [252] = 1511.870 ($p < 0.001$), CFI = 0.93, TLI= 0.92, and RMSEA = 0.08) for the initiation model demonstrated the goodness of fit of the data. Standardized effects of latent variables on the factor loading indicators were observed. The factor loadings of all the subscales of initiation are shown in Figure 2.

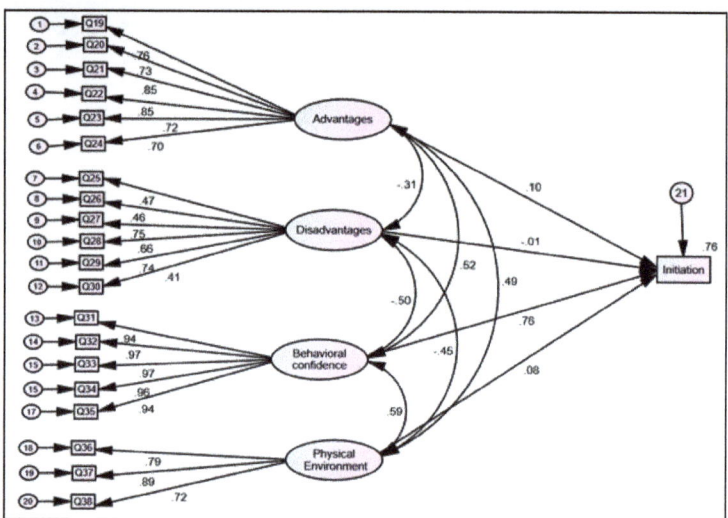

Figure 2. Structural equation modeling for initiation of sunscreen use behavior among Florida residents.

The sustenance model fit the data well (e.g., χ^2 [30] = 193.871 ($p < 0.001$), CFI = 0.98, TLI = 0.97, and RMSEA = 0.07). The factor loadings for emotional transformation, practice for change, and changes in the social environment were statistically significant. The factor loadings for all the subscales of sustenance are shown in Figure 3. The between construct correlations and standardized regression coefficients for emotional transformation showed moderate direct effects on the sustenance of sunscreen behavior, with β ranging from 0.12 to 0.51. However, both practice for change and changes in the social environment did not have any significant effects on the sustenance of sunscreen use behavior.

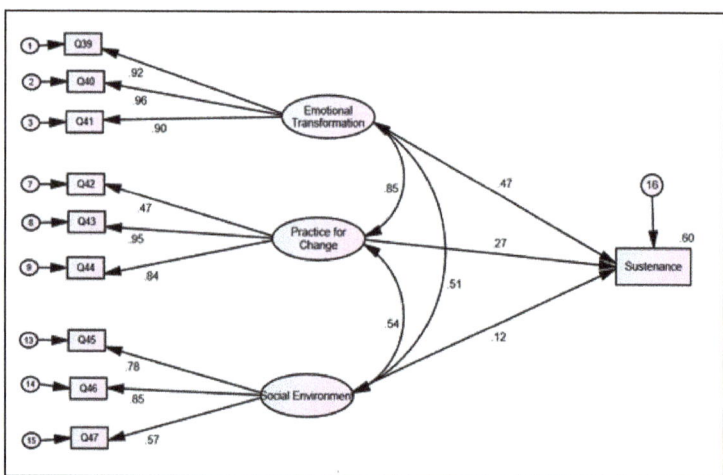

Figure 3. Structural equation modeling for sustenance of sunscreen use behavior among Florida residents.

4. Discussion

The purpose of this study was to identify the correlates of sunscreen use, based on the fourth-generation multi-theory model (MTM) of health behavior change among Florida residents. MTM has been tested or applied to explain various health behaviors in community settings [37–43]. The results of the study were encouraging; the contribution of MTM constructs in all four models tested were significant and accounted for a substantial proportion of variance in the dependent variables. In our sample, 40.7% of the respondents used sunscreen, which was higher than the national rate of 31.5% [21]. However, sunscreen behavior was still low, given the second highest rate of skin cancer in Florida [4,5]. Understanding the determinants of sunscreen behavior is an important first step in promoting sunscreen usage behavior.

In the group who indicated sunscreen usage, all three MTM constructs (participatory dialogue, behavioral confidence, and changes in the physical environment), along with gender, race, and a history of skin cancer, were found to be significant predictors. This accounted for 73.6% of the variance in the initiation of the use of sunscreen, which is substantive in behavioral and social sciences [30]. Likewise, for sustaining sunscreen behavior among those who were already using sunscreens, all three constructs of MTM (emotional transformation, practice for change, and changes in the social environment) were found to account for 59.0% variance in the continuation of sunscreen usage. Moreover, all three constructs of MTM (participatory dialogue, behavioral confidence, and changes in the physical environment), along with gender and race, were significant explanatory variables for initiating sunscreen usage behavior among those who were not currently using sunscreen and accounted for 50% of the variance in initiation. Equally important was the finding that all three constructs of MTM (emotional transformation, practice for change, and changes in the social environment), along with gender and race, significantly accounted for 23.9% of the variance in the intention to maintain sunscreen usage behavior. These findings lend support to MTM as a strong model for designing, implementing, and evaluating sunscreen promotion interventions in the general population.

Consistently with previous studies, males were less likely to initiate use of sunscreens, both among those who were sunscreen users and those who were not. Holman and colleagues (2018), in their national study with 31,162 respondents, found that 22.1% of men compared to 40.2% of women used sunscreens [21]. Gender differences associated with intentional UV exposure through indoor tanning were also studied by previous reports [44–46]. In a U.S. based study, a higher proportion of females reported using indoor tanning compared to their male counterparts; however, data describing the setting (indoor or outdoor) of sunscreen use were insufficient [44–46]. Another interesting finding of our study was that history of skin cancer was positively associated with initiation of sunscreen usage behavior among those who were sunscreen users, but was not significant among those who did not use sunscreens. This could be explained by the reasoning that non-users were not concerned as much about their getting skin cancer or did not have "cues to action." The MTM can play a vital role in motivating this group of non-users. This finding provides additional support for designing sunscreen promotion interventions based on MTM. Another intriguing finding was that family history of skin cancer was a positively associated significant factor for both initiation and sustenance of sunscreen usage among those who were sun screen users, indicating that users were indeed convinced of the benefits of wearing sunscreens. These findings provide the basis of developing MTM-based interventions to promote sunscreen use.

4.1. Strengths and Limitations

To our knowledge, this was the first study to apply MTM to explain sunscreen usage behavior. We collected data on a multitude of correlates and adjusted for those in our analysis to generate robust estimates. Despite these strengths, this study is not without limitations. First, the use of a cross-sectional design has the limitation of collecting information on independent variables and dependent variables at the same time, thereby precluding causal inferences. Future studies could test the validity of MTM in experimental designs, whereby actual manipulation of the variables is done in a longitudinal manner. Furthermore, self-reports are liable to several shortcomings, such as dishonesty, exaggerated responses, and so on. However, when measuring attitudes, one cannot choose another approach and these are indeed the only means. Finally, the study was done in Florida, thereby limiting the generalizability to other parts of the country.

4.2. Implications for Practice

The MTM offers a valuable prototype to design efficacious and effective sunscreen promotion interventions. Such interventions can be delivered in community settings, such as through recreational centers, faith-based organizations, community centers, community-based organizations, beach clubs, and other such venues. The promotional interventions could take the form of media campaigns; social media campaigns; one to one health education interventions, as well as in group forums; events and fairs; m-health interventions; counseling at clinics and patient care settings; and policy level efforts. For promotional interventions, the construct of participatory dialogue can be mobilized by underscoring the advantages, such as appeals to health, prevention of skin cancer, having peace of mind, not getting sunburn, and so on. At the same time, misperceptions about the disadvantages, such as staining, inconvenience, forgetfulness, cost, etc. can be clarified through discussion. The construct of behavioral confidence can be built through discussions on building assurance through self-reflection and other sources and overcoming potential barriers. The construct of changes in the physical environment can be developed through looking into the possibility of making sunscreen available to those who cannot afford it, discussing methods of application during travel and also looking into mobilizing policy support in this direction. Regarding the maintenance constructs, for emotional transformation, learning to identify feelings must be the first step in educational interventions. Then ways of converting these feelings, especially those that are negative, along with self-motivation and overcoming self-doubt must be undertaken. Regarding the practice for change construct, methods of monitoring sunscreen application behavior through apps or simple record keeping in a diary should be discussed. Troubleshooting lapses in practice and remedies must also be discussed. Finally, ways to mobilize support from family, friends, social media, health professionals, etc. must be discussed.

5. Conclusions

This was the first study undertaken to study the determinants of sunscreen usage behavior, using the fourth-generation, multi-theory model (MTM) of health behavior change. All the constructs of MTM were found to be significant predictors of sunscreen use among Floridians, thereby lending support to this model. All the constructs of MTM are modifiable, making it a practical approach for effecting behavior change. This study provides preliminary data to develop and test theory-based interventions to promote sunscreen usage among Florida residents.

Author Contributions: Conceptualization, M.S.; methodology, M.S., M.A., E.L.-W., J.M., M.B., R.L.; software, M.S., M.A., M.B.; validation, M.S., M.A., E.L.-W., J.M., M.B., R.L., K.B.; formal analysis, M.A.; investigation, M.S., M.A., E.L.-W., J.M., M.B., R.L., K.B.; resources, M.S., M.A., E.L.-W., J.M., M.B.; data curation, E.L.-W., J.M., M.B.; writing, M.S., M.A., E.L.-W., J.M., M.B., R.L., K.B.; writing—review and editing, M.S., M.A., E.L.-W., J.M., M.B., R.L., K.B.; visualization, M.S., M.A., K.B.; supervision, M.S.; project administration, M.S., E.L.-W., M.B. All authors have read and agreed to the published version of the manuscript.

Funding: This research received no external funding.

Institutional Review Board Statement: This study was conducted according to the guidelines of the Declaration of Helsinki and approved by the Institutional Review Board (or Ethics Committee) of the University of North Florida (1015079-8 dated 5 April 2021).

Informed Consent Statement: Informed consent was obtained from all subjects involved in the study.

Data Availability Statement: The data presented in this study are available on request from the corresponding author. The data are not publicly available due to ethical reasons.

Conflicts of Interest: The authors declare no conflict of interest.

References

1. Rogers, H.W.; Weinstock, M.A.; Feldman, S.R.; Coldiron, B.M. Incidence Estimate of Nonmelanoma Skin Cancer (Keratinocyte Carcinomas) in the US Population, 2012. *JAMA Dermatol.* **2015**, *151*, 1081–1086. [CrossRef] [PubMed]
2. American Academy of Dermatology/Milliman. Burden of Skin Disease. 2017. Available online: www.aad.org/BSD (accessed on 12 February 2021).
3. Fernandez, C.A.; McClure, L.A.; Leblanc, W.G.; Clarke, T.C.; Kirsner, R.S.; Fleming, L.E.; Arheart, K.L.; Lee, D.J. Comparison of Florida skin cancer screening rates with those in different US regions. *South. Med. J.* **2012**, *105*, 524. [CrossRef] [PubMed]
4. Centers for Disease Control and Prevention. Melanoma Dashboard. 2021. Available online: https://ephtracking.cdc.gov/Applications/melanomadashboard/ (accessed on 4 July 2021).
5. Nestor, M.S.; Zarraga, M.B. The Incidence of Nonmelanoma Skin Cancers and Actinic Keratoses in South Florida. *J. Clin. Aesthetic Dermatol.* **2012**, *5*, 20–24.
6. Perera, E.; Sinclair, R. An estimation of the prevalence of nonmelanoma skin cancer in the US. *F1000Research* **2013**, *2*, 107. [CrossRef] [PubMed]
7. Henrikson, N.B.; Morrison, C.C.; Blasi, P.R.; Nguyen, M.; Shibuya, K.C.; Patnode, C.D. *Behavioral Counseling for Skin Cancer Prevention: A Systematic Evidence Review for the U.S. Preventive Services Task Force*; Preventive Services Task Force, 2018. Available online: https://www.ncbi.nlm.nih.gov/books/NBK493693/ (accessed on 6 October 2021).
8. Fahradyan, A.; Howell, A.C.; Wolfswinkel, E.M.; Tsuha, M.; Sheth, P.; Wong, A.K. Updates on the Management of Non-Melanoma Skin Cancer (NMSC). *Health* **2017**, *5*, 82. [CrossRef]
9. Oh, C.-M.; Cho, H.; Won, Y.-J.; Kong, H.-J.; Roh, Y.H.; Jeong, K.-H.; Jung, K.-W. Nationwide Trends in the Incidence of Melanoma and Non-melanoma Skin Cancers from 1999 to 2014 in South Korea. *Cancer Res. Treat.* **2018**, *50*, 729–737. [CrossRef] [PubMed]
10. Arab, K.A.; AlRuhaili, A.; AlJohany, T.; AlHammad, R.S. Melanoma and non-melanoma skin cancer among patients who attended at King Khalid University Hospital in Riyadh, Saudi Arabia from 2007–2018. *Saudi Med. J.* **2020**, *41*, 709–714. [CrossRef] [PubMed]
11. Housman, T.S.; Feldman, S.; Williford, P.M.; Fleischer, A.B.; Goldman, N.D.; Acostamadiedo, J.M.; Chen, G. Skin cancer is among the most costly of all cancers to treat for the Medicare population. *J. Am. Acad. Dermatol.* **2003**, *48*, 425–429. [CrossRef]
12. Gandini, S.; Sera, F.; Cattaruzza, M.S.; Pasquini, P.; Zanetti, R.; Masini, C.; Boyle, P.; Melchi, C.F. Meta-analysis of risk factors for cutaneous melanoma: III. Family history, actinic damage and phenotypic factors. *Eur. J. Cancer* **2005**, *41*, 2040–2059. [CrossRef]
13. Livingstone, E.; Windemuth-Kieselbach, C.; Eigentler, T.K.; Rompel, R.; Trefzer, U.; Nashan, D.; Rotterdam, S.; Ugurel, S.; Schadendorf, D. A first prospective population-based analysis investigating the actual practice of melanoma diagnosis, treatment and follow-up. *Eur. J. Cancer* **2011**, *47*, 1977–1989. [CrossRef]
14. Bradford, P.T. Skin cancer in skin of color. *Dermatol. Nurs.* **2009**, *21*, 170–178.
15. Agbai, O.N.; Buster, K.; Sanchez, M.; Hernandez, C.; Kundu, R.V.; Chiu, M.; Roberts, W.E.; Draelos, Z.D.; Bhushan, R.; Taylor, S.C.; et al. Skin cancer and photoprotection in people of color: A review and recommendations for physicians and the public. *J. Am. Acad. Dermatol.* **2014**, *70*, 748–762. [CrossRef]
16. Dawes, S.M.; Tsai, S.; Gittleman, H.; Barnholtz-Sloan, J.; Bordeaux, J.S. Racial disparities in melanoma survival. *J. Am. Acad. Dermatol.* **2016**, *75*, 983–991. [CrossRef]
17. American Cancer Society. Can Melanoma Skin Cancer Be prevented? Available online: https://www.cancer.org/cancer/melanoma-skin-cancer/causes-risks-prevention/prevention.html (accessed on 21 March 2021).
18. Green, A.; Williams, G.; Neale, R.; Hart, V.; Leslie, D.; Parsons, P.; Marks, G.C.; Gaffney, P.; Battistutta, D.; Frost, C.; et al. Daily sunscreen application and betacarotene supplementation in prevention of basal-cell and squamous-cell carcinomas of the skin: A randomised controlled trial. *Lancet* **1999**, *354*, 723–729. [CrossRef]
19. Green, A.C.; Williams, G.; Logan, V.; Strutton, G.M. Reduced Melanoma After Regular Sunscreen Use: Randomized Trial Follow-Up. *J. Clin. Oncol.* **2011**, *29*, 257–263. [CrossRef]
20. Weig, E.A.; Tull, R.; Chung, J.; Brown-Joel, Z.O.; Majee, R.; Ferguson, N.N. Assessing factors affecting sunscreen use and barriers to compliance: A cross-sectional survey-based study. *J. Dermatol. Treat.* **2019**, *31*, 403–405. [CrossRef]
21. Holman, D.M.; Ding, H.; Guy, G.P.; Watson, M.; Hartman, A.M.; Perna, F.M. Prevalence of Sun Protection Use and Sunburn and Association of Demographic and Behavioral Characteristics with Sunburn Among US Adults. *JAMA Dermatol.* **2018**, *154*, 561–568. [CrossRef]
22. Kristjánsson, S.; Bränström, R.; Ullén, H.; Helgason, Á.R. Transtheoretical model: Investigation of adolescents' sunbathing behaviour. *Eur. J. Cancer Prev.* **2003**, *12*, 501–508. [CrossRef]
23. Jeihooni, A.K.; Rakhshani, T. The Effect of Educational Intervention Based on Health Belief Model and Social Support on Promoting Skin Cancer Preventive Behaviors in a Sample of Iranian Farmers. *J. Cancer Educ.* **2018**, *34*, 392–401. [CrossRef] [PubMed]
24. Crane, L.A.; Asdigian, N.L.; Barón, A.E.; Aalborg, J.; Marcus, A.C.; Mokrohisky, S.T.; Byers, T.E.; Dellavalle, R.P.; Morelli, J.G. Mailed Intervention to Promote Sun Protection of Children. *Am. J. Prev. Med.* **2012**, *43*, 399–410. [CrossRef] [PubMed]

25. Craciun, C.; Schüz, N.; Lippke, S.; Schwarzer, R. Facilitating Sunscreen Use in Women by a Theory-Based Online Intervention: A Randomized Controlled Trial. *J. Health Psychol.* **2011**, *17*, 207–216. [CrossRef] [PubMed]
26. Prentice-Dunn, S.; Mcmath, B.F.; Cramer, R. Protection Motivation Theory and Stages of Change in Sun Protective Behavior. *J. Health Psychol.* **2009**, *14*, 297–305. [CrossRef]
27. Sharma, M. Multi-theory model (MTM) for health behavior change. *WebmedCentral Behav.* **2015**, *6*, WMC004982. Available online: http://www.webmedcentral.com/article_view/4982 (accessed on 6 April 2021).
28. United States Census Bureau. Age and Sex Composition. Available online: https://www.census.gov/prod/cen2010/briefs/c2010br-03.pdf (accessed on 11 March 2021).
29. Sharma, M. *Theoretical Foundations of Health Education and Health Promotion*, 4th ed.; Jones and Bartlett: Burlington, MA, USA, 2021; pp. 250–262. ISBN 978-1284208627.
30. Sharma, M.; Petosa, R.L. *Measurement and Evaluation for Health Educators*; Jones and Bartlett: Burlington, MA, USA, 2014.
31. Arbuckle, J.L. *Amos 7.0 User's Guide*; SPSS: Chicago, IL, USA, 2006.
32. Byrne, B.M. *Structural Equation Modeling with AMOS: Basic Concepts, Applications, and Programming*, 2nd ed.; Routledge Taylor & Francis Group: New York, NY, USA, 2001; ISBN 978-0-8058-6372-7.
33. Hu, L.; Bentler, P.M. Cutoff criteria for fit indexes in covariance structure analysis: Conventional criteria versus new alternatives. *Struct. Equ. Model. Multidiscip. J.* **1999**, *6*, 1–55. [CrossRef]
34. Cohen, J. *Statistical Power Analysis for the Behavioral Sciences*, 2nd ed.; Lawrence Erlbaum Associates: Mahwah, NJ, USA, 1988; ISBN 0-8058-0283-5. Available online: http://utstat.toronto.edu/~{}brunner/oldclass/378f16/readings/CohenPower.pdf (accessed on 1 May 2021).
35. Faul, F.; Erdfelder, E.; Buchner, A.; Lang, A.-G. Statistical power analyses using G*Power 3.1: Tests for correlation and regression analyses. *Behav. Res. Methods* **2009**, *41*, 1149–1160. [CrossRef]
36. Tabachnick, B.G.; Fidell, L.S. *Using Multivariate Statistics*, 7th ed.; Pearson: Upper Saddle River, NJ, USA, 2018.
37. Sharma, M.; Batra, K.; Flatt, J. Testing the Multi-Theory Model (MTM) to Predict the Use of New Technology for Social Connectedness in the COVID-19 Pandemic. *Health* **2021**, *9*, 838. [CrossRef]
38. Yoshany, N.; Sharma, M.; Bahri, N.; Jambarsang, S.; Morowatisharifabad, M.A. Predictors in Initiating and Maintaining Nutritional Behaviors to Deal with Menopausal Symptoms Based on Multi-Theory Model. *Int. Q. Community Health Educ.* **2021**. [CrossRef]
39. Williams, J.L.; Sharma, M.; Mendy, V.L.; Leggett, S.; Akil, L.; Perkins, S. Using multi theory model (MTM) of health behavior change to explain intention for initiation and sustenance of the consumption of fruits and vegetables among African American men from barbershops in Mississippi. *Health Promot. Perspect.* **2020**, *10*, 200–206. [CrossRef]
40. Sharma, S.; Aryal, U.R.; Sharma, M. Testing the multi-theory model for initiation and sustenance of smoking cessation at Kathmandu Metropolitan, Nepal: A cross-sectional study. *J. Health Soc. Sci.* **2020**, *5*, 397–408. [CrossRef]
41. Asare, M.; Agyei-Baffour, P.; Lanning, B.A.; Owusu, A.B.; Commeh, M.E.; Boozer, K.; Koranteng, A.; Spies, L.A.; Montealegre, J.R.; Paskett, E.D. Multi-Theory Model and Predictors of Likelihood of Accepting the Series of HPV Vaccination: A Cross-Sectional Study among Ghanaian Adolescents. *Int. J. Environ. Res. Public Health* **2020**, *17*, 571. [CrossRef]
42. Bashirian, S.; Barati, M.; Ahmadi, F.; Abasi, H.; Sharma, M. Male students' experiences on predictors of waterpipe smoking reduction: A qualitative study in Iran. *Tob. Prev. Cessat.* **2019**, *5*, 30. [CrossRef]
43. Lakhan, R.; Turner, S.; Dorjee, S.; Sharma, M. Initiation and sustenance of small portion size consumption behavior in rural Appalachia, USA: Application of multi-theory model (MTM). *J. Health Soc. Sci.* **2019**, *4*, 85–100.
44. Julian, A.K.; Bethel, J.W.; Odden, M.C.; Thorburn, S. Sex differences and risk behaviors among indoor tanners. *Prev. Med. Rep.* **2016**, *3*, 283–287. [CrossRef] [PubMed]
45. Dodds, M.; Arron, S.T.; Linos, E.; Polcari, I.; Mansh, M.D. Characteristics and Skin Cancer Risk Behaviors of Adult Sunless Tanners in the United States. *JAMA Dermatol.* **2018**, *154*, 1066–1071. [CrossRef] [PubMed]
46. Fischer, A.H.; Wang, T.S.; Yenokyan, G.; Kang, S.; Chien, A.L. Association of Indoor Tanning Frequency with Risky Sun Protection Practices and Skin Cancer Screening. *JAMA Dermatol.* **2017**, *153*, 168. [CrossRef] [PubMed]

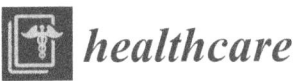

Systematic Review

Effect of Doll Therapy in Behavioral and Psychological Symptoms of Dementia: A Systematic Review

Angela Martín-García [1], Ana-Isabel Corregidor-Sánchez [2,*], Virginia Fernández-Moreno [3], Vanesa Alcántara-Porcuna [2] and Juan-José Criado-Álvarez [4]

1. Occupational Therapy Department, Altagracia Nursing Home, 28660 Madrid, Spain; angela71196@hotmail.com
2. Faculty of Health Sciences, University of Castilla la Mancha, 45600 Talavera de la Reina, Spain; vanesa.alcantara@uclm.es
3. HNSP–SESCAM, Health Service of Castilla la Mancha, 45600 Talavera de la Reina, Spain; vfernandezmoreno@sescam.jccm.es
4. Institute of Sciences Health, 45006 Talavera de la Reina, Castilla la Mancha, Spain; jjcriado@jccm.es
* Correspondence: anaisabel.corregidor@uclm.es; Tel.: +34-902904100

Abstract: (1) Background: Behavioral and psychological symptoms of dementia (BPSD) are a threat for people with dementia and their caregivers. Doll therapy is a non-pharmacological person-centered therapy to promote attachment, company, and usefulness with the aim of minimizing challenging behaviors. However, the results are not clear. (2) Objective: To know the effectiveness of doll therapy in reducing behavioral and psychological symptoms of people with dementia at a moderate-severe phase. (3) Methodology: The systematic review was informed according to the criteria established by the Preferred Reporting Items for Systematic Reviews and Meta-Analyses (PRISMA) statement. Searches were conducted in eight databases: Cochrane, PubMed, Web of Science, Cinahl, Embase, Lilacs, PeDro, and Scopus before October 2021. Studies were selected when they accomplished the simple majority of Consolidated Standards of Reporting Trials (CONSORT). The risk of bias was appraised with the Cochrane Collaboration Risk of Bias Tool. The review protocol was recorded in Inplasy:1539. (4) Results: The initial search strategy showed 226 relevant studies, 7 of which met the eligibility criteria. In the included studies, a total number of 295 participants (79% female) with a mean age of 85 years were enrolled. There was found to be a reduction in challenging and aggressive behaviors, the participants were less rough and irritable, and their communication skills and emotional state were also improved. (5) Conclusion: Our findings suggest that doll therapy improves the emotional state of people with dementia, diminishes disruptive behaviors, and promotes communication. However, randomized studies with a larger sample size and higher methodological rigor are needed, as well as follow-up protocols in order to reaffirm these results.

Keywords: doll-therapy; dementia; behavioral and psychological symptoms of dementia

1. Introduction

Dementia is one of the most common syndromes in old age with an evolution that follows an exponential pattern; it is estimated that by 2030 there will be 82 million people in the world diagnosed with dementia [1].

Alzheimer's disease (AD) is a neurodegenerative disease of unknown etiology characterized by a progressive deterioration of memory and cognitive function and represents between 60 and 80% of dementia cases [2]. In the initial phase, it appears as temporospatial disorientation and a tendency for frequent forgetfulness, in the intermediate phase, the disorientation and memory alterations intensify and provoke difficulties in communication and the need for help to carry out daily life activities. The third phase is characterized by obstacles in orientation, walking, communicating, or recognizing close family members.

The course of AD may be affected by the appearance of psychological and cognitive symptoms of dementia (SPCD) as well. In 90% of AD cases, symptoms such as agitation, psychosis, apathy, sleep disorders, appetite changes, euphoria, irritability, aberrant motor behavior, depression, and anxiety usually appear [3]. Aggression, agitation, delirium, and erratic wandering have been identified as one of the main reasons for the overload of informal caregivers [4,5]. The impact of BPSD is so intense and overwhelming that it provokes high exhaustion, stress, anxiety, and depression in the patient, as well as in the family and caregivers, triggering institutionalization in most cases. Among professional caretakers, several studies have found that SCPD, such as agitation, erratic wandering, and aggressive episodes, may cause negative feelings and discomfort [6], causing a painful experience [7,8] and reducing their work motivation [9].

The development of programs of non-pharmacological interventions such as reminiscence therapy, music therapy, therapy with animals, or sensory stimulation therapy seems to improve the emotional wellness of people with advanced dementia. The common denominator of these techniques is based on achieving positive emotions through pleasant memories, music, or contact with pets that minimize states of anxiety or anguish, diminishing the risk of BPSD.

Doll therapy (DT) is a non-pharmacological technique with the aim to promote attachment, company, and usefulness in people with dementia to increase their wellness and minimize the appearance of challenging behaviors [10,11]. It is based on the combination of three theories: the Attachment Theory, the Transitional Object Theory, and the Person-centered Theory. The attachment theory [12] postulates the need for a human being to establish affective bonds when facing unknown situations, fear, or danger. In this way, people with dementia usually have behaviors related to attachment and fixing phenomena with their parents, looking constantly for them. DT offers the possibility to establish the affective bond needed in stress situations, thus lowering agitation.

The Transitional Object Theory [13] is based on the calming properties that certain objects may have to alleviate and diminish the anguish. Two kinds of objects have been defined: transition objects (known by the subject) [13] and precursor objects (unknown by the subject) [14]. In the case of people with dementia, the doll might be a precursor object introduced in their environment by the caregiver to give comfort and alleviate and diminish the anguish generated by the SCPD [15,16].

The Person-centered Theory was developed by Carl Rogers in 1961 [17] and places the individual at the center of care, being supported and trained to be able to collaborate with the decision-making process. Uniting this approach to positive personal workouts developed by Kitwood [18], DT can offer the possibility of developing game interactions, facilitation, and validation, converting the interactions with the doll into a positive activity and a way to connect with others.

The dolls are designed to recreate the feeling of touching, staring, dressing up, and holding a baby in their arms and can bring to the present-day older roles related to maternity and generate feelings of utility and meaning which may substitute challenging behaviors with care behaviors towards the doll. In this way, the use of dolls with a baby-like appearance (newborn dolls, reborn, or empathy dolls) generated a higher commitment from the patients in comparison with the use of stuffed and other kinds of dolls [19]. Several authors have found benefits in the use of DT, observing a decrease of negative behaviors such as agitation, aggressiveness, or erratic wandering as well as an increase in communication with the environment and independence in daily life [10,11,20]. Systematic revisions in this regard conclude that DT has positive effects on the person with dementia as long as it improves communication with the environment, alleviates the SCPD, and improves quality of life [21–23]. Mitchell [24,25] discovered an increase in commitment levels, communication, and reduction of anguish episodes in addition to the potential of DT to improve independence in daily life. Ng [22] concluded that people with dementia could interact in a better way with their environment after obtaining benefits from the DT. Despite these positive findings on the effect of DT, the authors warn about the scarcity of empirical studies and the need for a future investigation that includes methodologically correct clinical trials. The objective of this systematic review is double. First, the best evidence available about DT will be examined, including only clinical trials that meet most of the CONSORT (Consolidated Standards of Reporting Trials) criteria. Secondly, the relevant information for the design of treatment protocols and investigation will be extracted to allow for the establishment of clear parameters and facilitating the design of future studies of DT.

2. Materials and Methods

The PRISMA (Preferred Reporting Items for Systematic Reviews and Meta-Analyses) statement was employed to report this review. The protocol was registered in INPLASY:1539.

2.1. Bibliographic Search and Inclusion Criteria

Searches were conducted in eight databases: Cochrane, PubMed, Web of Science, Cinahl, Embase, Lilacs, PeDro, and Scopus before October 2021. No limits of date, language, or study design were established in order to increase the number of registers obtained. The search strategy was made according to the PICO (Patient, Intervention, Comparation, Outcome) methodology with the help of an expert on bibliographical resources. The search strategy used was: TITLE-ABS-KEY (("lifelike doll" OR "baby doll" OR "doll therapy" OR "baby doll therapy" OR "doll therapy intervention" OR "doll" OR "empathy doll") AND ("Alzheimer Disease" OR "Dementia" OR "Alzheimer" OR "Alzheimer's" OR "Alzheimer dementia" OR "dementia sufferers" OR "nursing home resident" OR "long term care" OR "cognitive decline" OR "cognitive impairment")). Authors were contacted to retrieve non-reported data.

The inclusion criteria were: (1) dementia diagnosis according to DSM-V; (2) people over 65 years; (3) intervention with DT; (4) clinical trials; and (5) simple majority of the CONSORT (Consolidated Standards of Reporting Trials) checklist (Appendix A). The use of several types of dolls such as empathy dolls, newborn, or reborn was accepted. The exclusion criteria were: (1) participants with severe sensory disorders that may not count due to a minimum ability to communicate or those who used dolls before the beginning of the study; (2) studies that used dolls that did not have a realistic appearance or were stuffed dolls (most of the previous studies emphasize the importance that the appearance of the doll truly resembles a real baby).

2.2. Data Review, Selection, and Extraction

Two independent reviewers (AMG and AICS) reviewed the titles, abstracts, and full texts. Duplicates were identified and excluded. A third reviewer (VAP) handled the disagreements. The software Covidence was used for the management and selection of the records [26]. The data extraction form was based on the Cochrane Library recommendations [27] and included information about the study (type of study, objectives, design, measures of result, and results), the participants (age, sex, kind of housing, and inclusion and exclusion criteria), the different kinds of intervention and comparisons (number of sessions, duration of each session, type of doll, and personnel involved).

2.3. Assessment of Risk of Bias in Individual Studies

Two independent reviewers (JJCA and VFM) were in charge of the assessment of the risk of bias of each article using the items of the Review Manager (RevMan) tool (Review Manager (RevMan) [Computer program]. Version 5.4, The Cochrane Collaboration, 2020): randomization sequence, allocation concealment, blinding of participants, blinding of assessment, attrition bias, and information bias. The risk of bias of each one of these items was determined by the following premises:

- Low risk of bias: articles in which every item obtained a low risk of bias.
- Unclear risk of bias: those studies in which one or more items had an unclear risk of bias.

- High risk of bias: studies in which one or more items had a high risk of bias.

3. Results

The search strategy reported 226 records. Once duplicates were removed, 180 studies were screened by title and abstract according to eligibility criteria. A total of 35 articles were identified for full reading, of which 28 were excluded. Finally, seven articles were obtained for the present systematic review. The PRISMA flowchart synthesizing the study selection processes and the deletion reasons is shown in Figure 1.

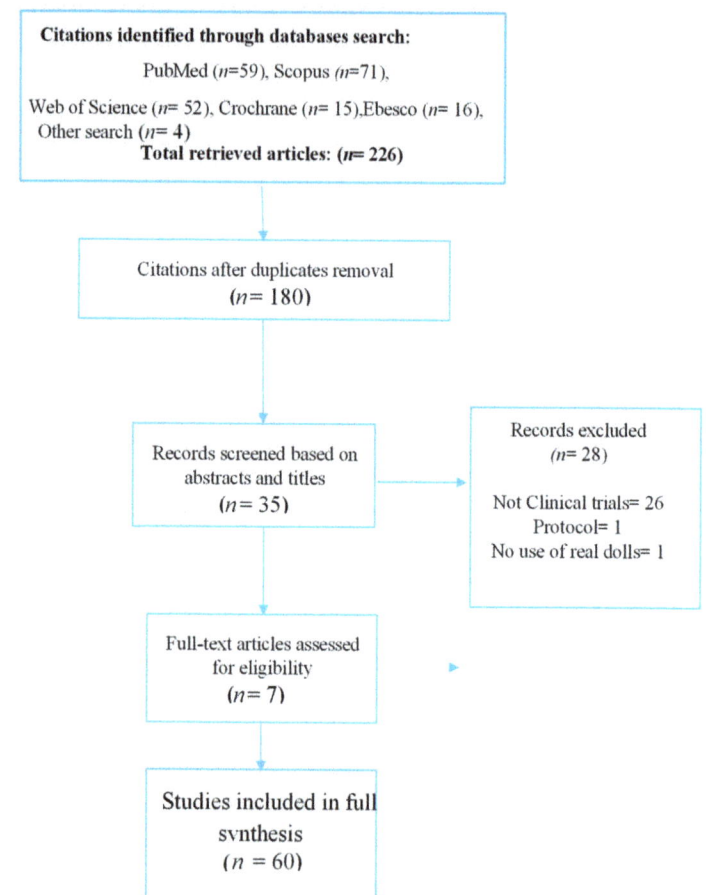

Figure 1. The PRISMA diagram for the records search and study selection.

3.1. Characteristics of the Studies and Participants Included

The articles were published between 2006 and 2020. The main objective of most of the articles was to know the efficacy and benefits of doll therapy in the neuropsychiatric symptomatology of elders with severe dementia. Three studies out of the seven were randomized clinical trials [28–30] one a non-randomized clinical trial [31], another an exploratory study [32] one a pilot study [33] and the last, a before-and-after study [20]. The characteristics of each study are described in Table 1.

Table 1. Characteristics of the studies included in the systematic review.

Author	Type of Study and Participants				Characteristics of the Intervention of Doll Therapy					
	Study	n	Age (Yrs)	Sex	Inclusion Criteria	Emplacement	Experimental Group	Control Group	Outcome Measure	Results
Moyle, 2018 [29]	RCT	35	<65 years	Female	<65 years, dementia diagnosis; documented history (in last four weeks) of anxiety, agitation, or aggressiveness.	Residents were recruited from five LTC facilities located within a 60 km radius of the Brisbane Central Business District (Queensland, Australia)	Doll Therapy	Usual treatment	Mini Mental CMAI-SF; OERS	Clinically significant improvements in the well-being of residents in comparison with the usual care, but there were no improvements in anxiety, agitation, and aggressiveness.
Balzoti 2018 [31]	Non-randomized clinical trial	30	<65 years	25 Females 10 Males	Severe to low cognitive impairment, behavioral disorders, <65 years, dementia.	Residenza Sociosanitaria Assistenziale per Anziani "Storelli" in Bisceglie (Italia)	1. Doll therapy 2. Gestural-verbal treatment	No intervention	NPI-Q	Doll therapy was effective for the reduction of agitated and irritable behaviors. No changes in apathy were found.
Cantarella, 2018 [28]	RCT	32	<70 years	26 Females 6 Males	Punctuation of ≥5 in the Short Portable Mental Status Questionnaire; <70 years; dementia diagnosis, post-traumatic stress disorder according to doctors; no participation in other non-pharmacological interventions before or during the study; without severe sensorial or perceptive deficiencies or ongoing mourning; and the capacity of understanding easy messages and producing sentences.	Residential facilities	Doll Therapy	Hand-warmer	SPMSQ EBS	Significant reduction in post-traumatic stress disorder, relief of negative feelings, fulfilling of attachment needs, and the reduction of the feeling of loneliness. Several aspects that influence food intake, such as anguish, improved but not enough to improve the eating behavior.

Table 1. Cont.

Author	Type of Study and Participants				Characteristics of the Intervention of Doll Therapy					
	Study	n	Age (Yrs)	Sex	Inclusion Criteria	Emplacement	Experimental Group	Control Group	Outcome Measure	Results
Yilmaz, 2020 [30]	RCT	29	82–89 years	15 Females 14 Males	Moderate-severe dementia, motor abilities needed to hold and caress a doll, adequate visual and auditive functions, and ability to communicate in Turkish.	A. KadirU¨ cyldız, elder facility	Doll Therapy	No intervention	SMMSE CMAI NPI-Q	Statistically significant improvements in agitation and behavior problems. Cognition did not improve.
Shin, 2015 [20]	pre-post	62	82.4 years	86.3% Females 74.5% Males	Slight-severe cognitive impairment, three months residing in the nursing home.	Korea nursing home	Doll Therapy	-	SMMSE QUALID	Statistically significant decrease in the use of swear words, shouts, aggressive episodes, and less obsessive behaviors. Erratic wandering episodes were reduced as well. There were found positive changes in moods and physical appearance, a decrease of depression, and an increment of the interactions with other individuals, but without significant differences.

Table 1. *Cont.*

Author	Type of Study and Participants				Characteristics of the Intervention of Doll Therapy				
	Study	n	Age (Yrs)	Sex	Inclusion Criteria	Emplacement	Experimental Group	Control Group	Outcome Measure	Results

Author	Study	n	Age (Yrs)	Sex	Inclusion Criteria	Emplacement	Experimental Group	Control Group	Outcome Measure	Results
Mackenzie, 2006 [33]	Pilot study	14	75–94 years	12 Females 2 Males	-	Nursing home	Doll Therapy	-	Ad hoc questionnaire	Increase in social interaction. The participants seemed to be happier and less agitated. They were also more receptive towards personal care activities; erratic wandering episodes were reduced.
Cohen-Mansfield, 2014 [32]	Exploratory study	93	85.9 years	73% Females	Three months residing at a nursing home, behavior disorders, <60, dementia diagnosis.	Maryland nursing home	Doll Therapy	-	MMSE CAR LMBS	There was a rejection of Doll Therapy; it is associated with a low social level. In spite of this, it was one of the most used therapies and obtained a relatively high rate for the impact on the behavioral symptoms.

CAR: Change Assessment Rating; CMAI-SF: Cohen-Mansfield Agitation Inventory-Short Form; EBS: Eating Behavior Scale; LMBS: Lawton's Modified Behavior Stream; LTC: Long term care; MMSE: Mini-Mental Status Examination; NPI-Q: Neuropsychiatric Inventory Questionnaire; OERS: Observed Emotion Rating Scale; QUALID: quality of life in late-stage dementia; SMMSE: Standardized Mini-Mental State Examination; SPMSQ: short portable mental status questionnaire; RCT: randomized controlled trial.

The studies included made the assessment of the appearance of SPCD through several tests, mainly the Neuropsychiatric Inventory Questionnaire (NPI-Q), Observed Emotions Rating Scale (OERS), and Eating Behavior Scale (EBS). The quality of life in late-stage dementia (QUALID) was used as well to assess life quality.

3.2. Risk of Bias of Individual Studies

The risk of bias for each trial is summarized in Figures 2 and 3. Most of the included studies completed the results with similar groups at the beginning and the end of the treatment, although this information was not clear in three of the studies [28,32,33].

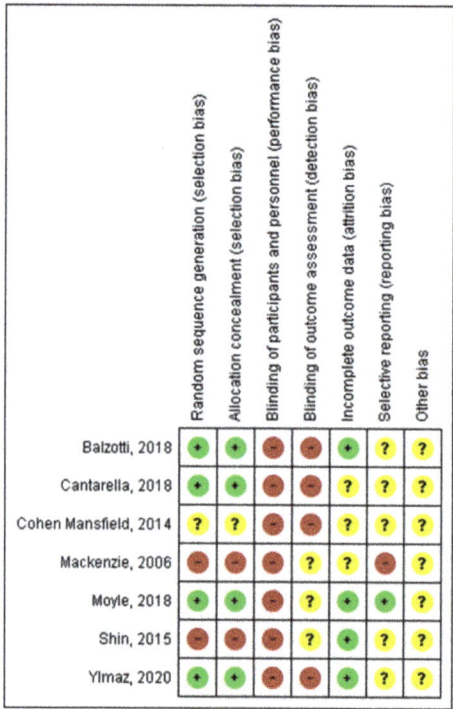

Figure 2. Risk of bias of studies included in the systematic review (Balzotti, 2018 [31], Cantarella, 2018 [28], Cohen Mansfield, 2014 [32], Mackenzie, 2006 [33], Moyle, 2018 [29], Shin, 2015 [20], Ylmaz, 2020 [30]).

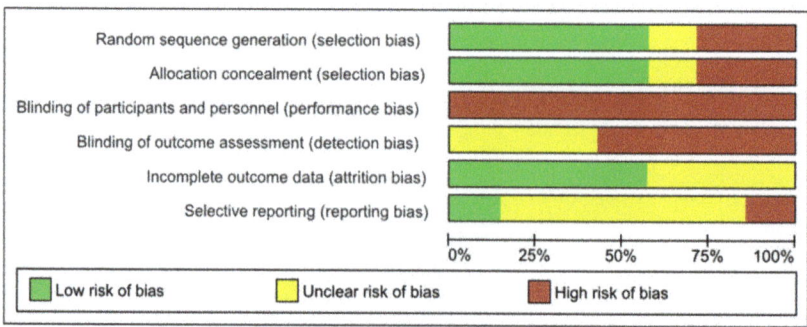

Figure 3. Risk of bias: systematic review authors' judgments about each risk of bias item presented as percentages across all included trials using the Cochrane risk of bias tool ($n = 7$).

Four studies had a low risk of bias in the randomization sequence and the allocation concealment. No study could blind the participants due to the characteristics of the intervention, and in four of the studies the assessment of the results was not blinded either. The report of data was only clear in one study [29].

3.3. Intervention with Doll Therapy

Every study used a doll with a realistic appearance with which the person with dementia could freely interact. The duration of the sessions mainly depended on two factors: how long the participant committed to the intervention and how long were they awake. Figure 4 shows the development of an intervention protocol based on the information extracted from the included studies. This protocol is structured in six phases: starting with an evaluation of the background of the individual (phase 1), establish a way of introducing the doll and assess of the reaction of the individual in order to continue with the process (phases 2, 3, and 4); encourage the care of the doll (phase 5), and finally the removal of the doll (phase 6). The full duration of the intervention was heterogeneous, from 1 to 24 weeks.

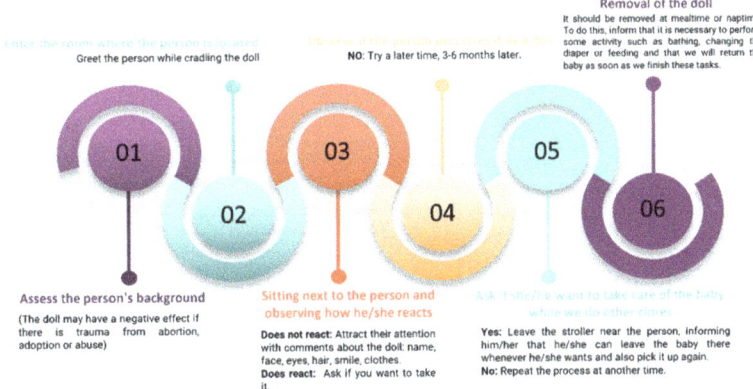

Figure 4. Intervention protocol with Doll Therapy.

3.4. Effectiveness of Doll Therapy on Behaviour

Four out of seven studies [20,29,30,32] reported a reduction in SCPD, observing the decrease of disruptive and aggressive behaviors. The participants were less agitated and irritable while holding the doll (Cantarella Mdiff: -0.025, $p < 0.001$; Shin: $t = 16.31$, $p < 0.01$; Balzotti $z = 2.66$, $p < 0.007$). They verbalized fewer swear words, fewer shouts, and fewer obsessive behaviors. Three studies [20,30,32] found a higher number of interactions with the environment, increasing social contact and verbalization ($t = -8.41$, $p < 0.01$). The episodes of erratic wandering decreased in two of the studies (Shin, $t: -17.46$, $p < 0.001$) [20,33]. Only one study [29] did not report significant evidence in reducing anxiety, agitation, and aggressiveness (Moyle, $p < 0.88$).

3.5. Effectiveness of Doll Therapy on Emotions

Four studies [20,29,31,32] reported benefits in the use of dolls to provide emotional support. Three of those studies found statistically significant improvements regarding the emotional component of people with dementia. Shin [20] reported statistically significant differences in positive mood and found a significant diminishment in depression ($p < 0.01$). In this way, Moyle's work [29] had a positive effect on well-being ($p < 0.05$), and Balzotti's study [31] reported mood changes at the third week of treatment: IC del 95% (-1.09 a 0.20) and the presence of anger (CI: -0.51 a 0.51). It also found improvements in depression ($Z = 2.02$, $p = 0.04$) and apathy ($Z = 2.01$, $p = 0.04$).

3.6. Effectiveness of Doll Therapy on the Basic Activities of Daily Living

Only one study evaluated the impact of DT on daily life activities. Cantarella et al. [28] studied the effect of DT on diet, one of the most problematic basic activities in people with dementia. Despite finding signs of improvement in this activity, the authors concluded that was necessary to increase the intervention time to obtain perceptible changes in the development of this activity.

4. Discussion

This systematic review analyzed the effectiveness of Doll Therapy to diminish the appearance of psychological and cognitive symptoms in people with dementia. This is the first updated systematic review that has selected clinical trials which met most of the CONSORT criteria and have been reported according to the PRISMA statement.

Previous systematic reviews [22,24] have included qualitative studies that were mainly narratives of professionals about their impressions about the effect of DT, not the group randomization measurement of the effect with valid evaluation tools. This led to reporting conclusions that could move away from real effectiveness due to methodological bias. To avoid this, our systematic review collected information from studies that methodologically met the randomization and objective evaluation of results criteria.

DT is a technique that started to be used in the 1980s. From its beginnings, it has provoked contrary opinions and an ethical dilemma in the professionals working with people with dementia. Several authors [11,34,35] express their concern about the ethical conflicts that may derive from this technique, considering it a practice that infantilizes and could potentially undermine the dignity of the person. On the other hand, there are other authors that defend the use of this technique, claiming the benefits of its applications [10,25,35]. For our part, the results obtained in this systematic review report that DT produces positive changes and statistically significant results in the diminishing of disruptive behaviors such as erratic wandering, aggressiveness, agitation, and negative verbalization. We have also found that most of the included studies report improvements in the emotional component of people with dementia, resulting in fewer episodes of suffering, and witnessing more positive moods. These changes may be due to the interaction and meaning that the person with dementia has with the doll, corroborating the emotional benefits generated by attachment and person-centered attention found in previous studies [25,36,37].

Related to the time of intervention, it was found that a prolonged duration contributes to the obtention of positive results, even producing changes in food intake. The study developed by Cohen [32] found that a 6-month intervention allows for the development of an initial test phase and familiarization with the doll in people with dementia, as well as their families; and a later phase in which the treatment was implemented to obtain more effective results on the behaviors of rejection towards the intervention and overall behavioral symptoms. Moreover, a prolonged intervention allows for a higher acceptance of DT, since caregivers and families can observe the benefits in a more complete way. On the other hand, it is also important to plan post-intervention follow-up in order to observe if the participants maintain the changes in behavior after applying the therapy. Most of the studies of this review do not include any follow-up after the end of the intervention with dolls.

Nevertheless, the interpretation of this data should be taken with caution and be considered in the context of several methodological problems. The randomization sequence and the concealment were only clear in half of the studies, and the blinding of the evaluation was not clear in any study, so the obtained results can lead to higher estimations than the real effect of DT over psychological and behavioral symptoms of dementia. Previous reviews [21,22] found similar methodological limitations to DT and that is why we suggest further studies that might design protocols that control possible confusion factors, as well as the planification during and after the intervention.

In relation to daily life activities, only one article [29] studied the impact of DT on the performance of daily life activities, finding benefits at the time of feeding.

Related to the limitations of this review, it is probable that not all the studies could have been identified, despite using exhaustive search strategies. The methodological demand of inclusion criteria is the reason for the small number of studies included in the review; this might be a limitation, but ensures the reliability of the obtained evidence. Additionally, the included studies had a small sample size, which could have conditioned the effect of the intervention. Furthermore, it has been not possible to know the lasting effect of DT on the psychological and behavioral symptoms of dementia, given the absence of subsequent follow-up in most of the studies.

The results obtained in this systematic review have important implications for socio-sanitary professionals that provide care to people with dementia, as it reports the benefits that DT entails in the improvement of behavioral symptoms and mood. At the same time, guidelines are provided for the implementation of this type of non-pharmacological therapy which can be summarized into four items:

- Doll therapy reduces psychological and behavioral symptoms of dementia.
- It is beneficial to follow a six phase protocol for treatment (evaluation, introduction of the doll, assessment of the reaction, presentation of the doll, care of the doll, and the removal of the doll).
- The prolonged duration of doll therapy allows for achieving more benefits.
- Future studies must include the randomization and the blinding of the assessment to increase the methodological quality.

5. Conclusions

Our findings suggest that doll therapy improved the emotional state, diminished disturbing behaviors, and enhanced communication with the environment in dementia patients. However, randomized studies with a greater sample size and methodological rigor are needed, as well as follow-up protocols to reaffirm these results.

Author Contributions: Conceptualization, A.M.-G. and A.-I.C.-S.; methodology, A.M.-G. and A.-I.C.-S.; formal analysis J.-J.C.-Á. and V.F.-M.; resources, V.A.-P.; writing—original draft preparation, A.M.-G., A.-I.C.-S. and V.A.-P.; writing—review and editing, V.F.-M.; visualization, V.F.-M.; supervision, A.M.-G. and A.-I.C.-S., project administration, A.-I.C.-S. All authors have read and agreed to the published version of the manuscript.

Funding: This research received no external funding.

Institutional Review Board Statement: The study was conducted in accordance with the Preferred Reporting Items for Systematic Reviews and Meta-Analyses (PRISMA). The systematic review protocol was registered in INPLASY with code: 1539.

Conflicts of Interest: The authors declare no conflict of interest.

Appendix A

The appendix is an optional section that can contain the methodological analysis of the studies according to the checklist Consolidated Standards of Reporting Trials (CONSORT).

	Balzotti [32]	Cantarella [29]	Cohen-Mansfield, [28]	Mackenzie, [30]	Moyle, [31]	Shin, [20]	Yilmaz, [36]
1A	NO	NO	NO	NO	X	NO	X
1B	X	X	X	NO	X	NO	X
2A	X	X	X	X	X	X	X
2B	X	X	X	X	X	NO	X
3A	NO	NO	NO	X	X	X	X
3B	NO	NO	NO	NO	NO	NO	NO
4A	X	X	X	NO	X	X	X
4B	X	X	X	X	X	X	X

	Balzotti [32]	Cantarella [29]	Cohen-Mansfield, [28]	Mackenzie, [30]	Moyle, [31]	Shin, [20]	Yilmaz, [36]
5	X	X	X	X	X	NO	X
6A	X	X	X	NO	X	X	X
6B	X	X	X	NO	NO	NO	NO
7A	NO	NO	NO	NO	X	X	X
7B	NO	X	NO	NO	X	NO	NO
8A	NO	NO	X	NO	X	NO	X
8B	NO	NO	NO	NO	NO	NO	NO
9	NO	NO	NO	NO	X	NO	X
10	NO	NO	NO	NO	X	NO	NO
11A	X	NO	NO	NO	X	N	X
11B	X	X	NO	NO	NO	NO	NO
12A	X	X	X	NO	X	NO	X
12B	X	NO	NO	NO	X	NO	NO
13A	NO	NO	X	NO	X	NO	X
13B	X	X	NO	NO	X	NO	X
14A	NO	NO	NO	NO	NO	X	NO
14B	X	X	X	X	X	X	X
15	X	X	NO	X	X	NO	X
16	X	X	NO	X	X	NO	X
17A	NO	X	X	NO	X	NO	X
17B	NO	X	NO	NO	X	NO	X
18	X	NO	X	NO	NO	NO	NO
19	NO	NO	X	X	X	X	X
20	X	X	X	X	X	X	X
21	X	NO	NO	NO	X	X	NO
22	X	X	X	X	X	X	X
23	X	X	X	X	X	X	X
24	NO	NO	NO	NO	NO	NO	NO
25	NO	NO	X	NO	X	NO	X

References

1. OMS | La Demencia: Una Prioridad Para La Salud Pública. Available online: http://www.who.int/mental_health/neurology/dementia/es/ (accessed on 23 March 2021).
2. Garre-Olmo, J. Epidemiology of Alzheimer's disease and other dementias. *Rev. Neurol.* **2018**, *66*, 377–386. [PubMed]
3. Radue, R.; Walaszek, A.; Asthana, S. Neuropsychiatric Symptoms in Dementia. *Handb. Clin. Neurol.* **2019**, *167*, 437–454. [CrossRef]
4. Etters, L.; Goodall, D.; Harrison, B.E. Caregiver Burden among Dementia Patient Caregivers: A Review of the Literature. *J. Am. Acad. Nurse Pract.* **2008**, *20*, 423–428. [CrossRef] [PubMed]
5. Chiao, C.-Y.; Wu, H.-S.; Hsiao, C.-Y. Caregiver Burden for Informal Caregivers of Patients with Dementia: A Systematic Review. *Int. Nurs. Rev.* **2015**, *62*, 340–350. [CrossRef] [PubMed]
6. Holst, A.; Skär, L. Formal Caregivers' Experiences of Aggressive Behaviour in Older People Living with Dementia in Nursing Homes: A Systematic Review. *Int. J. Older People Nurs.* **2017**, *12*, e12158. [CrossRef]
7. Miyamoto, Y.; Tachimori, H.; Ito, H. Formal Caregiver Burden in Dementia: Impact of Behavioral and Psychological Symptoms of Dementia and Activities of Daily Living. *Geriatr. Nur.* **2010**, *31*, 246–253. [CrossRef]
8. Song, J.-J. Virtual Reality for Vestibular Rehabilitation. *Clin. Exp. Otorhinolaryngol.* **2019**, *12*, 329–330. [CrossRef]
9. Lim, D.Y. Coping with dementia related behavior problems of the elderly and care providers. *J. Korea Acad.-Ind. Coop. Soc.* **2015**, *16*, 4805–4815. [CrossRef]
10. Bisiani, L.; Angus, J. Doll Therapy: A Therapeutic Means to Meet Past Attachment Needs and Diminish Behaviours of Concern in a Person Living with Dementia—A Case Study Approach. *Dement. Lond. Engl.* **2013**, *12*, 447–462. [CrossRef]
11. Mitchell, G.; O'Donnell, H. The Therapeutic Use of Doll Therapy in Dementia. *Br. J. Nurs.* **2013**, *22*, 329–334. [CrossRef]
12. Pezzati, R.; Molteni, V.; Bani, M.; Settanta, C.; Di Maggio, M.G.; Villa, I.; Poletti, B.; Ardito, R.B. Can Doll Therapy Preserve or Promote Attachment in People with Cognitive, Behavioral, and Emotional Problems? A Pilot Study in Institutionalized Patients with Dementia. *Front. Psychol.* **2014**, *5*, 342. [CrossRef]
13. Winnicott, D.W. Objetos transicionales. In *Realidad Y Juego*; Gedisa: Barcelona, Spain, 1974; pp. 17–45.
14. Gaddini, R. The Relationship of Reactions to Illness to Developmental Stages. *Bibl. Psychiatr.* **1979**, *159*, 96–106.
15. Stephens, A.; Cheston, R.; Gleeson, K. An Exploration into the Relationships People with Dementia Have with Physical Objects: An Ethnographic Study. *Dementia* **2013**, *12*, 697–712. [CrossRef]

16. LoboPrabhu, S.; Molinari, V.; Lomax, J. The Transitional Object in Dementia: Clinical Implications. *Int. J. Appl. Psychoanal. Stud.* **2007**, *4*, 144–169. [CrossRef]
17. Rogers, C.R. The Place of the Person in the New World of the Behavioral Sciences. *Pers. Guid. J.* **1961**, *39*, 442–451. [CrossRef]
18. Kitwood, T. Professional and Moral Development for Care Work: Some Observations on the Process. *J. Moral Educ.* **1998**, *27*, 401–411. [CrossRef]
19. Tamura, T.; Nakajima, K.; Nambu, M.; Nakamura, K.; Yonemitsu, S.; Itoh, A.; Higashi, Y.; Fujimoto, T.; Uno, H. Baby Dolls as Therapeutic Tools for Severe Dementia Patients. *Gerontechnology* **2001**, *1*, 111–118. [CrossRef]
20. Shin, J.H. Doll Therapy: An Intervention for Nursing Home Residents with Dementia. *J. Psychosoc. Nurs. Ment. Health Serv.* **2015**, *53*, 13–18. [CrossRef]
21. Chinnaswamy, K.; DeMarco, D.M.; Grossberg, G.T. Doll Therapy in Dementia: Facts and Controversies. *Ann. Clin. Psychiatry* **2021**, *33*, 58–66. [CrossRef]
22. Ng, Q.X.; Ho, C.Y.X.; Koh, S.S.H.; Tan, W.C.; Chan, H.W. Doll Therapy for Dementia Sufferers: A Systematic Review. *Complement. Ther. Clin. Pract.* **2017**, *26*, 42–46. [CrossRef]
23. Cai, X.; Zhou, L.; Han, P.; Deng, X.; Zhu, H.; Fang, F.; Zhang, Z. Narrative Review: Recent Advances in Doll Therapy for Alzheimer's Disease. *Ann. Palliat. Med.* **2021**, *10*, 4878–4881. [CrossRef] [PubMed]
24. Mitchell, G.; McCormack, B.; McCance, T. Therapeutic Use of Dolls for People Living with Dementia: A Critical Review of the Literature. *Dementia* **2016**, *15*, 976–1001. [CrossRef] [PubMed]
25. Mitchell, G. Use of Doll Therapy for People with Dementia: An Overview. *Nurs. Older People* **2014**, *26*, 24–26. [CrossRef] [PubMed]
26. Covidence—Better Systematic Review Management. Available online: https://www.covidence.org/ (accessed on 6 July 2021).
27. Chandler, J.; Higgins, J.P.; Deeks, J.J.; Davenport, C.; Clarke, M.J. *Cochrane Handbook for Systematic Reviews of Interventions*, 2nd ed.; John Wiley & Sons: Chichester, UK, 2019.
28. Cantarella, A.; Borella, E.; Faggian, S.; Navuzzi, A.; De Beni, R. Using Dolls for Therapeutic Purposes: A Study on Nursing Home Residents with Severe Dementia. *Int. J. Geriatr. Psychiatry* **2018**, *33*, 915–925. [CrossRef]
29. Moyle, W.; Murfield, J.; Jones, C.; Beattie, E.; Draper, B.; Ownsworth, T. Can Lifelike Baby Dolls Reduce Symptoms of Anxiety, Agitation, or Aggression for People with Dementia in Long-Term Care? Findings from a Pilot Randomised Controlled Trial. *Aging Ment. Health* **2019**, *23*, 1442–1450. [CrossRef]
30. Yilmaz, C.K.; Aşiret, G.D. The Effect of Doll Therapy on Agitation and Cognitive State in Institutionalized Patients With Moderate-to-Severe Dementia: A Randomized Controlled Study. *J. Geriatr. Psychiatry Neurol.* **2021**, *34*, 370–377. [CrossRef]
31. Balzotti, A.; Filograsso, M.; Altamura, C.; Fairfield, B.; Bellomo, A.; Daddato, F.; Vacca, R.A.; Altamura, M. Comparison of the Efficacy of Gesture-Verbal Treatment and Doll Therapy for Managing Neuropsychiatric Symptoms in Older Patients with Dementia. *Int. J. Geriatr. Psychiatry* **2019**, *34*, 1308–1315. [CrossRef]
32. Cohen-Mansfield, J.; Marx, M.S.; Dakheel-Ali, M.; Thein, K. The Use and Utility of Specific Nonpharmacological Interventions for Behavioral Symptoms in Dementia: An Exploratory Study. *Am. J. Geriatr. Psychiatry* **2015**, *23*, 160–170. [CrossRef]
33. Mackenzie, L.; James, I.A.; Morse, R.; Mukaetova-Ladinska, E.; Reichelt, F.K. A Pilot Study on the Use of Dolls for People with Dementia. *Age Ageing* **2006**, *35*, 441–444. [CrossRef]
34. Higgins, P. Using Dolls to Enhance the Wellbeing of People with Dementia in Residential Care. *Nurs. Times* **2010**, *106*, 18–20.
35. Salari, S.M. Intergenerational Partnerships in Adult Day Centers: Importance of Age-Appropriate Environments and Behaviors. *Gerontologist* **2002**, *42*, 321–333. [CrossRef]
36. Managing Challenging Behaviors in Patients with Dementia: The Use of Therapy Dolls | Article | NursingCenter. Available online: https://www.nursingcenter.com/journalarticle?Article_ID=5460106&Journal_ID=417221&Issue_ID=5459955 (accessed on 3 January 2022).
37. Santagata, F.; Massaia, M.; D'Amelio, P. The Doll Therapy as a First Line Treatment for Behavioral and Psychologic Symptoms of Dementia in Nursing Homes Residents: A Randomized, Controlled Study. *BMC Geriatr.* **2021**, *21*, 545. [CrossRef]

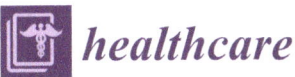

Article

HeartMath as an Integrative, Personal, Social, and Global Healthcare System

Stephen D. Edwards *, David J. Edwards and Richard Honeycutt

Department of Psychology, University of Zululand, Private Bag X1001, KwaDlangezwa 3886, South Africa; edwards.davidjohn@googlemail.com (D.J.E.); rhoneycutt@triad.twcbc.com (R.H.)
* Correspondence: profsdedwards@gmail.com

Abstract: COVID-19 is a recent major event, adding to planet Earth's contexts of chaos, crime, injustice, illness, and violence. The HeartMath system has produced research evidence for scientific interventions that alter contexts characterized by chaos and stress, promoting health, coherence, and interconnectedness. This study provides an updated overview of HeartMath as an interdisciplinary, scientific, coherent, integral heart-based healthcare system, operated locally through various initiatives and globally through the Global Coherence Initiative. The HeartMath approach integrates ancient and contemporary, indigenous and mainstream, popular and folk, Eastern, Western, and African forms of healing. The HeartMath interdisciplinary, personal, social, and global vision and mission have considerable theoretical and practical potential for promoting planetary health, education, and development.

Keywords: healthcare; HeartMath; Global Coherence Initiative; coherence; interconnectedness

1. Introduction

COVID-19 is only one recent example of a factor influencing planet Earth's contexts of chaos, incoherence, illness, and violence. In addition, endemic struggles for survival and subsistence stresses consume human energy, distort consciousness, and exacerbate inhumanity and disorder. All of this occurs within a planet in desperate need of healing. The compound word healthcare combines the quintessentially human notion of care with that of healing, in all its meanings: making whole, transferring from illness to health, and various forms of illness prevention and health promotion. At quantum information level, healthcare translates into dynamic human, social, and environmental energy patterns [1,2]. At a global level, healthcare needs to represent all inhabitants of planet Earth in their considerable diversity [1,2].

The HeartMath system has revealed various coherent, interconnected energetic patterns within and between human persons and populations [2]. As a concept, HeartMath may be operationally defined as the math of heart rate variability [HRV], particularly, heart rhythm variability, which varies coherently in optimal health and becomes disordered under stress as well as in various disorders and forms of illness [3]. HRV is recognized as key to unlocking the profound significance and meaning of the Morse-code-like information patterns communicated by the heart in its interactions with other bodily systems, particularly the brain. Healthcare information transfer is optimally facilitated during states of psychophysiological, personal, social, and global coherence, associated with stable, regular, rhythmic heart rate activity. In simple terms, independent of fast or slow heart rate, optimal heart rate variability and coherent heart rhythms indicate health and performance [2,3].

The HeartMath system was specifically created and developed by Doc Childre, a stress researcher who gathered an expert, interdisciplinary, multi-professional research team to reduce stress through the study and development of heart intelligence [1,3]. The special vision and mission of the HeartMath system is to promote personal, social, and global coherence and health [3]. Pioneering research has revealed profound patterns of heart communication

Citation: Edwards, S.D.; Edwards, D.J.; Honeycutt, R. HeartMath as an Integrative, Personal, Social, and Global Healthcare System. *Healthcare* **2022**, *10*, 376. https://doi.org/10.3390/healthcare10020376

Academic Editors: Manoj Sharma and Kavita Batra

Received: 12 January 2022
Accepted: 31 January 2022
Published: 15 February 2022

Publisher's Note: MDPI stays neutral with regard to jurisdictional claims in published maps and institutional affiliations.

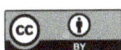

Copyright: © 2022 by the authors. Licensee MDPI, Basel, Switzerland. This article is an open access article distributed under the terms and conditions of the Creative Commons Attribution (CC BY) license (https://creativecommons.org/licenses/by/4.0/).

involving human, energetic, electromagnetic, neurochemical, biophysical, and hormonal information [2,4,5]. Other studies have developed practical methods and techniques for stress reduction, health promotion, and performance enhancement [6], as well as biofeedback technology for heart rate variability (HRV) coherence training [3,7–9].

An overview follows of HeartMath as a scientific, coherent, integral heart-based, healthcare system that postulates and promotes planetary interconnectedness [10–13]. This system, its model, and perspectives are in line with some of the phenomenological insights of the ancient sages, meditative and contemplative traditions, as well as with integral theory [14,15] in a creatively evolving cosmos [7,13,16,17].

Goal of This Study

This article was specifically motivated by the theoretical considerations and considerable evidence-based studies available in the HeartMath research library as to the scientific foundations and effectiveness of the HeartMath Institute in promoting coherent personal, social, and global healthcare. It is intended as an updated overview for instructional purposes.

2. The Math behind Heart Rate/Rhythm Variability Patterns

Figure 1 graphically illustrates the HeartMath method of heart rhythm calculation. Figure 2 indicates synchronized entrainment, a healthcare intervention that can be brought about in minutes by the HeartMath Quick Coherence Technique [1–9].

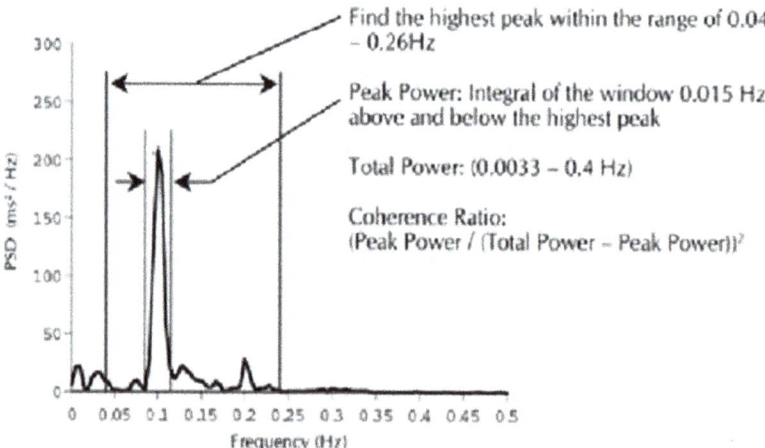

Figure 1. Indicates the HeartMath method of heart rhythm calculation [9]. The maximum peak is identified in the 0.04–0.26 Hz range in which coherence occurs. Peak power is determined by calculating the integral in a window that is 0.030 Hz wide. The total power of the entire spectrum is then calculated. The coherence ratio is formulated as: (Peak Power/(Total Power—Peak Power)) [2].

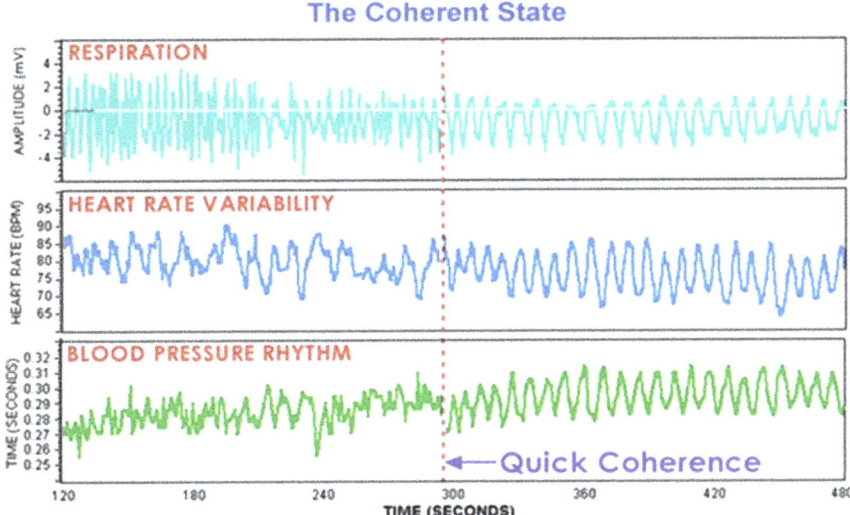

Figure 2. The Coherent State as reflected in synchronized entrainment of respiration, heart rate variability, and blood pressure rhythms brought about by the Quick Coherence technique.

3. The HeartMath System Is Unique in Its Recognition of the Integral Heart in All Its Physical, Emotional, Mental, Social, Ecological, and Spiritual Relatedness

From a transcultural perspective, the heart has received perennial recognition as the font of sentience, awareness, and consciousness; it is considered to be the center of the spiritual, intellectual, and emotional life. Various scientific disciplines provide evidence [18] that heart wisdom has developed over many millennia in central and southern Africa, predating the migrations of Homo sapiens through Asia and the subsequent development of the Vedanta, Yoga, and Chakra systems.

The integral heart appears to have dimensions of increasing depth: physical, emotional, transpersonal, and transcultural [3]. For example, in isiZulu, meanings of the heart include the physical organ, the seat of emotions, and the conscience [19]. Yoga views life-energy as flowing up and down the spine in three main pathways: the Ida, Pingala, and the Sushumna. These chakras are associated with particular anatomical locations of the nervous, endocrine, and other human functional systems [20,21]. The heart chakra expresses love and compassion [20,22]. Traditional Chinese medicine, especially Taoist chi-gung, is based on subtle consciousness/breath/energy work related to oscillating pacemaker cell rhythms that can be altered intentionally [21]. The Buddhist term for heart, sutra, is associated with ultimate enlightenment through the union of form and emptiness. Judaic energy centers (sefirot) include the harmony of the heart (tiferet). In the Kabbalah, the heart forms the central sphere [3]. In Christian Hesychastic and Sufi traditions, the Prayer of the Heart, which consists of the repetition of a phrase or the name of a deity, is intentionally accompanied by breath-paced heart focus. Centering prayer refers to a contemporary form of the Prayer of the Heart, which is very similar to the HeartMath Lock-In technique. In this context, Bourgeault [23] (p. 5) refers to the integral heart as a "homing magnetic center", which is associated with a neurological shift in the mechanics of perception towards a unified field, where one becomes enabled to "see from wholeness"; this is discussed further in Section 7.

For millennia, the major great wisdom traditions, including Islam, Christianity, Buddhism, Hinduism, Taoism, and ancestral reverence [13,24,25], have espoused heart love. However, meaningful planetary effects have been slow, as the traditions have been engaged in continual disputes amongst themselves. Although many wisdom traditions advocate love, the practice of respect may be a more realistic goal for temporary transformation;

Native American and many other indigenous traditions teach respect for all one's relatives, namely, all of creation, as a primary duty. However, predictably endemic human destructiveness, greed, and power motivations will probably continue, especially since most people are still struggling to survive and satisfy their basic needs, let alone care for other, higher needs such as belongingness, love, and connection to greater Being [26].

Improved healthcare innovations concerning coherent, heartfelt intentions and actions are in short supply.

4. HeartMath Healthcare Research

HeartMath is an interdisciplinary approach that bridges the natural, human, social, spiritual, and ecological sciences in its focus on heart-based research [9]. Coherence is a central concept. The fundamental vision and mission is to promote healthcare through research and education in personal, social, and global coherence.

Healthcare research findings from over 8000 researchers are freely downloadable from the research library 8000 compiled by HeartMath researchers. Over 400 additional studies undertaken by independent researchers have provided extensive external validity for the effectiveness of the HeartMath system, its methods, tools, and techniques. This is to be expected, as findings are generally based on evidence related to: 1. Physics; 2. Electromagnetics; 3. Cardiorespiratory activity, especially related to communication networks involving the vagus nerve; 4. The natural mechanism of respiratory sinus arrhythmia (RSA), whereby heart rate increases during inhalation and decreases during exhalation; 5. Coherent and incoherent heart rhythms, associated with positive and negative emotion, respectively; 6. Correlated heart rhythm mathematics; 7. Biofeedback conditioning principles and practices.

Pribram's [17] holonomic, dynamic systems theory provides the theoretical, scientific model for much of the HeartMath research. For example, the model proposes complex pattern identification brain functioning, with special reference to emotion, the amygdala, and the cardiovascular system, especially the vagus nerve. In the model, experiential imprints stored as sets of familiar patterns in the neural architecture are continually monitoring and interacting with internal environmental inputs from many rhythmic physiological processes, such as heartbeat, respiration, and digestion, as well as with external environmental and social processes that help organize sensory perception, cognition, feelings, and behavior. According to the model, emotions are energetic happenings generated immediately from the occurrence of discontinuities, or novel patterns that do not match familiar, ongoing, and recurring inputs. Emotions, especially negative emotions, are known to highjack cognition via stress-induced, amygdala-generated fight/flight/freeze responses [3]. It is therefore postulated that a direct effect of utilizing HeartMath tools and techniques is the intentional facilitation of a heart-based re-patterning effect from physiological coherence [9]. It is also hypothesized that this operates at the physiological, emotional, and cognitive levels through afferent cardiac signals, a positive feeling pattern match, and the associated cortical electrophysiological activity. Rigorous research has provided empirical support for these hypotheses. After appropriate practice, their great value is the ability to transform the energy of negative emotions into their polar opposites, e.g., anger into assertiveness, overwhelming panic into centered motivation, overexcitement into relaxed release, sadness into contentment; hatred into love [2].

5. HeartMath Coherence Model

Theoretically, the HeartMath coherence model includes all the usual meanings of the term coherence, as implied in such terms as relationship, harmony, order, stability, consistency, synchrony, logic, and by the idea of the whole being more than the sum of its parts [8]. In academia, coherence refers to the internal integrity of an argument or thesis. Linguistically, it refers to intelligibility. Physiologically, the concept of coherence includes the synchrony of the circulatory and respiratory rhythms associated with overlapping sine wave patterns. In physics, it implies phase relationships. Auto-coherence, or auto-correlation, indicates stability in a single wave form; cross-coherence, among multiple waveforms, while phase locking and resonance include the concept of harmony in various rhythmic activities. In math and statistics, the term coherence implies correlation. In dynamic systems theory, it means connectedness, alignment, resonance, and optimal energy utilization.

From a psychophysiological perspective, coherence interconnects positive emotions with the cardiovascular, respiratory, immune, and nervous systems [9]. From a human as well as a social perspective, coherence applies to couples, teams, groups, organizations, and communities. Coherent relationships promote communication, synchronized behavior in rowing teams, and groups with similar goals. From a global perspective, communities and countries working cooperatively can cause ecological and planetary peace and harmony. Experientially, HeartMath praxis is accompanied by the sentient, increasing awareness of the synchronization of pulsation, respiration, and the renewing of positive feelings, whereby emotions such as peace and love are cumulatively experienced as radiating throughout the body, and among people and the wider world in harmonious interconnectedness.

Various HRV-related psychophysiological theories resonate with the HeartMath coherence model. Resonance theory is founded on heart rate variability biofeedback (HRVB) studies, which indicate that optimal heart rate oscillations occur via paced respiration at a frequency of about 0.1 Hz. Polyvagal theory, which hypothesizes social evolutionary mechanisms, advocates RSA and enhanced HRV for improved health and well-being. The neurovisceral integration model postulates a central autonomic network (CAN) related to social, cognitive, affective, and physiological regulation [9].

5.1. Psychophysiological Coherence

Psychophysiological studies indicate that bidirectional heart–brain communication has been recognized for over a century [27]. The heart possesses an intrinsic nervous system, capable of autonomous, functional decisions [9]. The heart communicates more with the brain than with any other organ [9]. Intricate heart rate variability patterns provide vital communicative links within the body, as well as between and among people, the ecology, and the cosmos. The sympathetic and parasympathetic (vagal) branches of the autonomic nervous system (ANS) function similarly to an accelerator and a brake, reflecting dynamic, resonant HRV patterns, signaling adaptation, resilience, and general health for diverse forms of healthcare assessment and intervention. HRV oscillations are typically categorized into very low frequency (VLF) bands between 0.0033 and 0.04 Hz, low frequency (LF) bands between 0.04 and 0.15 Hz, and high frequency (HF) bands from 0.15 to 0.4 Hz [28]. The psychophysiological coherence experience of zoned performance is closely related to Antonovsky's [29] sense of coherence construct of the world as meaningful, manageable, and comprehensible, which also provides healthcare initiatives with a valid, unifying, theoretical, and practical rationale [30].

5.2. Social Coherence

Social coherence refers to harmonious relationships that facilitate efficient energy communication, cohesion, and action [8]. Effective multi-professional team functioning is ideal in many healthcare contexts. When nursing personnel, physiotherapists, medical practitioners, clinical psychologists, social workers, and occupational therapists effectively pool their particular areas of expertise in diagnostic and therapeutic contexts, patients heal. Hospitals implementing HeartMath programs have seen increased personal, team, and organizational functioning, as well as significant decreases in anxiety, depression, and anger. Studies provide evidence of functioning bioenergetics communication systems in highly coherent group contexts. Individuals with high heart coherence readily facilitate group coherence [8,31]. These findings have important implications for interpersonal group, family, and community psychotherapy. Studies indicate that emotional self-regulation skills and heart rhythm coherence training are associated with significant improvements in communication, employee satisfaction, productivity, problem solving, and significant returns on financial and social investments [8,31,32]. Numerous studies show that HRV coherence feedback facilitates self-regulation techniques and a wide range of health and performance outcomes.

5.3. Global Coherence

Ample evidence indicates that the Earth's magnetic field generates and facilitates an interconnecting global information network [8,33,34]. Global Coherence Initiative (GCI) interconnectedness research from the Institute of HeartMath has established that there is a global network of magnetic field detectors around the planet, yielding information on human, planetary, and cosmic relationships. The GCI and the Global Consciousness Project (GCP) [34,35] provide a field view of human interconnectedness. Other related, emerging interdisciplinary field trends include neuroscience and cosmology [36]; the psychology of global consciousness [37] and co-created embodied spirituality [38]. The study of Timofejeva et al. [39] found synchronization between local magnetic field data, HRV wave rhythms, and interpersonal relationships. An integral Heart Based Resonant Frequencies [HBRF] theory of consciousness was postulated [40]. These findings support and extend those of many older studies concerned with transformations of consciousness, as particularly evident in moral behavior, creativity, and health promotion [41–43]. Conceptual and practical implications of this initiative, with special reference to global healthcare, are available from the websites: www.Heartmath.org and www.glcoherence.org (accessed on 4 April 2021). These websites also contain information on various online courses, for example, courses for any individual needing HeartMath Coach/Mentor training.

In a similar initiative, based upon his work researching the measurable effects of human intention [Steps for Moving Psychoenergetics Science Research Into the Hands of Interested General Public Researchers (filesusr.com accessed on 4 April 2021) and Steps for Moving Psychoenergetics Science Research Into the Hands of Interested General Public Researchers (filesusr.com accessed on 4 April 2021)], Stanford University Emeritus Professor William Tiller has initiated the Global Intention project through which concerned individuals the world over can create focused intention to improve our world. An example of this is the use of the intention suggested on the Global Intention | The Tiller Foundation website for healing the world from the effects of the COVID-19 virus. While in a meditative (coherent) state, participants create a positive intention that is "broadcast" worldwide.

6. HeartMath's Healthcare Practice

HeartMath techniques and tools promote practical energetics, transform stress, strengthen resilience, and improve health. They typically emphasize heartfelt breathing in a ten-second cardio-respiratory rhythm, which facilitates RSA, rhythmic pulsation, and a focus on positive, renewing feelings [6]. Some traditional techniques include:

Depletion to Renewal Grid The visualization of an energy graph of the hormonal system along the horizontal axis and the autonomic nervous system along the vertical axis facilitates the limiting of the negative effects of stress hormones such as cortisol and the increase of healthy hormones such as DHEA.

Heart Focused Breathing is an effective, very brief meditation technique for slowing down fight, flight, and freeze reactions in order to focus on positive and renewing emotions, such as appreciation, peace, or love.

Prep-Shift-Reset assists in resetting the energy system and building resilience for the rest of the day.

Freeze-Frame consists in recognizing and "freeze-framing" any stressful feeling as if it were one static movie image, then practicing heart focused breathing, recalling a positive feeling, and finding a deep heart answer.

Heart Lock-In facilitates deeper levels of heart experience. This technique is similar to other heart-based meditation, prayer and contemplation methods such as the Prayer of the Heart and the Arka Dhyana Intuitive Meditation, which will receive further discussion shortly.

Cut-Thru addresses negative emotions triggered by situations, thoughts, and actions, and is typically associated with treating depression, anxiety, or anger [3].

Coherent Communication improves relationships by cultivating personal coherence, clearly apprehending the other's communication, and confirming the essence of that communication. When practiced regularly, coherent communication immediately increases empathy and Ubuntu and I-Thou relationships [44].

Additional HeartMath (2020) tools are freely available at: https://www.heartmath.org/resources/downloads/12-heartmath-tools/, accessed on 4 April 2021.

Biofeedback instruments that have been scientifically developed to provide heart rate variability and heart rhythm coherence include:

The emWave2, which gives readings of and feedback on heart rate, heart rate variability, and physiological coherence. The instrument can be handheld for field use.

The emWave Pro is a sophisticated coherence biofeedback program for use by professional specialists in education, psychology, medicine, etc.

The Inner Balance Application (app) for personal coherence training is available to iPhone or smartphone users who download HeartMath programs from the internet.

The Global Coherence (GC) app records mean coherence levels at individual, group and global levels. The app is freely downloadable from the internet. A HeartMath Pulse sensor provides biofeedback.

7. The HeartMath Website

The HeartMath website can be found at https://www.hearthmath.org/, accessed on 4 April 2021. The website and annual report provide further practical healthcare information. For example, it lists programs, including Add Heart and Children's Heart Smarts and the 100,000 Coherent Kids Initiative, active in 93 countries. Since its inception, the HeartMath Institute has facilitated links with other health, educational, and research institutions. These established linkages are combined with the interdisciplinary originality and operational autonomy to lead to ground-breaking research in interdisciplinary fields such as biofield physiology and vibroengineering, which have impressed with their robust, scientific grounding [36].

8. HeartMath Global Healthcare Meditation

As concerns in-depth personal healthcare, the Heart Lock-In is one of the earliest HeartMath techniques developed. In a recently published study, 104 participants from five countries completed 15 days of ambulatory HRV monitoring. Analysis of participants HRV before, during, and after a Heart Lock-In meditation period indicated significantly increased coherence, as well as correlation with magnetic field activity on the day of the meditation [45].

This study may be regarded as cutting-edge quantitative scientific evidence for the claims of many earlier mass meditation studies to decrease violence and facilitate moral consciousness and behaviour, creativity, and health promotion [46]. From a qualitative perspective, an in-depth coherence experience has been described as follows [9,47]:

"Beyond the unique nature of each event, with their individual integrity and superficial differences, the essential structure of the coherence experience initially appears as some variation on the conscious practise of the cardiorespiratory, rhythmic process of breath connecting heart beats, warming and softening the heart, heralding a sense of stillness, alignment, harmony and peace, as scattered energy is felt to collect in the heart area, bringing deepening heart awareness and, typically, at some point a sense of "lift off" to unlimited self or space. This gathering energy seems to be distributed throughout the body and beyond, resonating with increasing subtlety and/or refinement into a higher, vibrational level typically experienced as love, accompanied by finer feelings of centeredness, wholeness, oneness and interconnectedness. Unique, individual experiences vary. They may be concrete, abstract, diffuse, definite, ordinary, mixed, mystical and/or paradoxical, of, for example, homecoming, unboundedness, spaciousness, timelessness, emptiness, freedom, happiness, bliss, joy and infinite creativity. Experiences typically have local, social or global action implications, insights, intuitions and moral directions, as, for example, for "making the world a better place" through writing, healing and teaching".

From this qualitative experiential perspective, it is instructive to note the great wisdom traditions of Judaism, Christianity, and Islam view the heart as the principal organ of spiritual perception. The great healing value of the Prayer of the Heart is commonly extolled by Christian and Sufi mystics [23,48]. HeartMath technology has also recently indicated highly significant increases in both coherence and achievement in the use of a similar heart-based method called Arka Dhyana, or Intuitive Meditation. Authors postulate that the HeartMath Coherence Model cast new light on the ancient Yogic idea of yoking in relation to embodied spirituality, both with regard to integration of the diverse bodily energies in immanent spirituality and holistic divine heart-based transcendence.

9. Conclusions

The HeartMath Institute formally reviews its activities in the form of annual reports. A variety of these activities regularly feature in update formal reviews by independent researchers, more of which are needed [49,50]. The specific goal of this study was to provide an inclusive, update, overview of HeartMath as an integrative, personal, social, and global healthcare system. Various research studies have consistently endorsed the practical value of diverse HeartMath tools, techniques, and electronics as excellent in transforming negativity into positivity and renewing the patterns of energy typically experienced in the forms of such feelings as peace and love. Considerable scientific evidence points to vast, energetic, interconnectivity at the human, planetary, and solar systemic levels. It is reasonable to conclude that the many HeartMath practitioners and GCI ambassadors from over 150 countries [2,3] who practice heart focused care, compassion, and love with an aim towards improving global coherence provide substantial human and planetary healthcare.

The present study has provided an overview of HeartMath as a coherent, integral heart-based healthcare system. Various forms of evidence have been presented to support this contention. There does not appear to be any contradictory evidence to this effect, although further gold-standard, empirically orientated, randomized controlled trials are needed [50]. Future conceptual, theoretical, and paradigmatic studies are also needed. In practical healthcare terms, positive emotions and heart focused breathing may facilitate vast interconnectivity. In addition to the pursuit of scientific programs and interventions, global healthcare amongst the general public needs vigorous promotion, especially when aimed towards facilitating the coherent collaboration of all related healthcare organizations and their associated stakeholders.

Author Contributions: Conceptualization, S.D.E.; methodology, S.D.E.; validation, S.D.E. and D.J.E.; formal analysis, S.D.E.; investigation, S.D.E.; resources, S.D.E. and R.H.; data curation, S.D.E.; writing—original draft preparation, S.D.E.; writing—review and editing, R.H. and D.J.E.; visualization, S.D.E.; supervision, D.J.E.; project administration, D.J.E.; funding acquisition, S.D.E. and D.J.E. All authors have read and agreed to the published version of the manuscript.

Funding: This research received no external funding, beyond University of Zululand.

Institutional Review Board Statement: The study was approved by the Research Committee, University of Zululand project number S894/97. Figures are reproduced with the permission of HeartMath Institute.

Informed Consent Statement: Not applicable.

Data Availability Statement: Not applicable.

Acknowledgments: The authors would like to thank Rollin McCraty, the Director of Research at the HeartMath Institute, for his immeasurable contribution to healthcare.

Conflicts of Interest: The authors declare no conflict of interest.

References

1. Edwards, S.D. The Global Coherence Initiative: A Global Psychology Paradigm for Health Promotion. *J. Psychol. Afr.* **2016**, *26*, 194–198. [CrossRef]
2. Childre, D.L.; Martin, H.; Rozman, D.; McCraty, R. *Heart Intelligence. Connecting with the Intuitive Guidance of the Heart*; Water Front Press: Boulder Creek, CA, USA, 2016.
3. Childre, D.L.; Martin, H. *The HeartMath Solution*; Harper Collins: New York, NY, USA, 2000.
4. Alabdulgader, A.A.; McCraty, R.; Atkinson, M.; Dobyns, Y.; Vainoras, A.; Ragulskis, M. Long-term study of heart rate variability responses to changes in the solar and geomagnetic environment. *Sci. Rep.* **2018**, *8*, 2663–2777. [CrossRef] [PubMed]
5. Edwards, S.D. HeartMath: A Positive Psychology Paradigm for Promoting Psychophysiological and Global Coherence. *J. Psychol. Afr.* **2015**, *25*, 367–374. [CrossRef]
6. McCraty, R.; Zayas, M.A. Cardiac Coherence, Self-Regulation, Autonomic Stability and Psychosocial Well-Being. *Front. Psychol.* **2014**, *5*, 1090. [CrossRef] [PubMed]
7. Edwards, S.D. Ubuntu Heartmath Programme Efficacy for Social Coherence and Work Spirit: Preliminary Evidence. *J. Psychol. Afr.* **2018**, *28*, 420–425. [CrossRef]
8. McCraty, R. New Frontiers in Heart Rate Variability and Social Coherence Research: Techniques, Technologies, and Implications for Improving Group Dynamics and Outcomes. *Front. Public Health* **2017**, *5*, 267. [CrossRef]
9. McCraty, R.; Atkinson, M.; Tomasino, D.; Bradley, R.J. The Coherent Heart. Heart-Brain Interaction, Psychophysiological Coherence and the Emergence of a System Wide Order. *Integral Rev.* **2009**, *2*, 10–115. Available online: https://www.integral-review.org/issues/vol_5_no_2_mccraty_et_al_the_coherent_heart.pdf (accessed on 4 April 2021).
10. Bohm, D. *Wholeness and the Implicate Order*; Routledge & Kegan Paul: New York, NY, USA, 1980.
11. Bourgeault, C. *The Wisdom Way of Knowing. Reclaiming an Ancient Tradition to Awaken the Heart*; Jossey-Bass: San Francisco, CA, USA, 2003.
12. Joye, S. *The Pribram–Bohm Holoflux Theory of Consciousness: An Integral Interpretation of the Theories of Karl Pribram, David Bohm, and Pierre Teilhard De Chardin*; Unpublished Dissertation for the Degree Doctor in Philosophy, Cosmology, and Consciousness; California Institute of Integral Studies: San Francisco, CA, USA, 2016.
13. Wilber, K. *Integral Meditation*; Shambhala Publications: Boulder, CO, USA, 2016.
14. Wilber, K. *Integral Psychology*; Shambhala Publications: Boulder, CO, USA, 2000.
15. Varela, F.J.; Thompson, E.T.; Rosch, E. *The Embodied Mind: Cognitive Science and Human Experience*; MIT Press: Cambridge, MA, USA, 1991.
16. McCraty, R. *Science of the Heart*; HeartMath Institute: Boulder Creek, CA, USA, 2016; Volume 2.
17. Pribram, K.H. *Brain and Perception. Holonomy and Structure in Figural Processing*; Routledge: New York, NY, USA, 2011.
18. Jobling, M.A.; Hurles, M.E.; Tyler-Smith, C. *Human Evolutionary Genetics*; Garland Publishing: New York, NY, USA, 2004.
19. Doke, C.M.; Vilakazi, B.M. *Zulu-English Dictionary*; Witwatersrand University Press: Johannesburg, Gauteng, South Africa, 1972.
20. Judith, A. *Eastern Body, Western Mind: Psychology and the Chakra System as a Path to the Self*; Celestial Arts: Berkeley, CA, USA, 2004.
21. Reid, D. *Chi-Gung: Harnessing the Power of the Universe*; Simon and Schuster: New York, NY, USA, 1998.
22. Graham, H. *Time, Energy and the Psychology of Healing*; Jessica Kingsley: London, UK, 1990.
23. Bourgeault, C. *The Heart of Centering Prayer. Nondual Christianity in Theory and Practice*; Shambhala: Boulder, CO, USA, 2016.
24. Louchakova, O. Spiritual Heart and Direct Knowing in the Prayer of the Heart. *Existent. Anal.* **2007**, *18*, 81–102. Available online: https://www.academia.edu/2364546/Louchakova_O_2007_Spiritual_heart_and_direct_knowing_in_the_Prayer_of_the_Heart_Existential_Analysis_18_1_81_102 (accessed on 4 April 2021).
25. Mutwa, V.C. *Zulu Shaman. Dreams, Prophecies and Mysteries*; Destiny Books: Rochester, VT, USA, 2003.
26. Maslow, A.H. *The Further Reaches of Human Nature*; Viking Press: New York, NY, USA, 1972.
27. MacKinnon, S.; Gevirtz, R.; McCraty, R.; Brown, M. Utilizing Heartbeat Evoked Potentials to Identify Cardiac Regulation of Vagal Afferents During Emotion and Resonant Breathing. *Appl. Psychophysiol. Biofeedback* **2013**, *38*, 241–255. [CrossRef]
28. Lehrer, P.; Gevirtz, R. Heart Rate Variability Biofeedback: How and Why Does It Work? *Front. Psychol.* **2014**, *5*, 756. [CrossRef]
29. Antonovsky, A. The Salutogenic Model as a Theory to Guide Health Promotion. *Health Promot Int.* **1996**, *11*, 11–18. [CrossRef]
30. Field, L.; Edwards, S.D.; Edwards, D.J.; Dean, S. Influence of Heartmath Training Programme on Physiological and Psychological Variables. *Glob. J. Health Sci.* **2018**, *10*, 126. [CrossRef]
31. Morris, S.M. Achieving Collective Coherence: Group Effects on Heart Rate Variability Coherence and Heart Rhythm Synchronization. *Altern. Ther. Health Med.* **2010**, *16*, 62–72. Available online: https://www.heartmath.org/assets/uploads/2015/01/achieving-collective-coherence.pdf (accessed on 4 April 2021).
32. Feldman, R. The Development of Regulatory Functions from Birth to 5 Years: Insights from Premature Infants. *Child Dev.* **2009**, *80*, 544–561. [CrossRef] [PubMed]
33. László, E. *Science and the Akashic Field: An Integral Theory of Everything*; Inner Traditions: Rochester, VT, USA, 2007.
34. Nelson, R. Detecting Mass Consciousness: Effects of Globally Shared Attention and Emotion. *J. Cosmol.* **2011**, *14*, 1.
35. McCraty, R.; Alabdulgader, A. A Consciousness, the Human Heart and the Global Energetic Field Environment. *Cardiol. Vasc. Res.* **2021**, *5*, 1–19. Available online: https://scivisionpub.com/pdfs/consciousness-the-human-heart-and-the-global-energetic-field-environment-1529.pdf (accessed on 4 April 2021). [CrossRef]

36. Hammerschlag, R.; Levin, M.; McCraty, R.; Bat, N.; Ives, J.A.; Lutgendorf, S.K.; Oschman, J.L. Biofield Physiology: A Framework for an Emerging Discipline. *Glob. Adv. Health Med.* **2015**, *4*, 35–41. [CrossRef]
37. Liu, J.H.; Macdonald, M. Towards a Psychology of Global Consciousness through an Ethical Conception of Self in Society. *J. Theory Soc. Behav.* **2016**, *46*, 310–334. [CrossRef]
38. Ferrer, J. Participation, Metaphysics, and Enlightenment. Reflections on Ken Wilber's Recent Work. *Approaching Relig.* **2015**, *5*, 42–66. [CrossRef]
39. Timofejeva, I.; McCraty, R.; Atkinson, M.; Joffe, R.; Vainoras, A.; Alabdulgader, A.A.; Ragulskis, M. Identification of a Group's Physiological Synchronization with Earth's Magnetic Field. *Int. J. Environ. Res. Public Health* **2017**, *14*, 998. [CrossRef]
40. Alabdulgader, A.A. Quantum consciousness and the heart based resonant frequencies theory. *Arch. Neurol. Neurosci.* **2021**, *9*, 1–10. [CrossRef]
41. Orme-Johnson, D.W. Application of Maharishi Vedic Science to Collective Consciousness and Peace Studies. *J. Soc. Behav. Personal.* **2005**, *17*, 277–283.
42. Horan, R. The Neuropsychological Connection Between Creativity and Meditation. *Creat. Res. J.* **2009**, *21*, 199–222. [CrossRef]
43. Nidich, S.I.; Nidich, R.J.; Alexander, C.N. Moral Development and Higher States of Consciousness. *J. Adult Dev.* **2000**, *7*, 217–225. [CrossRef]
44. Rogers, C. *A Way of Being*; Houghton Mifflin: Boston, MA, USA, 1980.
45. Timofejeva, I.; McCraty, R.; Atkinson, M.; Alabdulgader, A.A.; Vainoras, A.; Landauskas, M.; Šiaučiūnaitė, V.; Ragulskis, M. Global Study of Human Heart Rhythm Synchronization with the Earth's Time Varying Magnetic Field. *Appl. Sci.* **2021**, *11*, 2935. [CrossRef]
46. Alexander, V.K. Applications of Maharishi Vedic Science to Developmental Psychology. *J. Soc. Behav. Personal.* **2005**, *17*, 9–20. Available online: https://gawc.edu.in/uploads/attachments/a83594cb5ba517ea683b166e011b1b06/applications-of-maharishi-vedic-science-to-developmental-psychology.pdf (accessed on 4 April 2021).
47. Edwards, S.D. Heart Intelligence: Heuristic phenomenological investigation into the coherence experience using HeartMath methods. *AI Soc.* **2017**, *34*, 677–685. [CrossRef]
48. Bourgeault, C. Eye of the Heart. Bouldrer, CO. Shambala. 2020. Available online: https://www.contemplative.org/eye-of-the-heart-cynthia-bourgeault-shares-the-imaginal-roadmap/ (accessed on 4 April 2021).
49. Hancock, L. The Heart-Led Counselling Programme (HLC) Developing a Programme to Reduce Anxiety, Using Heart-Led Interventions and Positive Psychology Techniques in a Counselling Context. 2021. Available online: https://www.heartmath.org/assets/uploads/2021/12/heart-led-counselling-programme.pdf (accessed on 4 April 2021).
50. Field, L.; Forshaw, M.; Poole, H. Systematic Review of HeartMath© Interventions to Improve Psychological Outcomes in Individuals with Psychiatric Conditions. *Integral Rev.* **2021**, *17*, 69–89.

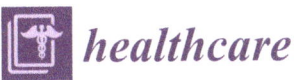

Article

The Effectiveness of Neroli Essential Oil in Relieving Anxiety and Perceived Pain in Women during Labor: A Randomized Controlled Trial

Cristiano Scandurra [1,*], Selene Mezzalira [2], Sara Cutillo [1], Rosanna Zapparella [1], Giancarlo Statti [3], Nelson Mauro Maldonato [1,*], Mariavittoria Locci [1,†] and Vincenzo Bochicchio [2,†]

1 Department of Neuroscience, Reproductive Sciences and Dentistry, University of Naples Federico II, 80133 Naples, Italy; saracutillo99@gmail.com (S.C.); info@rosannazapparella.it (R.Z.); m.locci@unina.it (M.L.)
2 Department of Humanistic Studies, University of Calabria, 87036 Rende, Italy; selene.mezzalira@unical.it (S.M.); vincenzo.bochicchio@unical.it (V.B.)
3 Department of Pharmacy, Health and Nutritional Sciences, University of Calabria, 87036 Rende, Italy; g.statti@unical.it
* Correspondence: cristiano.scandurra@unina.it (C.S.); nelsonmauro.maldonato@unina.it (N.M.M.); Tel.: +39-081-746-34-58 (C.S.)
† These authors contributed equally to this work.

Abstract: Childbirth is a stressful and physically painful event in a woman's life and aromatherapy is one of the most used non-pharmacological methods that is effective in reducing anxiety and perceived pain. This randomized controlled study aimed at determining the effect of neroli oil aromatherapy on anxiety and pain intensity perception in 88 women during labor, randomly assigned to either an intervention group ($n = 44$) or control group ($n = 44$). Anxiety and perceived pain were assessed through the visual analogue scale during the latent, early, and late active phases of labor. Data analyses included the t-test, Chi-square test, and repeated measures ANOVA. Perceived pain and anxiety in the group receiving aromatherapy were significantly lower than in the control group at all stages of labor ($p < 0.05$). Specifically, as the labor progressed, pain and anxiety increased in all participants, but the increase was milder in the experimental group than in the control group. The multiparas showed higher average anxiety scores, but not perceived pain, than the primiparas in all phases of labor ($p < 0.05$). Ultimately, neroli oil aromatherapy during labor can be used as an alternative tool to relieve anxiety and perceived pain in women during all stages of labor.

Keywords: aromatherapy; neroli oil; anxiety; pain; labor; randomized controlled trial

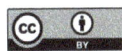

1. Introduction

During childbirth, fear and anxiety go hand in hand with anticipation and joy [1]. Indeed, childbirth is a stressful and physically painful event in a woman's life, to the point that labor pain has been defined as one of the most severe types of human pain [2]. Perception of pain during labor is due to uterus' contractions, uterine extension, and cervical dilation [3]. Inadequate pain management may affect diverse outcomes, such as psychological health, sexual functioning, or the infant–mother bond [4]. Previous studies stressed the association between pain and anxiety [5]. Anxiety activates the sympathetic nervous system releasing stress-related hormones (e.g., cortisol and adrenaline), which, as a consequence, may increase the severity of labor pain [6]. Therefore, it is imperative for midwives and obstetricians/gynecologists (Ob/Gyns) to find effective ways to relieve labor pain and anxiety.

Non-pharmacological methods such as relaxation techniques, massage, acupuncture, and aromatherapy are considered nowadays a promising area in midwifery thanks to their ease of use, low cost, and effectiveness [1,7–10]. Among them, aromatherapy represents one of the most used non-pharmacological methods for women in labor. It refers to the employment of the power of plant-sourced essential oils to treat and heal the individual's body and psyche [11], and represents a strategy of care that utilizes essentials oils by massaging them into the skin, adding them to bath water, or inhaling their odor when added to a steam infusion [12].

Aromatherapy has been used to enhance women's well-being during post-partum, as well as to facilitate mother–infant interactions [13]. It is often referred to as a useful means to alleviate anxiety and pain, thus fostering the individuals' well-being [14]. Furthermore, aromatherapy has been shown to decrease anxiety and perceived pain during labor [15], as well as increase comfort and satisfaction [14,16]. Aromatherapy has been also successfully utilized jointly with massage to decrease stress and enhance immune function during pregnancy [12], as well as to reduce body tension and emotional stress [17].

Even though aromatherapy and essential oils such as orange scent, geranium, and lavender have been employed to reduce anxiety and perceived pain during labor [1,18–20], no studies have been carried out utilizing neroli oil to alleviate pain and anxiety during childbirth.

Neroli oil is extracted from the *Citrus aurantium* L. blossoms, commonly named bitter orange, which is a tree belonging to the *Rutaceae* family. It has antimicrobial and antioxidant properties [21], and has been shown to possess active constituents that play a significant role against inflammation, thus resulting useful for pain management [22]. Other therapeutic properties include sedative, calming, tonic, cytophylactic, aphrodisiac, anti-depressant, and antispasmodic action [23]. Most importantly, neroli oil can be utilized as an anxiolytic [24]. Therefore, neroli oil is frequently used for medicinal purposed, in particular for treating gastrointestinal disorders, tachycardia, and rheumatism, for minimizing central nervous system disorders [25], and as a sedative [26]. *Citrus Aurantium L.* flowers produce the orange blossom water, also utilized for therapeutic purposes [27]. Originally employed as a cardiac stimulant, for carminative purposes, and to help babies fall asleep, this water has been suggested to be useful in detoxification programs or when quitting addiction habits such as smoking [23]. Besides the aromatic water, the distillation of sour orange flowers produces neroli, a rare aromatic oil that contains a fragrance and represents the core of one of the world's most used perfumes, "eau de cologne," which is also used in pharmacy as a flavoring agent [21], as well as in some medicines approved by the American Food and Drug Administration.

Based on these premises, this study aimed at determining the effect of neroli oil aromatherapy on anxiety and pain intensity perception in a group of women in labor.

2. Materials and Methods

2.1. Essential Oil Chemical Characterization

Neroli essential oil was purchased by Gya Labs. The essential oil chemical characterization was performed on 100% pure oil. In the final product, instead, the essential oil was used in a 5% formulation.

The investigated essential oil was characterized through a Hewlett-Packard 6890 gas chromatograph equipped with a 100% dimethylpolysiloxane SE-30 capillary column (30 m length, 0.25 mm in diameter, 0.25 μm film thickness), coupled with a Hewlett Packard 5973 mass spectrometer. A programmed temperature ranging from 60 to 280 °C, with a rate of 16 °C/min was used; the analysis was performed by using helium (0.00167 cm/s linear velocity) as carrier gas.

Essential oil constituents were identified by matching the obtained spectra with those listed in the Wiley 138 mass spectral library.

2.2. Study Design and Procedures

This was a prospective, interventional, non-pharmacological, and randomized controlled study, with a repeated-measure design.

Participants were randomly distributed in the experimental or in the control group according to a randomization with a 1:1 ratio obtained through a web-based computer system (randomization.com). The pregnant women in the control group received only routine prenatal care, which included emotional support from a midwife, the ability to take free positions during labor, massage and/or the application of hot packs in the lumbosacral area. The pregnant women in the intervention group received routine prenatal care plus the aromatherapy with vapor diffusion.

The essential neroli oil was diffused continuously through an aroma diffuser and using standard concentration at four drops of aroma oil per 300 mL of diffused water. The aromatherapy lasted the whole time of labor. Anxiety and pain intensity perception were assessed during 3 stages of labor: the latent phase (cervical dilatation of 3–4 cm), early active phase (cervical dilatation of 5–7 cm), and late active phase (cervical dilatation of 8–10 cm).

To better promote the spread of the active ingredients of neroli oil, a water (50%) and alcohol (32%) based formulation was made in which a percentage of 5% of the essential neroli oil was added. The formulation was completed by a phenolic antioxidant agent, BHT or butylhydroxytoluene, used at 0.1% and finished with the addition of PEG-40 hydrogenated castor oil, which has emulsifying functions, and propylene glycol, a carrier that makes the fragrance more lasting.

All participants provided written informed consent. The study was approved by the Ethical Committee of Psychological Research of the University of Naples Federico II (protocol number 2/2021; date of approval: 9 February 2021), designed with respect of the principles of the Declaration of Helsinki, and conducted following the EU General Data Protection Regulation. The clinical trial was retrospectively registered on the Deutsches Register Klinischer Studien (n° DRKS00027563).

2.3. Participants and Sample Size

Participants were recruited from May to October 2021 at the prenatal clinic of the University Public Hospital Federico II of Naples, which is also an obstetric emergency department.

All pregnant women, aged between 18 and 40 years, with a low-risk full-term pregnancy (between the 37th and 42nd week of amenorrhea) undergoing labor and with the fetus in cephalic presentation were included in the study. Pregnant women with maternal and/or fetal pathologies, subjected to drug induction to labor, or who had resorted to epidural analgesia, were excluded from the study.

A statistical power analysis was performed for sample size estimation through G*Power program (Heinrich Heine University, Düsseldorf, Germany). Based on parameters used by Tanvisut et al. [28], the effect size was set at 0.05, the α at 0.05 (two-tailed), and the power at 90%. Results indicated that a sample size of at least 42 participants for each group was needed.

During the study period, 1258 women were admitted to the delivery room at the hospital. Among them, a total of 96 women met the inclusion criteria. They were randomly assigned to either the intervention group (n = 48) or control group (n = 48). Four women for each group were then excluded because they needed to take drugs to induce labor or to undergo epidural analgesia. Thus, analyses were conducted on 44 women in the experimental group and 44 in the control group. The CONSORT flow diagram is shown in Figure 1.

2.4. Measures
2.4.1. Clinical and Demographic Information

Clinical and demographic variables assessed in this study included age, parity (primiparas vs. multiparas), duration of labor, and the Apgar index.

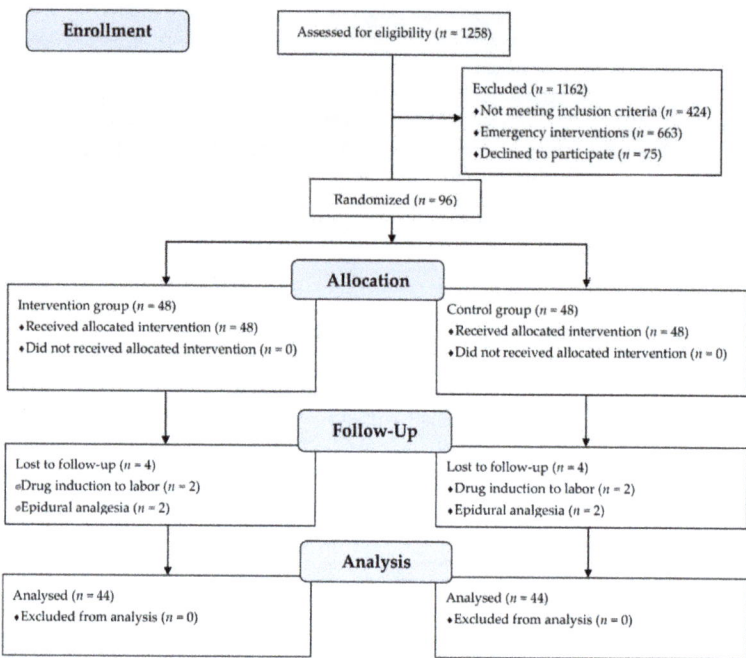

Figure 1. CONSORT diagram of study participants in control and intervention groups.

2.4.2. Anxiety

Anxiety was assessed through two measures: the Visual Analogue Scale for Anxiety (VAS-A [29]; Italian adaption by Facco et al. [30]) and the State-Trait Anxiety Inventory Form Y (STAI-Y [31]; Italian adaption by Pedrabissi and Santinello [32]).

VAS-A is a measure assessing perceived levels of anxiety which is particularly effective in those situations where answering many questions may be burdensome for participants, as well as it is for women during labor. The VAS-A is a line 10 centimeters in length with zero representing "not at all anxious" and 10 "very anxious". Participants are asked to mark their subjective anxious status on a visual scale by putting a cross. Different studies demonstrated the validity of the VAS-A (for a review, see Rossi and Pourtois [33]). VAS-A was assessed during latent, early active, and late active phases of labor.

STAI-Y is a measure consisting of 20 items that assess transitory feelings of tension, worry, and nervousness at a given moment. The answer options range from 1 ("not at all") to 4 ("very much so"), with higher scores indicating greater state anxiety. In our sample the values of Cronbach's alpha at the moment of the recruitment and immediately after the birth were 0.81 and 0.80, respectively. This measure was administered at the moment of the recruitment (i.e., before the childbirth), and immediately after the childbirth.

2.4.3. Pain Intensity

Pain was assessed through the Visual Analogue Scale (VAS [34]; Italian adaptation by De Benedittis et al. [35]), a widely used scale assessing the perceived intensity of pain. The VAS is a continuous unidimensional scale comprised of a horizontal line 10 centimeters in length with zero representing "no pain" and 10 "worst pain". Participants are asked to mark their perceived pain intensity on a visual scale by putting a cross. Different studies demonstrated the validity of the VAS (for a review, see Bijur et al. [36]). As the VAS-A, even the pain VAS was assessed during latent, early active, and late active phases of labor.

2.5. Statistical Analyses

Statistical analyses were conducted using SPSS version 27 (IBM, Armonk, NY, USA) and setting the level of significance at 0.05.

First, Student's t-test for continuous variables or chi-square (χ^2) for frequencies were used to evaluate any socio-demographic or clinical differences between experimental and control group and assess whether the two groups were comparable.

Then, Student's t-test was performed to evaluate the differences between the experimental and control groups in the mean scores on perceived pain and anxiety during different stages of labor. The effect size was calculated with Cohen's d [37] (small effect size = 0.01, medium effect size = 0.06, and large effect size = 0.14).

Finally, a repeated measures ANOVA was performed to evaluate the effect of "Study Group" (experimental vs. control), "Time" (i.e., the three phases of labor), and "Childbirth Group" (primiparas vs. multiparas) on pain and anxiety. The effect size, in this case, was calculated with Cohen's η^2 [37] (small effect size = 0.01, medium effect size = 0.06, and large effect = size 0.14).

3. Results

3.1. Gas Chromatography–Mass Spectrometry (GC-MS) Analysis

Major constituents of neroli essential oil were investigated through gas chromatography–mass spectrometry (GC-MS) analysis (Table 1). The monoterpene Linalool represents the most abundant compound in the essential oil composition (10.70 ± 0.55 %), followed by anthranilic acid, limonene, α-terpineol, and geranil acetate, with value percentage of 6.43 ± 0.60, 3.91 ± 0.12, 3.31 ± 0.15, and 3.21 ± 0.23, respectively. Other compounds, such as 4-carene and α-ocimene, were found in trace amounts.

Table 1. Gas chromatography–mass spectrometry (GC-MS) analysis.

N.	Compound [a]	Rt [b]	RAP [c]
1	α-Pinene	6.33	2.72 ± 0.09
2	Camphene	6.63	0.12 ± 0.01
3	β-Pinene	7.20	0.85 ± 0.07
4	β-Myrcene	7.47	1.50 ± 0.10
5	3-Carene	7.81	1.85 ± 0.14
6	Isocineole	7.88	0.26 ± 0.01
7	Limonene	8.16	3.91 ± 0.12
8	4-Carene	8.24	Tr [d]
9	α-Ocimene	8.40	Tr
10	Linalool	9.25	10.70 ± 0.55
11	1-p-menthol	9.83	0.47 ± 0.02
12	Acetophenone	10.27	0.13 ± 0.01
13	α-terpineol	10.43	3.31 ± 0.15
14	Citronellol	10.86	1.73 ± 0.09
15	Anthranilic acid	10.95	6.43 ± 0.60
16	Geraniol	11.09	1.52 ± 0.20
17	1,4-dimethyl-4-vinylciclohexene	11.29	1.30 ± 0.08
18	Fenchyl acetate	11.35	0.49 ± 0.02
19	Indole	11.66	0.21 ± 0.01
20	Geranyl acetate	12.15	3.21 ± 0.23
21	Tridecanol	12.80	2.28 ± 0.18
22	Nerolin	13.44	1.47 ± 0.16
23	Nerolidol	13.63	0.29 ± 0.01
24	Farnesol	14.62	1.20 ± 0.05

Notes: [a] Major compounds listed in order of elution from SE30 MS column; [b] Retention time (as min); [c] Relative area percentage (peak area relative to total peak area in total ion current (TIC) %); [d] Tr: Traces percentages < 0.1%. Data are expressed as mean ± standard deviation (n = 3) of 3 independent experiments.

3.2. Participants' Characteristics

Fifty-one participants were primiparas (26 in the experimental group and 25 in the control group) and 37 multiparas (18 in the experimental group and 19 in the control group). No statistical differences in sample terms were detected ($\chi^2 = 0.04$, $p = 0.84$).

The average age of the participants was 31 years ($SD = 5.64$) in the experimental group and 32.11 years ($SD = 5.60$) in the control group, and the difference was not significant ($t = -0.43$, $p = 0.67$).

The mean duration of labor was 2.47 hours ($SD = 1.51$) in the experimental group and 2.32 hours ($SD = 1.59$) in the control group, and the difference was not significant ($t = 0.21$, $p = 0.84$).

The averages of the Apgar index at 1 min (experimental group: $M = 8.00$, $SD = 0.82$; Control group: $M = 8.11$, $SD = 1.27$; $t = -0.23$, $p = 0.82$) and at 5 min (experimental group: $M = 8.90$, $SD = 0.32$; Control group: $M = 9.00$, $SD = 0.50$; $t = -0.53$, $p = 0.60$) did not differ significantly between groups.

The absence of statistically significant differences on the variables reported made the groups comparable.

3.3. Effect of Neroli Oil Aromatherapy on Pain Intensity

The results showed that participants undergoing aromatherapy had lower perceived pain intensity than participants in the control group at all stages of labor (Table 2).

Table 2. Comparisons between experimental and control groups on pain intensity during the stages of labor.

	Experimental Group ($n = 44$) M (SD)	Control Group ($n = 44$) M (SD)	t	95% CI	d
Latent phase	5.70 (1.42)	7.44 (1.33)	−2.75 *	−3.08, −0.41	1.26
Early active phase	6.50 (1.27)	8.44 (1.42)	−3.15 **	−3.25, −0.64	1.44
Late active phase	8.00 (1.56)	9.33 (1.12)	−2.11 *	−2.66, −0.01	0.98

Notes: M = mean; SD = standard deviation; t = Student's t-test; CI = confidence intervals; d = Cohen's d. * $p < 0.05$; ** $p < 0.01$.

Repeated measures ANOVA revealed that the main effect of the "Study Group" (experimental vs. control) was significant ($F = 7.55$, $p = 0.01$, $\eta^2 = 0.32$), indicating that there was an overall difference in the mean pain scores of the experimental group compared to those of the control group, with a large effect size. Similarly, the "Time" effect (i.e., the three phases of labor) was also significant and with a large effect size ($F = 6.98$, $p = 0.003$, $\eta^2 = 0.30$). On the contrary, no significant effect was found for the "Childbirth Group", indicating that the results obtained did not depend on being primiparas or multiparas.

Overall, as shown in Figure 2, as labor progressed, women in both groups perceived pain as getting stronger, but the increase was milder in the experimental group than in the control group.

3.4. Effect of Neroli Oil Aromatherapy on Anxiety

The results relating to anxiety assessed through the VAS-A were similar to those obtained for pain. Indeed, they showed that participants undergoing aromatherapy perceived lower levels of anxiety than participants in the control group at all stages of labor (Table 3).

Repeated measures ANOVA revealed that the main effect of the "Study Group" (experimental vs. control) was significant ($F = 11.41$, $p = 0.004$, $\eta^2 = 0.42$), indicating that there was an overall difference in mean anxiety scores reported by the experimental group compared to those of the control group, with a large effect size. Similarly, the "Time" effect (i.e., the three phases of labor) was also significant and with a large effect size ($F = 7.66$, $p = 0.014$, $\eta^2 = 0.32$). However, as opposed to the results concerning pain intensity, in this case even the effect of the "Childbirth Group" (primiparas vs. multiparas) on anxiety was significant and with a large effect size ($F = 16.19$, $p = 0.001$, $\eta^2 = 0.50$). Specifically, the multiparas showed higher average anxiety scores than the primiparas in all phases of labor, as follows: latent phase (primiparas: M = 2.91, SD = 2.12; multiparas: M = 5.87, SD = 1.12; t = −3.59, p = 0.002), early active phase (primiparas: M = 4.09, SD = 2.47; multiparas: M = 7.00, SD = 1.07; t = −3.11, p = 0.006), and late active phase (primiparas: M = 5.00, SD = 2.65; multiparas: M = 8.25, SD = 1.67; t = −3.05, p = 0.007). Again, as shown in Figure 3, with the progress of labor, anxiety increased in all participants, but the increase was milder in the experimental group than in the control group.

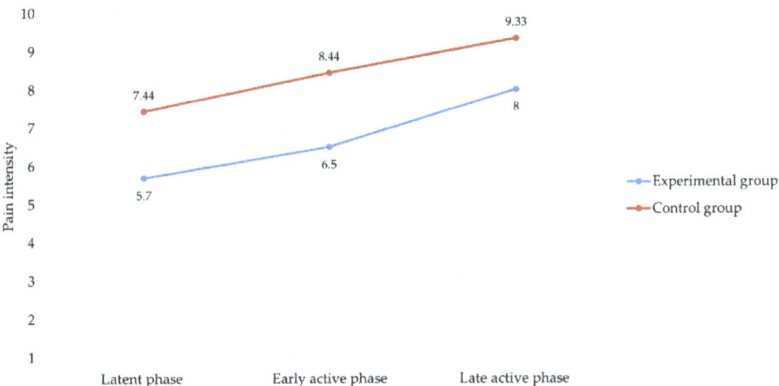

Figure 2. Changes in pain intensity scores along the stages of labor in experimental and control group.

Table 3. Comparisons between experimental and control groups on anxiety measured with VAS-A during the stages of labor.

	Experimental Group (n = 44) M (SD)	Control Group (n = 44) M (SD)	t	95% CI	d
Latent phase	3.10 (2.13)	5.33 (1.94)	−2.38 *	−4.21, −0.25	1.09
Early active phase	4.10 (2.68)	6.67 (1.22)	−2.63 *	−4.63, −0.50	1.23
Late active phase	5.00 (3.02)	7.89 (1.45)	−2.61 *	−5.23, −0.55	1.22

Notes: VAS-A = Visual Analogue Scale for Anxiety; M = mean; SD = standard deviation; t = Student's t-test; CI = confidence intervals; d = Cohen's d. * p < 0.05.

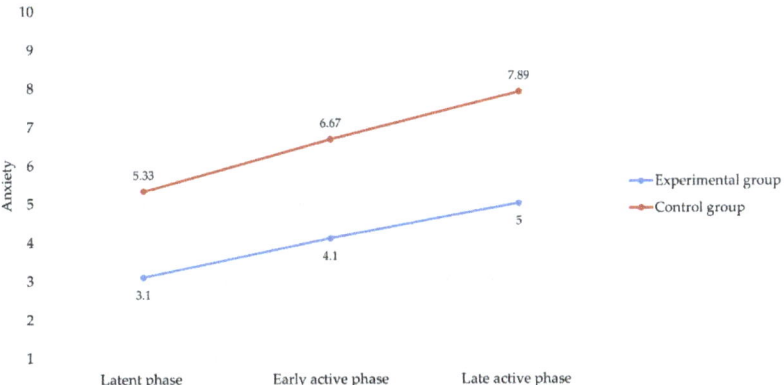

Figure 3. Changes in anxiety scores measured with the Visual Analogue Scale for Anxiety along the stages of labor in experimental and control group.

Finally, with regard to state anxiety assessed through the STAI-Y, it clearly emerged that the average anxiety scores measured before labor did not differ between the experimental and control groups, while differed significantly after childbirth, indicating that neroli oil aromatherapy had a positive effect on anxiety (Table 4).

Table 4. Comparisons between experimental and control groups on anxiety measured with STAI-Y before and after the childbirth.

	Experimental Group (n = 44) M (SD)	Control Group (n = 44) M (SD)	t	95% CI	d
Before the childbirth	2.07 (0.15)	2.08 (0.18)	−0.04	−0.16, 0.16	1.09
After the childbirth	2.01 (0.06)	2.32 (0.19)	−4.69 ***	−4.44, −0.17	1.23

Notes: STAI-Y = State–Trait Anxiety Inventory Form Y; M = mean; SD = standard deviation; t = Student's t-test; CI = confidence intervals; d = Cohen's d. *** p < 0.001.

4. Discussion

The current randomized controlled study was aimed at evaluating the effectiveness of neroli essential oil aromatherapy in relieving anxiety and perceived pain in women in labor. Results showed that neroli oil aromatherapy significantly and positively impacts women's experience of perceived pain and anxiety during labor, representing a further confirmation of the effectiveness of non-pharmacological methods in making the childbirth a less stressful experience.

Specifically, our findings showed that neroli oil reduced women's perception of pain and anxiety, which appeared less intense than in the women that did not receive aromatherapy treatment. Specifically, as the labor progressed, pain and anxiety increased in all participants, but the increase was milder in the experimental group when compared to the control group. Furthermore, since the average anxiety and perceived pain scores measured before labor did not differ between the experimental and control groups, while differed significantly after childbirth, we can conclude that neroli oil aromatherapy had a positive effect on anxiety and perceived pain. These findings confirm the results obtained in previous studies using other essential oils [16,28,38,39]. For instance, the use of essential oils in aromatherapy, thanks to their validated analgesic, anti-inflammatory, calming, and relaxing effects, has been proven to alleviate physical and emotional disorders in cancer patients [40]. This makes it reasonable to infer that aromatherapy represents a helpful alternative method for anxiety and pain control [41–43].

A second finding showed that the mean anxiety scores were higher in the multiparas than in the primiparas in all stages of labor. This might be explained by taking into account the role that previous experience might play in pregnant women's experience [44]. Provided that childbirth is a physically painful experience, we might hypothesize that having already gone through labor can be a predisposing factor for greater expectations of perceived pain, therefore explaining the differences in perceived anxiety in the two groups (i.e., primiparas vs. multiparas). However, this is a speculative and hypothetical explanation, as other studies have shown that primiparas experience more anxiety than multiparas during labor [44–47]. Thus, future studies should collect data about the quality of previous childbirth experiences in multiparas and assess whether negative experiences can affect anxiety during labor.

Findings should be read in light of some limitations. First, this study assessed only one mode of aromatherapy and one essential oil, and did not compare different techniques of aromatherapy administration or other essential oils. Future research should replicate this study assessing whether other techniques of aromatherapy and other essential oils are more or less effective than that used in this study. Second, the stressful condition under which participants had to answer the questionnaires may have confounded their responses to the pain and anxiety assessment. However, we tried to overcome this intrinsic limitation by administering not stressful and easy to use questionnaires (i.e., VAS and VAS-A). Third, we did not collect information about previous childbirth experiences or any other experience (e.g., previous negative medical experiences) that could have affected anxiety.

Despite these limitations, the findings obtained in the current study point to the fact that available non-pharmacological remedies such as aromatherapy are effective in relieving pain and anxiety in women during the most difficult phase of pregnancy, that is, labor and childbirth [48]. They also represent a viable alternative to a strict medicalization of labor [49], providing midwifes and Ob/Gyns with natural methods that can be easily used [10]. The relevance of our results also consists in the fact that when pain and anxiety are less severe, labor progresses more easily and with less difficulties. Therefore, neroli oil can and should be used as an alternative tool to relieve anxiety and perceived pain in women during all stages of labor.

5. Conclusions

Neroli oil aromatherapy during labor significantly impacts women's experience of perceived pain and anxiety, which seem to be reduced in their severity during all stages of labor. Since neroli oil is a non-pharmacological remedy, which is efficacious in relieving perceived pain and anxiety in women during labor and childbirth, it represents an extremely useful alternative to pharmacological drugs. In fact, neroli oil aids in the progress of labor by decreasing perceived pain and anxiety, thus rendering labor and childbirth easier and less problematic.

Author Contributions: Conceptualization, C.S., S.M., S.C., M.L. and V.B.; methodology, C.S., S.M., S.C., M.L. and V.B.; formal analysis, C.S.; investigation, C.S., S.M., S.C., R.Z., G.S., N.M.M., M.L. and V.B.; resources, S.C., R.Z., G.S. and N.M.M.; data curation, C.S. and S.C.; writing—original draft preparation, C.S. and S.M.; writing—review and editing, M.L. and V.B.; supervision, M.L. and V.B.; project administration, C.S., M.L. and V.B.; M.L. and V.B. equally contributed as last authors. All authors have read and agreed to the published version of the manuscript.

Funding: This research received no external funding.

Institutional Review Board Statement: The study was conducted in accordance with the Declaration of Helsinki, and approved by Ethical Committee of Psychological Research of the University of Naples Federico II (protocol number 2/2021; date of approval: 9 February 2021). The clinical trial was retrospectively registered on the Deutsches Register Klinischer Studien (n° DRKS00027563).

Informed Consent Statement: Informed consent was obtained from all subjects involved in the study. Written informed consent has been obtained from the patients to publish this paper.

Data Availability Statement: The data and materials that support the findings of this study are available from the corresponding authors upon reasonable request.

Conflicts of Interest: The authors declare no conflict of interest.

References

1. Liao, C.C.; Lan, S.H.; Yen, Y.Y.; Hsieh, Y.P.; Lan, S.J. Aromatherapy intervention on anxiety and pain during first stage labour in nulliparous women: A systematic review and meta-analysis. *J. Obstet. Gynaecol.* **2021**, *41*, 21–31. [CrossRef] [PubMed]
2. Rai, R.; Uprety, D.; Pradhan, T.; Bhattarai, B.; Acharya, S. Subcutaneous sterile water injection for labor pain: A randomized controlled trial. *Nepal. J. Obstet. Gynecol.* **2014**, *8*, 68–70. [CrossRef]
3. Gholipour Baradari, A.; Firouzian, A.; Hasanzadeh Kiabi, F.; Emami Zeydi, A.; Khademloo, M.; Nazari, Z.; Sanagou, M.; Ghobadi, M.; Fooladi, E. Bolus administration of intravenous lidocaine reduces pain after an elective caesarean section: Findings from a randomised, double-blind, placebo-controlled trial. *J. Obstet. Gynaecol.* **2017**, *37*, 566–570. [CrossRef]
4. Goodman, P.; Mackey, M.C.; Tavakoli, A.S. Factors related to childbirth satisfaction. *J. Adv. Nurs.* **2004**, *46*, 212–219. [CrossRef]
5. Lang, A.J.; Sorrell, J.T.; Rodgers, C.S.; Lebeck, M.M. Anxiety sensitivity as a predictor of labor pain. *Eur. J. Pain* **2006**, *10*, 263–270. [CrossRef]
6. Lowe, N.K.; Corwin, E.J. Proposed biological linkages between obesity, stress, and inefficient uterine contractility during labor in humans. *Med. Hypotheses* **2011**, *76*, 755–760. [CrossRef]
7. Jones, L.; Othman, M.; Dowswell, T.; Alfirevic, Z.; Gates, S.; Newburn, M.; Jordan, S.; Lavender, T.; Neilson, J.P. Pain management for women in labour: An overview of systematic reviews. *Cochrane Database Syst. Rev.* **2012**, *2012*, CD009234.
8. Muñoz-Sellés, E.; Vallès-Segalés, A.; Goberna-Tricas, J. Use of alternative and complementary therapies in labor and delivery care: A cross-sectional study of midwives' training in Catalan hospitals accredited as centers for normal birth. *BMC Complement. Altern. Med.* **2013**, *13*, 318. [CrossRef]

9. Simkin, P.; Bolding, A. Update on nonpharmacologic approaches to relieve labor pain and prevent suffering. *J. Midwifery Womens Health* **2004**, *49*, 489–504. [CrossRef]
10. Tabatabaeichehr, M.; Mortazavi, H. The effectiveness of aromatherapy in the management of labor pain and anxiety: A systematic review. *Ethiop. J. Health Sci.* **2020**, *30*, 449–458. [CrossRef]
11. Tournaire, M.; Theau-Yonneau, A. Complementary and alternative approaches to pain relief during labor. *Evid. Based Complement. Alternat. Med.* **2007**, *4*, 409–417. [CrossRef] [PubMed]
12. Chen, P.J.; Chou, C.C.; Yang, L.; Tsai, Y.L.; Chang, Y.C.; Liaw, J.J. Effects of aromatherapy massage on pregnant women's stress and immune function: A longitudinal, prospective, randomized controlled trial. *J. Altern. Complement. Med.* **2017**, *23*, 778–786. [CrossRef] [PubMed]
13. Imura, M.; Misao, H.; Ushijima, H. The psychological effects of aromatherapy-massage in healthy postpartum mothers. *J Midwifery Womens Health* **2006**, *51*, e21–e27. [CrossRef] [PubMed]
14. Cenkci, Z.; Nazik, E. The effect of aromatherapy on pain, comfort and satisfaction during childbirth. *New Trends Issues Proc. Humanit. Soc. Sci.* **2017**, *4*, 11–19. [CrossRef]
15. Tillett, J.; Ames, D. The uses of aromatherapy in women's health. *J. Perinat. Neonatal Nurs.* **2010**, *24*, 238–245. [CrossRef]
16. Burns, E.; Zobbi, V.; Panzeri, D.; Oskrochi, R.; Regalia, A. Aromatherapy in childbirth: A pilot randomised controlled trial. *BJOG* **2007**, *114*, 838–844. [CrossRef]
17. Wu, J.J.; Cui, Y.; Yang, Y.S.; Kang, M.S.; Jung, S.C.; Park, H.K.; Yeun, H.Y.; Jang, W.J.; Lee, S.; Kwak, Y.S.; et al. Modulatory effects of aromatherapy massage intervention on electroencephalogram, psychological assessments, salivary cortisol and plasma brain–derived neurotrophic factor. *Complement. Ther. Med.* **2014**, *22*, 456–462. [CrossRef]
18. Rashidi-Fakari, F.; Tabatabaeichehr, M.; Mortazavi, H. The effect of aromatherapy by essential oil of orange on anxiety during labor: A randomized clinical trial. *Iran. J. Nurs. Midwifery Res.* **2015**, *20*, 661–664.
19. Azima, S. The effect of lavender aromatherapy on pain perception and intrapartum outcome in nulliparas women. *Br. J. Midwifery* **2014**, *22*, 125–128.
20. Makvandi, S.; Mirteimoori, M.; Najmabadi, K.M.; Sadeghi, R. A review of randomized clinical trials on the effect of aromatherapy with lavender on labor pain relief. *Nurse Care Open Access J.* **2016**, *1*, 42–47. [CrossRef]
21. Ammar, A.H.; Bouajila, J.; Lebrihi, A.; Mathieu, F.; Romdhane, M.; Zagrouba, F. Chemical composition and in vitro antimicrobial and antioxidant activities of *Citrus aurantium* L. flowers essential oil (Neroli). *Pak. J. Biol. Sci.* **2012**, *15*, 1034–1040. [CrossRef]
22. Khodabakhsh, P.; Shafaroodi, H.; Asgarpanah, J. Analgesic and anti–inflammatory activities of *Citrus aurantium* L. blossoms essential oil (neroli): Involvement of the nitric oxide/cyclic–guanosine monophosphate pathway. *J. Nat. Med.* **2015**, *69*, 324–331. [CrossRef]
23. Jeannot, V.; Chahboun, J.; Russell, D.; Baret, P. Quantification and determination of chemical composition of the essential oil extracted from natural orange blossom water (*Citrus aurantium* L. ssp. aurantium). *Int. J. Aromather.* **2005**, *15*, 94–97. [CrossRef]
24. Chen, Y.J.; Cheng, F.; Shih, Y.; Chang, T.M.; Wang, M.F.; Lan, S.S. Inhalation of neroli essential oil and its anxiolytic effects. *J. Complement. Integr. Med.* **2008**, *5*, 13. [CrossRef]
25. Moraes, T.M.; Kushima, H.; Moleiro, F.C.; Santos, R.C.; Rocha, L.R.; Marques, M.O.; Vilegas, W.; Hiruma-Lima, C.A. Effects of limonene and essential oil from *Citrus aurantium* on gastric mucosa: Role of prostaglandins and gastric mucus secretion. *Chem. Biol. Interact.* **2009**, *180*, 499–505. [CrossRef]
26. Pultrini Ade, M.; Galindo, L.A.; Costa, M. Effects of the essential oil from *Citrus aurantium* L. in experimental anxiety models in mice. *Life Sci.* **2006**, *78*, 1720–1725. [CrossRef]
27. Ayadi, A.; Ayed, N.; Karmous, T.; Bessière, J.M.; Talou, T. Tunisian aromatic waters profile. *J. Essent Oil–Bear Plants* **2013**, *7*, 136–145. [CrossRef]
28. Tanvisut, R.; Traisrisilp, K.; Tongsong, T. Efficacy of aromatherapy for reducing pain during labor: A randomized controlled trial. *Arch. Gynecol. Obstet.* **2018**, *297*, 1145–1150. [CrossRef]
29. Hornblow, A.R.; Kidson, M.A. The visual analogue scale for anxiety: A validation study. *Aust. N. Zealand J. Psychiatry* **1976**, *10*, 339–341. [CrossRef]
30. Facco, E.; Stellini, E.; Bacci, C.; Manani, G.; Pavan, C.; Cavallin, F.; Zanette, G. Validation of visual analogue scale for anxiety (VAS–A) in preanesthesia evaluation. *Minerva Anestesiol.* **2013**, *79*, 1389–1395.
31. Spielberger, C.D.; Gorsuch, R.L.; Lushene, R.; Vagg, P.R.; Jacobs, G.A. *Manual for the State–Trait Anxiety Inventory*; Consulting Psychologists Press: Palo Alto, CA, USA, 1983.
32. Pedrabissi, L.; Santinello, M. *Verifica Della Validità Dello STAI Forma Y di Spielberger [Verification of the validity of the STAI, Form Y, by Spielberger]*; Giunti Organizzazioni Speciali: Firenze, Italy, 1989.
33. Rossi, V.; Pourtois, G. Transient state–dependent fluctuations in anxiety measured using STAI, POMS, PANAS or VAS: A comparative review. *Anxiety Stress Coping* **2012**, *25*, 603–645. [CrossRef]
34. Downie, W.W.; Leatham, P.A.; Rhind, V.M.; Wright, V.; Branco, J.A.; Anderson, J.A. Studies with pain rating scales. *Ann. Rheum. Dis.* **1978**, *37*, 378–381. [CrossRef]
35. De Benedittis, G.; Massel, R.; Nobili, R.; Pieri, A. The Italian Pain Questionnaire. *Pain* **1988**, *33*, 53–62. [CrossRef]
36. Bijur, P.E.; Silver, W.; Gallagher, E.J. Reliability of the visual analog scale for measurement of acute pain. *Acad. Emerg. Med.* **2001**, *8*, 1153–1157. [CrossRef]
37. Cohen, J. *Statistical Power Analysis for the Behavioral Sciences*, 2nd ed.; Lawrence Erlbaum: Mahwah, NJ, USA, 1988.

38. Namazi, M.; Amir Ali Akbari, S.; Mojab, F.; Talebi, A.; Alavi Majd, H.; Jannesari, S. Effects of *Citrus aurantium* (bitter orange) on the severity of first-stage labor pain. *Iran. J. Pharm. Res.* **2014**, *13*, 1011–1018.
39. Yazdkhasti, M.; Pirak, A. The effect of aromatherapy with lavender essence on severity of labor pain and duration of labor in primiparous women. *Complement. Ther. Clin. Pract.* **2016**, *25*, 81–86. [CrossRef]
40. Sharma, M.; Grewal, K.; Jandrotia, R.; Batish, D.R.; Singh, H.P.; Kohli, R.K. Essential oils as anticancer agents: Potential role in malignancies, drug delivery mechanisms, and immune system enhancement. *Biomed. Pharm.* **2022**, *146*, 112514. [CrossRef]
41. Bochicchio, V.; Winsler, A. The psychology of olfaction: A theoretical framework with research and clinical implications. *Psychol. Rev.* **2020**, *127*, 442–454. [CrossRef]
42. Bochicchio, V.; Scandurra, C.; Vitelli, R.; Valerio, P.; dell'Orco, S.; Maldonato, N.M. Epistemology of olfaction: Emotion, cognition, and decision making. In Proceedings of the 9th IEEE International Conference on Cognitive Infocommunications (CogInfoCom), Budapest, Hungary, 22–24 August 2018; pp. 267–270.
43. Bochicchio, V.; Maldonato, N.M.; Vitelli, R.; Scandurra, C. "Emotional nose": The hedonic character of olfaction and its epistemological and clinical implications. In Proceedings of the 10th IEEE International Conference on Cognitive Infocommunications (CogInfoCom), Naples, Italy, 23–25 October 2019; pp. 143–146.
44. Jokić-Begić, N.; Zigić, L.; Nakić Radoš, S. Anxiety and anxiety sensitivity as predictors of fear of childbirth: Different patterns for nulliparous and parous women. *J. Psychosom. Obstet. Gynaecol.* **2014**, *35*, 22–28. [CrossRef]
45. Alehagen, S.; Wijma, K.; Wijma, B. Fear during labor. *Acta Obstet. Gynecol. Scand.* **2001**, *80*, 315–320. [CrossRef]
46. Rouhe, H.; Salmela-Aro, K.; Halmesmäki, E.; Saisto, T. Fear of childbirth according to parity, gestational age, and obstetric history. *BJOG* **2009**, *116*, 67–73. [CrossRef] [PubMed]
47. Toohill, J.; Creedy, D.K.; Gamble, J.; Fenwick, J. A cross-sectional study to determine utility of childbirth fear screening in maternity practice—An Australian perspective. *Women Birth* **2015**, *28*, 310–316. [CrossRef]
48. Di Vito, M.; Cacaci, M.; Martini, C.; Barbanti, L.; Mondello, F.; Sanguinetti, M.; Mattarelli, P.; Bugli, F. Is aromatherapy effective in obstetrics? A systematic review and meta-analysis. *Phytother. Res.* **2021**, *35*, 2477–2486. [CrossRef]
49. Scandurra, C.; Zapparella, R.; Policastro, M.; Continisio, G.I.; Ammendola, A.; Bochicchio, V.; Maldonato, N.M.; Locci, M. Obstetric violence in a group of Italian women: Socio-demographic predictors and effects on mental health. *Cult. Health Sex.* **2021**; Advance Online Publication. [CrossRef]

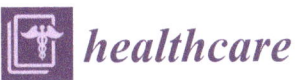

Article

Effect of Acupuncture on Movement Function in Patients with Parkinson's Disease: Network Meta-Analysis of Randomized Controlled Trials

Miri Kwon [1], Moon Joo Cheong [2], Jungtae Leem [3,*] and Tae-hun Kim [1,4,*]

[1] Department of Clinical Korean Medicine, College of Korean Medicine, Graduate School, Kyung Hee University, Seoul 02447, Korea; dove58@naver.com
[2] Rare Diseases Integrative Treatment Research Institute, Wonkwang University, Jangheung Integrative Medical Hospital, Iksan 59338, Korea; sasayayoou@naver.com
[3] Research Center of Traditional Korean Medicine, Wonkwang University, Iksan 54538, Korea
[4] Korean Medicine Clinical Trial Center, Korean Medicine Hospital, Kyung Hee University Medical Center, Seoul 02447, Korea
* Correspondence: julcho@naver.com (J.L.); taehunkim@khu.ac.kr (T.-h.K.); Tel.: +82-063-850-5114 (J.L.); +82-02-958-9194 (T.-h.K.)

Abstract: We aimed to compare the effectiveness of some different acupuncture modalities on motor function using the unified Parkinson disease rating scale (UPDRS)-III scores of idiopathic Parkinson's disease (PD) via pairwise and network meta-analyses (NMA) of randomized controlled trials (RCTs). The Cochrane risk of bias assessment tool was used to assess the methodological quality of the included RCTs. A frequentist approach-based random effect model NMA was performed. Seventeen RCTs with 1071 participants were included. The five following modalities were identified: combination of conventional medication (levodopa) with (1) electroacupuncture (ELEC), (2) manual acupuncture (MANU), (3) bee venom acupuncture (BEEV), (4) sham acupuncture (SHAM), and (5) conventional medication alone (CONV). In NMA on UPDRS-III, BEEV was the best modality compared to CONV (mean difference [MD] −7.37, 95% confidence interval [−11.97, −2.77]). The comparative ranking assessed through NMA was suggested to be BEEV, MANU, ELEC, SHAM, and CONV. Regarding daily activity assessment (UPDRS-II), the magnitude of effectiveness was in the order of BEEV, ELEC, MANU, SHAM, and CONV. Combination treatment with BEEV (MANU or ELEC) and CONV can be recommended to improve motor function in PD patients. Due to the limited number of included RCTs, further NMA with more rigorous RCTs are warranted.

Keywords: network meta-analysis; meta-analysis; Parkinson's disease; motor symptom; systematic review; acupuncture

Citation: Kwon, M.; Cheong, M.J.; Leem, J.; Kim, T.-h. Effect of Acupuncture on Movement Function in Patients with Parkinson's Disease: Network Meta-Analysis of Randomized Controlled Trials. Healthcare 2021, 9, 1502. https://doi.org/10.3390/healthcare9111502

Academic Editors: Manoj Sharma and Kavita Batra

Received: 7 October 2021
Accepted: 2 November 2021
Published: 5 November 2021

Publisher's Note: MDPI stays neutral with regard to jurisdictional claims in published maps and institutional affiliations.

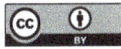

Copyright: © 2021 by the authors. Licensee MDPI, Basel, Switzerland. This article is an open access article distributed under the terms and conditions of the Creative Commons Attribution (CC BY) license (https://creativecommons.org/licenses/by/4.0/).

1. Introduction

Parkinson's disease (PD) is a degenerative neurological disorder associated with dopaminergic cell loss in the substantia nigra and other brain structures characterized by several movement symptoms, such as tremor, rigidity, tremor at rest, and postural instability [1]. PD is the second most common neurodegenerative disorder after Alzheimer's dementia. The prevalence of PD is increasing faster than in other neurological diseases [1,2]. The prevalence increases with age, and in most cases, the cause is unknown [3,4]. Approximately 6.1 million people worldwide were diagnosed with PD in 2016, which is more than double that of 1990 [5]. The movement symptoms of PD are managed using a combination of conventional medications, such as levodopa, carbidopa, dopamine agonists, and monoamine oxidase B inhibitors [5]. On the other hand, if levodopa is administered for a long period, treatment may not be continued due to side effects, such as the on-off phenomenon [6]. Levodopa-induced dyskinesia also impairs the quality of life of patients with PD, making effective treatment difficult [7]. In a previous study, more than 40% of patients with PD experienced wear-off and levodopa-induced dyskinesia, which lowered drug adherence [8]. If conventional drugs are ineffective, several surgical strategies, such as deep brain stimulation (DBS) or radiofrequency ablation, could be considered [9]. However, there are a number of complications associated with a surgical approach, and patient expectations after surgery are sometimes not fulfilled [10]. In addition, as the disease progresses, the burden on caregivers increases because of frequent nursing home visits, longer hospital stays, and higher rates of emergency room visitation [11]. Therefore, in addition to conventional management, alternative therapeutic options are needed to manage various symptoms considering the characteristics of PD, which has a long disease duration.

Recently, various complementary and integrative medicine (CIM) therapies, such as acupuncture, herbal medicine, qi-gong, massage, yoga, meditation, and music therapy, have been widely utilized in clinical practice for PD symptom management [12]. Acupuncture is one of the most commonly used CIM interventions for the management of patients with PD [13]. In previous studies, acupuncture improved motor symptoms, non-motor symptoms, quality of life, and disease progression, and decreased the adverse events and dosage of anti-parkinsonian medication [13]. Several clinical studies and systematic reviews have shown the effects of various types of acupuncture treatment combined with conventional medication on motor symptom improvement using the unified PD rating scale (UPDRS) [14–17].

However, it is unknown which type of acupuncture treatment is the preferred option because the acupuncture treatment applied in each study is different. Most clinical research and systematic reviews have compared two interventions at a time. Multiple intervention comparison research designs are not common. However, in clinical practice, physicians are curious about which treatment is more effective among the various widely used treatments. However, in terms of time and cost, it is difficult to conduct direct comparative (head-to-head) studies on various acupuncture treatments, and the need to compare multiple interventions at a time is increasing. Nowadays, a novel methodology named 'network meta-analysis (NMA)' is used to simultaneously estimate the relative effect of various interventions [18,19]. NMA results help stakeholders to make decisions by providing a combined quantitative effect size acquired from direct and indirect comparisons of different interventions [20].

This study aimed to compare the effect on movement symptom improvement in patients with PD about several acupuncture types combined with conventional medication (CM), such as manual acupuncture (MA), electroacupuncture (EA), and bee venom acupuncture (BVA), compared with placebo acupuncture or conventional medication only. We adopted conventional systematic review, pairwise meta-analysis (PMA), and NMA methodology to compare the effect size of various acupuncture types to help with decision making regarding the management of patients with PD.

2. Materials and Methods

We followed the preferred reporting items for systematic reviews and meta-analyses for network meta-analysis checklist (PRISMA-NMA) [21]. This review protocol was registered with the Open Science Framework on 7 August 2021 (https://osf.io/q8n7z/).

2.1. Search Strategy

Eligible studies were systematically searched from their inception to June 2021 using Medline (via PubMed), Cochrane Library, Embase (via Elsevier), China National Knowledge Infrastructure, Korea Citation Index (KCI), NDSL, Research Information Sharing Service, and Oriental Medicine Advanced Searching Integrated System. A mixture of free words and medical subject headings were used for PD and acupuncture. There were no language restrictions. The search strategy in Medline (via PubMed) is as follows:
#1 parkinson disease [Mesh] OR parkinson disease OR Idiopathic Parkinson's Disease OR Lewy Body Parkinson's Disease OR Parkinson's Disease, Idiopathic OR Parkinson's Disease, Lewy Body OR Parkinson Disease, Idiopathic OR Parkinson's Disease OR Idio-

pathic Parkinson Disease OR Lewy Body Parkinson Disease OR Primary Parkinsonism OR Parkinsonism, Primary OR Paralysis Agitans.

#2 acupuncture [Mesh] OR Acupuncture OR Pharmacopuncture OR Acupuncture Treatment OR Acupuncture Treatments OR Treatment, Acupuncture OR Therapy, Acupuncture OR Pharmacoacupuncture Treatment OR Treatment, Pharmacoacupuncture OR Pharmacoacupuncture Therapy OR Therapy, Pharmacoacupuncture OR Acupotomy OR Acupotomies OR Electroacupuncture OR Bee Venoms OR Venoms, Bee OR Bee Venom OR Venom, Bee OR Apis Venoms OR Venoms, Apis OR Apitoxin OR Honeybee Venoms OR Venoms, Honeybee OR Honeybee Venom OR Venom, Honeybee OR Fire needle therapy OR Fire acupuncture.

#3 #1 AND #2: A detailed explanation of the search terms used in each database is provided in Supplementary Materials Digital Content 1.

2.2. Eligible Criteria

2.2.1. Type of Studies

Only randomized controlled clinical trials (RCTs) were included. We did not include cluster randomized clinical trials. Other study designs, such as animal studies, uncontrolled tests, or case reports, were excluded. Multi-armed trials ($\geq$ three arms) were included if they did not violate the eligibility criteria.

2.2.2. Type of Participants

Patients diagnosed with idiopathic PD were included without limitation of age, sex, race, severity, or duration of disease. Patients other than those with idiopathic PD, such as Parkinson's syndrome, were excluded.

2.2.3. Type of Intervention Used in the Experimental and Control Groups

The experimental group intervention consisted of different types of acupuncture treatment combined with CM. In the control group, we selected L-dopa, which has been an effective gold standard dopamine-based medication for movement symptom management for approximately 60 years, as an essential medication for the control group (CM) [22,23]. Studies were included if the combination of L-dopa and other drugs was equally applied to the acupuncture and control groups. However, studies in which treatment medication therapy was performed only with other drugs without L-dopa were excluded. Acupuncture treatments included electroacupuncture (EA), MA, or BVA. We excluded combined acupuncture treatments, such as EA + BVA or MA + BVA, to evaluate the therapeutic effect of each acupuncture intervention type. The intervention in the control group was defined as CM therapy alone or CM + sham acupuncture treatment. We did not restrict the duration, dosage, or frequency of treatment.

2.2.4. Type of Outcome Measure

The primary outcome of our study was the motor function of patients with PD evaluated using the UPDRS-III scale [24]. The secondary outcomes were daily life activity scores using the UPDRS-II [24]. The Movement Disorder Society UPDRS (MDS-UPDRS) was excluded because it is different from UPDRS [25]. The timing of the outcome assessment was selected immediately after the end of the acupuncture treatment session. Data acquired during the follow-up assessment were not considered.

2.3. Study Selection and Data Extraction

Two reviewers (M.K. and J.L.) independently conducted the study selection and data extraction.

Disagreement between the two researchers was resolved by discussion with a third independent reviewer (M.J.). Duplicate publications, patients diagnosed with Parkinsonism syndrome, and cases in combination with other treatments were excluded. A standardized data collection form developed during the pilot process using Excel was utilized during the data extraction process. The extracted items were as follows: sample size and the number of dropouts, first author, year of publication, location, age, sex, disease severity, disease duration, treatment intervention, control group intervention, treatment period, and outcome variables. We contacted the corresponding author to acquire sufficient data if there was insufficient information in the published article via e-mail. EndNote X9 (EndNote version X9, Thomson Reuters, CA, USA) was used for article selection and management.

2.4. Risk of Bias Assessment

Two independent researchers (J.L., M.K.) used the Cochrane risk of bias assessment tool to evaluate the quality of the research methods of the included studies [26]. Random sequence generation; allocation concealment; blinding of participants, personnel, and outcome assessors; incomplete outcome data; selective outcome reporting; and other sources of bias were graded as low, unclear, and high. Disagreement between the two researchers was resolved by discussion with a third independent reviewer (M.J.). Review Manager (RevMan) version 5.4 software was used to illustrate the risk of bias.

2.5. PMA

In the PMA, we conducted a conventional direct comparison of the two study arms. Data synthesis was performed using the Review Manager (RevMan) ([Computer program]. Version 5.4, The Cochrane Collaboration, 2020). The random effect model was adopted because it was judged that there was heterogeneity due to differences in the study design, such as baseline characteristics, number of interventions, and methods among the included studies. The mean difference (MD) for the continuous variables and 95% confidence interval (CI) were used to assess the effect size of the intervention on UPDRS-III and II. Heterogeneity was determined by both the chi-square ($\chi 2$) test and Higgins' I^2 statistic. The heterogeneity interpretation based on the I^2 statistic is considered not to be important (0 to 40%), moderate heterogeneity (30% to 60%), substantial heterogeneity (50% to 90%), and considerable heterogeneity (75% to 100%) [27]. A *p*-value of ≤ 0.1 was considered to indicate significant heterogeneity [28].

2.6. NMA

2.6.1. Assumptions of the NMA

The frequentist model was utilized for the NMA, combining direct and indirect evidence using R version 4.1.0 (A language and environment for statistical computing. R Foundation for Statistical Computing, Vienna, Austria)) using the Netmeta package [29]. There are several assumptions for NMA, such as connectivity, homogeneity, transitivity, and consistency [30]. Connectivity was visually verified by connecting each network node with a line using a network plot. Homogeneity was assessed using the Cochrane Q statistic or the I^2 score. In our study, a random effect model was applied, as it was judged that there was heterogeneity between studies due to differences in study design or interventions [30,31]. When evaluating transitivity, it is necessary to explore the distribution of effect modifiers and determine their effects on the effect size. In our study, we qualitatively compared the sample size, age, sex, disease duration, severity, treatment dosage, and period for transitivity assessment [30]. Consistency is a quantitative statistical evaluation of transitivity. Consistency was statistically evaluated using the net-splitting method [32].

2.6.2. Statistical Assessment

The network forest plot presented with MD and 95% CI of each intervention was used to rank each treatment strategy for visual and statistical verification. The P-score was also used to rank treatment, which assesses certainty that a specific intervention is better than competing inventions. The P-score is nearly identical to the numerical values of SUCRA in the Bayesian model NMA [33]. For the consistency assumption, we checked both global (network level) and local approaches (particular contrast of intervention level) [21]. In the global approach, we used the 'decomp.design' function of R software to assess consistency under the assumption of a full design-by-treatment interaction random effect model [34]. Q statistics were used to assess inconsistency in the global approach. If the *p*-value for the Q statistics was below 0.05, it was assumed that significant inconsistency (disagreement) existed in the global network. In the local approach, we adopted the net-splitting method to split the network estimation of the effect size on each intervention into direct and indirect evidence using the Facenetsplit function of R software. It calculates the difference between direct and indirect estimates and assesses whether the difference is statistically significant [34]. Net-split plots were also provided for visual inspection of inconsistencies between direct and indirect comparisons. If the *p*-value for the net-split analysis was below 0.05, it was assumed that significant inconsistency (disagreement) existed in a specific local loop, which indicates a considerable difference between indirect and direct effect size estimation. If there were significant disagreements in the local or global approach, we conducted a sensitivity analysis by sequentially excluding studies one by one. If we identified which studies were inconsistent, we excluded studies from the NMA. A net league table is also presented. The upper right triangle presents the effect size estimated by only direct comparison, which is similar to the pairwise comparison. As direct comparison does not exist in all treatment comparisons, there are several blanks in the upper triangle. The lower left triangle provides a pooled estimation of the direct and indirect comparisons of the effect size.

2.6.3. Sensitivity Analysis

NMA was performed by sequentially removing each study one by one to confirm whether a specific study excessively affected the overall result. The results were visually and statistically checked to determine whether the results were consistent with the overall trend.

2.7. Publication Bias

We used a conventional funnel plot for visual inspection of the publication bias. We also used Egger's test to statistically assess publication bias [35]. If the *p*-value for Egger's test was greater than 0.05, it indicated no evidence of publication bias.

3. Results

3.1. Characteristics of the Included Studies and Network Geometry

A total of 2505 articles were screened from eight databases. After careful review of the title and abstract, 17 articles were finally included (Figure 1). In 17 RCTs, 1071 participants were included. A list of the 28 studies excluded after reviewing the full text is provided in Supplementary Materials Digital Content 2. Eight articles were written in English [36–43], one article was written in Japanese [44], two in Korean [15,45], and six articles were written in Chinese [14,46–50]. Detailed characteristics of the included studies including publication year, first author, country, sample size (initial and final), age, sex, disease severity, disease duration, CM dosage (mg/day), treatment and control group intervention, and treatment period are described in Table 1.

Five types of arms were identified: (1) manual acupuncture + conventional drug (MANU), (2) electroacupuncture + conventional drug (ELEC), (3) BVA + conventional drug (BEEV), (4) sham acupuncture + conventional drug (SHAM), and (5) conventional drug alone (CONV). Fifteen RCTs had two armed designs, and only two RCTs had three armed designs (one RCT included MANU vs. SHAM vs. CONV [38], and one RCT included BEEV vs. MANU vs. CONV [41]). Seven trials included the ELEC arm, nine trials included the MANU arm, and two included the BEEV arm. Therefore, a total of 18 comparisons (36 treatment arms) were included in the 17 RCTs. Six RCTs compared ELEC vs. CONV [14,40,42,46,48,49]; five RCTs compared MANU vs. CONV [38,41,44,47,50]; one RCT compared ELEV vs. SHAM [36]; five RCTs compared MANU vs. SHAM [15,37,38,43,45]; and one RCT compared BEEV vs.

SHAM [39]. Detailed descriptions of each intervention, including the acupuncture point, needle stimulation, retention time, treatment duration, and frequency, are described in Table 2.

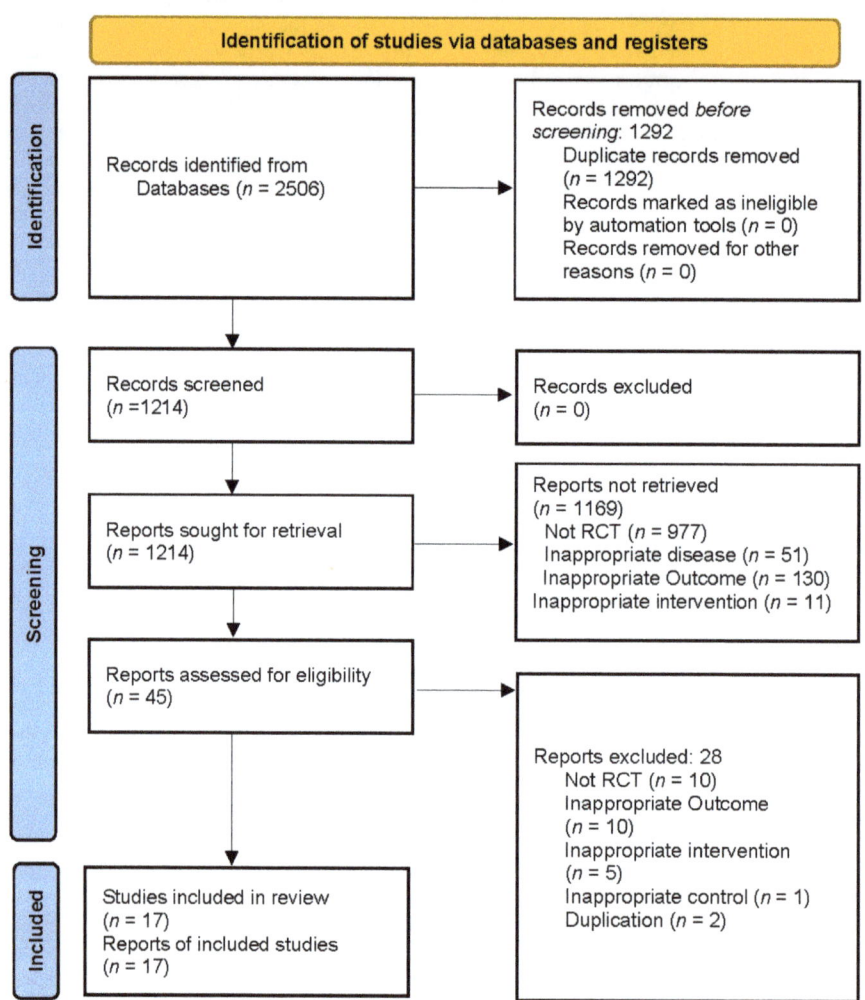

Figure 1. PRISMA flow diagram.

3.2. Risk of Bias of the Included Studies

In random sequence generation, five studies were graded as unclear [36,40,46,48,49]. In allocation concealment, 10 studies were graded as unclear [14,15,36,40,44–46,48–50]. Nine studies were graded as high in blinding of participants because several articles were add-on study designs that cannot blind participants [14,38,41–43,46,48–50]. Furthermore, four studies were graded as unclear. In the blinding of outcome assessment, 11 studies were graded as unclear [14,15,39,43–50]. In incomplete outcome data, two studies were graded as unclear [15,44]. Six studies were graded as high as the DR was more than 10% [36–39,41,45]. One study was graded as high in selective reporting because it did not report the outcome variables previously described in the protocol [36]. Detailed visualization of each study with the risk of bias graph is presented in Supplementary Materials Digital Content 3.

Table 1. Characteristics of the included studies.

First Author, Year (Location)	Sample Size (A:B) (Initial →Final)	Age (Year), Mean ± SD	Sex (M:F)	Disease Severity: H-Y Stage	Disease Duration (Year)	(A) Treatment Intervention (Conventional Drug Therapy Dosage, mg/d)	(B) Control Intervention (Conventional Drug Therapy Dosage, mg/day)	Treatment/Follow-Up Period (Week)
Electroacupuncture + Conventional drug therapy								
Chen 2012 [14] (China)	30:30 →30:30	(A) 65.60 ± 3.79 (B) 61.93 ± 3.67	(A) 19:11 (B) 17:13	(A) 2.18 ± 0.26 (B) 2.04 ± 0.30	(A) 5.40 ± 1.75 (B) 6.40 ± 2.15	ELEC (432 ± 139)	CONV (435 ± 154)	6/None
Gu 2013 [48] (China)	23:25 →23:25	(A) 66 ± 8 (B) 70 ± 8	(A) 10:13 (B) 15:10	NR	(A) 4.44 ± 3.32 (B) 4.56 ± 3.11	ELEC (250)	CONV (250)	12/None
Huang 2009 [46] (China)	15:15 →15:15	(A) 65.60 ± 3.78 (B) 60.80 ± 3.63	(A) 8:7 (B) 6:9	(A) 2.18 ± 0.26 (B) 2.04 ± 0.30	(A) 5.40 ± 1.75 (B) 6.4 ± 2.14	ELEC (375–750)	CONV (375–750)	5/None
Lei 2016 [36] (USA)	10:5 →10:5	(A) 69.8 ± 4.5 (B) 71.0 ± 11.7	(A) 6:4 (B) 2:3	(A) 3.0 ± 1.0 (B) 2.9 ± 0.7	(A) 6.2 ± 5.9 (B) 5.2 ± 4.7	ELEC (614 ± 381)	SHAM (324 ± 295)	3/None
Liu 2016 [49] (China)	39:35 →39:35	(A) 65.65 ± 4.15 (B) 65.59 ± 4.18	(A) 21:18 (B) 19:16	NR	(A) 4.41 ± 2.01 (B) 4.33 ± 2.04	ELEC (NR)	CONV (NR)	12/None
Wang 2015 [40] (China)	30:20 →28:20	(A) 62.1 ± 8.7 (B) 59.1 ± 12.4	(A) 13:15 (B) 9:11	(A) 2.0 ± 0.7 (B) 2.0 ± 0.8	(A) 2.9 ± 2.9 (B) 2.7 ± 2.3	ELEC (104.1 ± 253.2)	CONV (160.6 ± 260.0)	Two months/None
Xu 2020 [42] (China)	38:38 →33:37	(A) 61.73 ± 10.28 (B) 61.95 ± 9.77	(A) 15:18 (B) 21:16	Stage 1 (A) 9 (B) 8 Stage 1.5 (A) 4 (B) 12 Stage 2 (A) 5 (B) 6 Stage 2.5 (A) 9 (B) 5 Stage 3 (A) 4 (B) 4 Stage 4 (A) 2 (B) 2	(A) 3.52 ± 2.78 (B) 3.26 ± 2.32	ELEC (187.5–375)	CONV (187.5–375)	8/4
MA + Conventional drug therapy								
Jung 2006 [15] (Korea)	NR →16:21	(A) 59.69 ± 9.6 (B) 61.00 ± 9.7	(A) 11:5 (B) 10:11	NR	(A) 5.66 ± 4.23 (B) 6.07 ± 4.82	MANU (NR)	SHAM (NR)	4/None
Kluger 2016 [43] (USA)	47:47 →47:47	(A) 64.4 ± 10.3 (B) 63.0 ± 13.0	(A) 30:17 (B) 29:18	Stage 1 (A) 4 (B) 2 Stage 1.5 (A) 6 (B) 3 Stage 2 (A) 11 (B) 17 Stage 2.5 (A) 18 (B) 12 Stage 3 (A) 6 (B) 10 Stage 4 (A) 0 (B) 4	NR	MANU (558.9 ± 379.3)	SHAM (628.6 ± 482.9)	6/None

Table 1. Cont.

First Author, Year (Location)	Sample Size (A:B) (Initial →Final)	Age (Year), Mean ± SD	Sex (M:F)	Disease Severity: H-Y Stage	Disease Duration (Year)	(A) Treatment Intervention (Conventional Drug Therapy Dosage, mg/d)	(B) Control Intervention (Conventional Drug Therapy Dosage, mg/day)	Treatment/Follow-Up Period (Week)
Kong 2017 [37] (Singapore)	20:20 →19:17	(A) 66.4 ± 6.5 (B) 62.9 ± 9.7	(A) 6:14 (B) 7:13	NR	(A) 87.2 ± 53.2 (B) 50.1 ± 26.4	MANU (637.8 ± 394.3)	SHAM (592.6 ± 303.1)	5/4
Li 2018 [38] (China)	14:13:14 →14:12:11	(A) 62.17 ± 7.66 (B) 65.79 ± 6.07 (C) 62.85 ± 5.00	(A) 9:3 (B) 8:6 (C) 7:6	NR	NR	(A) MANU (367.86 ± 146.24)	(B) SHAM (338.46 ± 112.09) (C) CONV (345.83 ± 173.81)	12/None
Lu 2020 [50] (China)	20:20 →20:20	(A) 66.50 ± 8.81 (B) 65.90 ± 8.92	(A) 10:10 (B) 12:8	NR	(A) 15.10 ± 1.72 (B) 15.25 ± 2.04	MANU (250)	CONV (250)	4/None
Mizushima 2011 [44] (Japan)	NR →103:95	(A) 63.9 ± 8.2 (B) 64.7 ± 9.8	(A) 45:58 (B) 50:45	NR	(A) 1.6 ± 0.6 (B) 1.8 ± 1.2	MANU (186.0 ± 134.0)	CONV (251.0 ± 172.8)	Five years/5 years
Park 2007 [45] (Korea)	NR →21:13	(A) 60.00 ± 9.0 (B) 61.26 ± 9.81	(A) 12:9 (B) 2:11	(A) 1.7619 ± 0.95 (B) 1.8846 ± 0.68	(A) 5.63 ± 5.29 (B) 5.84 ± 3.3	MANU (NR)	SHAM (NR)	4/None
Ren 2011 [47] (China)	90:90 →90:90	(A) 59.1 ± 12.1 (B) 58.2 ± 11.9	(A) 52:38 (B) 49:41	NR	(A) 1.8 ± 0.3 (B) 1.9 ± 0.4	MANU (750)	CONV (750)	30 days/None
BVA + Conventional drug therapy								
Cho 2012 [41] (Korea)	18:17:14 →13:13:9	(A) 57.0 (B) 55.0 (C) 57.0	(A) 5:8 (B) 5:8 (C) 3:6	NR	(A) 5.0 (B) 6.0 (C) 5.0	(A) BEEV (NR) (B) MANU (NR)	(C) CONV (NR)	8/None
Hartmann 2016 [39] (France)	20:20 →15:20	(A) 60.3 ± 15 (B) 63.3 ± 8	(A) 8:12 (B) 12:8	Stage 2 (A) 6 (B) 7 Stage 2.5(A) 14 (B) 11 Stage 3 (A) 0 (B) 2	(A) 6.2 ± 5 (B) 6.3 ± 5.1	BEEV (391→64 ± 127 Baseline median→Result mean, SD	SHAM (512→98 ± 156 Baseline median→Result mean, SD	11 months

(A) Treatment intervention; (B) Control intervention (in 2 arm design); (C) Control intervention in 3 arm design; SD, standard deviation; H-Y stage, Hoehn and Yahr stage; NR, not reported. Intervention: ELEC, electroacupuncture + conventional drug therapy; SHAM, sham acupuncture + conventional drug therapy; MANU, manual acupuncture + conventional drug therapy; CONV, single conventional drug therapy; BEEV, bee-venom acupuncture + conventional drug therapy. Outcomes) UPDRS: Unified PD rating scale; AE: Rate of the number of participants with adverse events between groups; DR, dropout rate. Li 2018: MANU vs. SHAM vs. CONV; Cho 2012: BEEV vs. MANU vs. CONV.

Table 2. Detailed description of the acupuncture treatment.

First Author, Year (Location)	Acupuncture Point	Depth of Insertion	Needle Stimulation, Electrical Stimulation	Needle Retention Time	Treatment Frequency, Total Number of Treatment Session	Duration of Treatment Sessions
Electroacupuncture + Conventional drug therapy						
Chen 2012 [14] (China)	GV20, EX-HN1, EX-HN3	NR	2 Hz frequency	1 h	3 times a week, 18 total sessions	6 weeks
Gu 2013 [48] (China)	Bilateral anterior parietal-temporal oblique lines (motor areas) GB20, LI11, LI4, LR3, KI3, GB34	NR	2 Hz frequency, The strength the patient can tolerate	20 min	3 times a week, 36 total sessions	12 weeks
Huang 2009 [46] (China)	MS6, MS4, MS8, MS9, MS14	NR	Continuous waves, 100 Hz frequency, 2–4 mA	30 min	6 times a week, 30 total sessions	5 weeks
Lei 2016 [36] (USA)	Foot motor sensory area, balance area, GV20, GV14, LI4, ST36, GB34, BL40, SP6, KI3, LR3	NR	Amplitude (intensity) 3.5 and 4.5, Frequency 100 Hz or 4 Hz	30 min	Once a week, 3 total sessions	3 weeks
Liu 2016 [49] (China)	Anterior parietal and temporal oblique lines (motor areas) on both sides, LR3, KI3, LI11, GB20, GB34, LI4	NR	2 Hz frequency, The strength the patient can tolerate	20 min	Three times a week, 36 total sessions	12 weeks
Wang 2015 [40] (China)	Bilateral GB20, LI4, Central Du14, Du16	2–2.5 cm	Pulses of 9 V, 1 A, 9 W, 100 Hz	30 min	Once every three days, 20 total sessions	2 months
Xu 2020 [42] (China)	GV17, GB19, Sishenzhen, and temporal three-needle	0.8–1.5 cm	Twisting, lifting and thrusting, continuous waves at alternating low 100 Hz frequency	30 min	Four days per week, 32 total sessions	8 weeks
MA + Conventional drug therapy						
Cho 2012 [41] (Korea)	Bilateral GB20, LI11, GB34, ST36, LR3	1.0–1.5 cm	Twisting at 2 Hz for 10 s	20 min	Twice a week, 16 total sessions	8 weeks
Jung 2006 [15] (Korea)	Bilateral LR3, GB34	NR	None	15 min	Twice a week, 8 total sessions	4 weeks
Kluger 2016 [43] (USA)	GV20, GV24, CV6, Bilateral LI10, HT7, ST36, SP6	0.5–1 cm	Twisting three times in a clockwise direction	30 min	Twice a week (at least one day apart), 12 total sessions	6 weeks
Kong 2017 [37] (Singapore)	Bilateral PC6, LI4, ST36, SP6, KI3, CV6	0.5–1 inch	None	20 min	Twice a week (at least three days apart), 10 total sessions	5 weeks

Table 2. Cont.

First Author, Year (Location)	Acupuncture Point	Depth of Insertion	Needle Stimulation, Electrical Stimulation	Needle Retention Time	Treatment Frequency, Total Number of Treatment Session	Duration of Treatment Sessions
Li 2018 [38] (China)	DU20, Bilateral GB20, Chorea-Tremor Controlled Zone	2–3 cm	Twist every 10 min	30 min	Twice a week, 24 total sessions	12 weeks
Lu 2020 [50] (China)	LR3, LR2, LR8, KI3, KI7, KI10, SP6, ST36, LI11, PC6, LI4	20–30 mm	After 15 min, the needle is lifted, inserted, and twisted once	30 min	Once a day, 28 total sessions	28 days
Mizushima 2011 [44] (Japan)	Individualized point according to meridian diagnosis	Individualized depth	Individualized way according to diagnosis	NR	Two to four times a month, NR	5 years
Park 2007 [45] (Korea)	One side LR3, GB34, ST36	NR	None	15 min	Twice a week, 8 total sessions	4 weeks
Ren 2011 [47] (China)	Bilateral BL18, BL23, GB20, LI11, LI4, GB34, KI3, LR3	NR	Flattening and relieving	30 min	Once a day, 30 total sessions	30 days
BVA + Conventional drug therapy						
Cho 2012 [41] (Korea)	Bilateral GB20, LI11, GB34, ST36, LR3	NR	0.1 mL BEEV diluted to 0.005% in distilled water	-	Twice a week, 16 total sessions	8 weeks
Hartmann 2016 [39] (France)	NR	s.C	BEEV (Alyostal®100 μg in 1 mL of NaCl 0.9%)	-	Once a month, 11 total sessions	11 months

NR, Not reported; SC, subcutaneous; The control group, including the placebo acupuncture group, received the same frequency and total number of acupuncture treatments as the treatment group.

3.3. Primary Outcome (Movement Function, UPDRS-III): PMA

In PMA of movement function evaluated by UPDRS-III, statistical significance was shown between the following comparisons presented with MD and 95% CI **(in favor of bold marks)**: (1) **electroacupuncture + CM (ELEC)** vs. CM (CONV) (MD −3.63, 95% CI −6.05 to −1.21); (2) **manual acupuncture + CM (MANU)** vs. CONV (MD −3.90, 95% CI −6.24 to −1.57); (3) **electroacupuncture + CM (ELEC)** vs. sham acupuncture + CM (SHAM) (MD −18.10, 95% CI −30.31 to −5.89). In other comparisons, such as BVA + CM (BEEV) vs. CONV, MANU vs. SHAM, and BEEV vs. SHAM, the acupuncture modality tended to be more effective than the control group, but the difference was not statistically significant. Detailed descriptions of the effect size and each trial-based forest plot are provided in Supplementary Materials Digital Content 4.

3.4. Secondary Outcome (Daily Life Activity, UPDRS-II): PMA

In PMA of daily life activity evaluated by UPDRS-II, statistical significance was shown between the following comparisons presented with MD and 95% CI **(in favor of bold marks)**: (1) **ELEC** vs. CONV (MD −4.50, 95% CI −6.19 to −2.80); (2) **MANU** vs. CONV (MD −4.07, 95% CI −4.87 to −3.27). In other comparisons, such as BEEV vs. CONV, ELEC vs. SHAM, and MANU vs. SHAM, the acupuncture modality showed a tendency to be more effective than the control group, but this was not statistically significant. Detailed descriptions of the effect size and each trial-based forest plot are provided in Supplementary Materials Digital Content 4.

3.5. Primary Outcome (Movement Function, UPDRS-III): NMA

3.5.1. Assumption of NMA and Network Geometry

As explained in the Methods section, we decided to adopt a random effect model in the homogeneity assumption. In the transitivity assumption, the research team agreed on the transitivity of the included studies using Tables 1 and 2. We assessed the consistency assumption using a global and local approach. In the global approach, we found significant inconsistencies ($p < 0.05$). In the local approach, we found inconsistency due to a study that compared ELEC and CONV (Lei 2016 [36]). After we excluded the study (Lei 2016 [36]) according to the study protocol, the consistency assumption was satisfied at the local and global levels. Net-split graphs that include direct estimates, indirect estimates, and network estimates for consistency assessment are provided in Supplementary Materials Digital Content 5. The connectivity assumption was confirmed through network geometry (net graph), which is a visual presentation of the links in the included studies (Figure 2). After excluding the study (Lei 2016 [36]), in the network analysis of the primary outcome, there were five nodes (ELEC, BEEV, MANU, CONV, SHMA) from 16 studies and 20 pairwise comparisons from seven types of comparison pairs (edges). The number of included comparisons in each edge is shown in Figure 2.

3.5.2. Comparative Effectiveness of the Acupuncture Modality in UPDRS-III

The probabilities of treatment ranking (P-score) among the included interventions were as follows: BEEV (0.9509), MANU (0.6325), ELEC (0.5349), SHAM (0.3685), and CONV (0.0132). According to the P-score, BEEV is most likely the best acupuncture modality for movement function assessed by the UPDRS-III (Figure 3 and Table 3). Mixed effect estimates (combining direct and indirect estimates) for each intervention compared with CONV were as follows **(in favor of bold marks)**: **BEEV** (MD −7.37, 95% CI −11.97 to −2.77); **MANU** (MD −4.13, 95% CI −5.78 to −2.47); **ELEC** (MD −3.66, 95% CI −6.29 to −1.03); SHAM (MD −2.71, 95% CI −5.92 to 0.50). BEEV, MANU, and ELEC were superior to CONV in UPDRS-III. However, SHAM was not statistically significant. No difference was observed in the comparison between the different acupuncture modalities (Table 3).

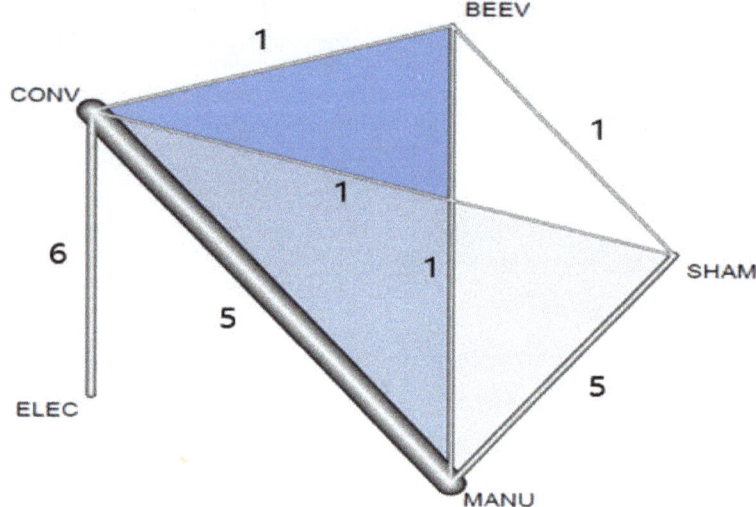

Figure 2. Network geometry of the included studies on UPDRS-III (Net graph). BEEV, bee venom acupuncture + conventional drug therapy; CONV, single conventional drug therapy; ELEC, electroacupuncture + conventional drug therapy; MANU, manual acupuncture + conventional drug therapy; SHAM, sham acupuncture + conventional drug therapy; UPDRS, Unified PD rating scale.

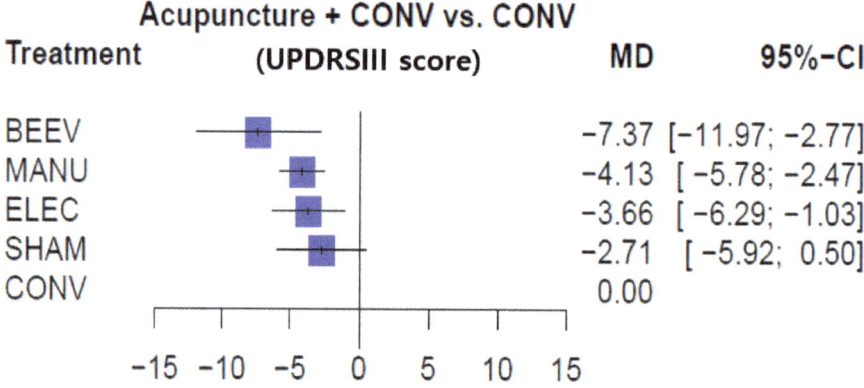

Figure 3. Treatment level network meta-analysis forest plot (UPDRS-III). BEEV, bee venom acupuncture + conventional drug therapy; CONV, single conventional drug therapy; ELEC, electroacupuncture + conventional drug therapy; MANU, manual acupuncture + conventional drug therapy; SHAM, sham acupuncture + conventional drug therapy; UPDRS, Unified PD rating scale.

Table 3. League table on UPDRS-III.

BEEV	−3.31(−8.91;2.29)			−7.13(−16.98;2.72)	−5.44(−12.53;1.65)
−3.24(−7.72;1.23)	MANU			−1.41(−4.38;1.57)	−4.07(−5.72;−2.41;)
−3.71(−9.01;1.59)	−0.47(−3.57;2.64)	ELEC		-	−3.66(−6.29;−1.03)
−4.66(−9.63;0.31)	−1.42(−4.24;1.41)	−0.95(−5.10;3.20)	SHAM		−7.48(−17.54;2.58)
−7.37(−11.97;−2.77)	−4.13(−5.78;−2.47)	−3.66(−6.29;−1.03)	−2.71(−5.92;0.50)	CONV	

BEEV, bee venom acupuncture + conventional drug therapy; CONV, single conventional drug therapy; ELEC, electroacupuncture + conventional drug therapy; MANU, manual acupuncture + conventional drug therapy; SHAM, sham acupuncture + conventional drug therapy; UPDRS, Unified PD rating scale.

The part highlighted in BOLD with underlining is a comparison with statistically significant results. The upper right triangle presents the effect size estimated using only direct comparison. As direct comparison does not exist in all treatment comparisons, there are several blanks in the upper right triangle. The lower left triangle provides a pooled estimation of the direct and indirect comparisons of the effect size.

3.5.3. Sensitivity Analysis

After excluding one study in the sensitivity analysis, (1) BEEV showed a tendency to be most effective in all 16 analyses; (2) in three sensitivity analyses (when excluding [40,44,47]), the ranking between MANU and ELEC was changed, with ELEC showing a better effect; and (3) CONV tended to have the smallest effect size throughout the analysis (Supplementary Materials Digital Content 6).

3.6. Secondary Outcome (Daily Life Activity, UPDRS-II): NMA

3.6.1. Assumption of NMA and Network Geometry

Homogeneity and transitivity assumptions are the same as those described in Section 3.5.1. We assessed the consistency assumption via a global and local approach and found no evidence of inconsistency after excluding the study by Lei [36]. The connectivity assumption was confirmed through network geometry (Supplementary Materials Digital Content 7). There were five nodes (ELEC, BEEV, MANU, CONV, and SHMA) from 10 studies and 14 pairwise comparisons from six types of comparison pairs (edges).

3.6.2. Comparative Effectiveness of the Acupuncture Modality in UPDRS-II

The probability of treatment as the best treatment option was presented through a measure called the P-score. The P-scores of the included modalities were as follows: BEEV (0.8971), ELEC (0.6685), MANU (0.5527), SHAM (0.3801), and CONV (0.0016). According to the P-score, BEEV was found to most likely be the best acupuncture modality for activities of daily life assessed by the UPDRS-II. The estimated effect size of each acupuncture modality compared to CONV via the NMA is presented in a treatment level forest plot and league table (Supplementary Materials Digital Content 7). In the treatment level forest plot and league table, the network estimate of the effect size (combining direct and indirect estimates) compared to CONV was as follows (in favor of bold marks): **BEEV** (MD −6.07, 95% CI −9.41 to −2.72); **ELEC** (MD −4.50, 95% CI −6.19 to −2.80); **MANU** (MD −4.08, 95% CI −4.84 to −3.32); **SHAM** (MD −3.21, 95% CI −5.72 to −0.70). BEEV, MANU, ELEC, and SHAM were superior to CONV in the UPDRS-II. As UPDRS-II is a secondary outcome, we did not conduct an additional sensitivity analysis.

3.7. Adverse Events (AEs)

AEs were also assessed in the present study. Based on the comparisons, AE rates are summarized as follows. Reported AEs according to RCT design are as follows: (1) ELEC vs. CONV design: 3/30 AEs in the ELEC group vs. 12/30 AEs in the CONV group were reported (Chen 2012 [14]); (2) MANU vs. CONV: not reported; (3) BEEV vs. CONV: 1/18 AEs in the BEEV group were reported (Cho 2012 [41]); (4) ELEC vs. SHAM: not reported; (5) MANU vs. SHAM: 1/47 in the MANU group was reported (Kluger 2016 [43]); and (6) BEEV vs. SHAM: 4/20 AEs in the BEEV group were reported (Hartmann 2016 [39]).

3.8. Publication Bias

A network funnel plot of the primary outcome (UPDRS-III) was constructed. There was no significant asymmetry seen in the visual inspection of the funnel plot (Figure 4). The Egger's test did not find any significant evidence of publication bias ($p = 0.269$). In the secondary outcome (UPDRS-II), there was no evidence of publication bias (Supplementary Materials Digital Content 7).

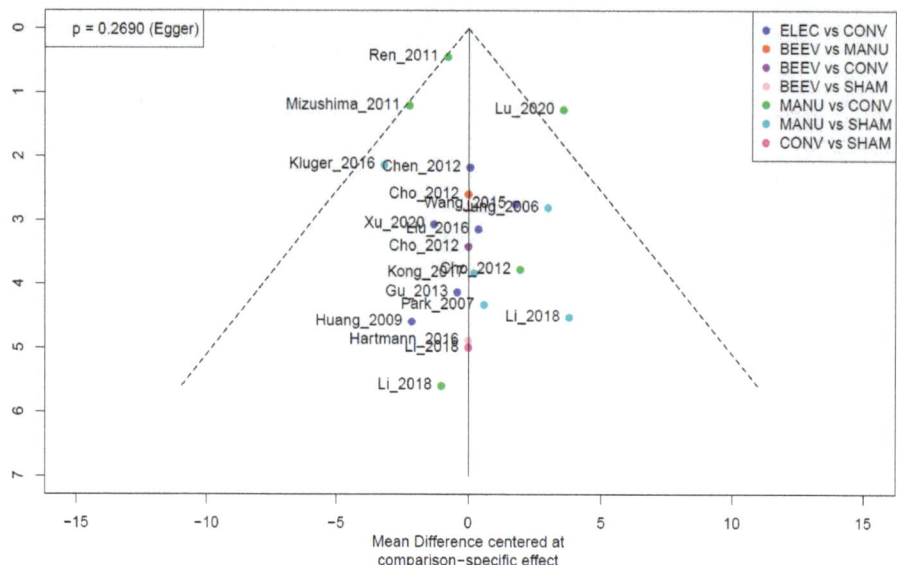

Figure 4. Network funnel plot: UPDRS-III score.

4. Discussion

4.1. Summary of Findings

The purpose of this PMA and NMA was to explore which acupuncture treatment modality combined with conventional drug therapy is more effective than conventional drug therapy alone for the improvement of motor symptoms (UPDRS-III) and activity of daily living (UPDRS-II) in PD. In NMA on motor symptoms (UPDRS-III), the order of effect size was BEEV, MANU, ELEC, SHAM, and CONV. BVA combination therapy is most likely the best modality for movement symptoms. In NMA on activities of daily living (UPDRS-II), the order of the effect size was BEEV, ELEC, MANU, SHAM, and CONV. BVA combination therapy is most likely to be the best modality for activities of daily living. No serious AEs were observed.

4.2. Implications for Clinical Practice and Suggestions for Further Research

The mechanism and therapeutic effect of acupuncture on PD have been elucidated in several studies. In a PD animal model, the expression of tropomyosin receptor kinase B (trkB) was increased in the ipsilateral substantia nigra, and a neuroprotective effect on neuronal cell death was revealed [51]. It also exhibits dopaminergic neuroprotective effects by inducing hypothalamic melanin-concentrating hormone biosynthesis [52]. As a result, it is possible to improve motor behavior while reducing the loss of dopaminergic neurons [51]. In a mechanistic study with functional MRI, acupuncture treatment for patients with PD demonstrated that the putamen and primary motor cortex were activated, and motor function was improved [51]. The mechanism of BVA has also been studied. Apamin toxin contained in BEEV is a polypeptide neurotoxin that blocks Ca2+ activated K + (SK) channels and induces hyperpolarization of dopaminergic neurons, thereby partially rescuing dopaminergic neurons in dissociated midbrain cell cultures [53]. BVA increases the size and number of neurons and striatal dopamine and protects dopaminergic neurons. Therefore, when BEEV is used alone or in combination with conventional drugs for PD, neuronal degeneration is alleviated, and movement disorders are reduced [54]. Several systematic reviews and meta-analyses of RCTs have also been published about the effect and safety of several acupuncture treatment modalities on PD [13,16,17,55].

However, it is unclear which acupuncture modality has a better effect and should be considered in clinical practice and research on PD. Therefore, we performed this NMA to help clinicians and researchers decide which acupuncture modality to use for PD. Although several NMA studies on acupuncture for various diseases have been reported [56–58], this is the first NMA study of acupuncture on PD. In our study, BEEV seems to be the best therapeutic option for motor symptoms and activities of daily living in patients with PD. However, the 95% CI overlapped different acupuncture modalities. Therefore, caution should be exercised when applying the results of this study to clinical practice and clinical research. In terms of effect size, the minimal clinical important differences (MCIDs) of the UPDRS motor scores were 2.5 points (minimal effect), 5.2 points (moderate effect), and 10.8 points (large effect) [59]. It was similar (approximately 5–7) in other MCID studies on the UPDRS III scores in patients with PD [60–62]. Considering the previous results of the MCID study, our results for the BEEV group showed a clinically significant moderate effect. The effect sizes of ELEC and MANU existed between minimal and moderate effects.

From a clinical perspective, even though BEEV might be the best option for motor symptoms and activities of daily living, MANU/ELEC might be an appropriate option for several motor symptoms [63]. In the presence of severe tremors, it may be difficult to use ELECs in the distal extremities. Therefore, physicians can try electroacupuncture treatment using acupuncture points on the scalp. BEEV might be inappropriate in some cases due to the risk of AEs, such as anaphylaxis [64]. In our results, MANU and ELEC had the best effect after BEEV in UPDRS-II and III. Therefore, if it is difficult to apply BEEV due to Aes, MANU or ELEC could be used as an alternative approach. However, the superiority between MANU and ELEC could not be determined in our study. In the sensitivity analysis, after excluding a long-term follow-up manual acupuncture study [44], ELEC was found to be better than MANU in UPDRS-III. Therefore, it might be possible that the treatment dose (number of sessions) might be an important factor for the therapeutic effect, but as the number of RCTs included in this study was relatively small, we could not conduct further analysis. As head-to-head comparison studies on ELEC and MANU are not common, meta-regression analysis or real-world evidence-based research with health insurance data are needed to address this issue. In summary, when deciding on the acupuncture treatment strategy for patients with PD in clinical practice, we need to consider several factors, such as applicability, adherence, AEs, and target symptoms. In real-world clinical practice, as an overlap of 95% CI of the effect size is clearly visible, it is recommended that BEEV combined with MA with/without electrical stimulation is recommended. Based on the results of this study, in clinical practice, we recommend using electroacupuncture on GB20 (Fengchi) and GB34 (Yanglingquan) for approximately 20–30 min in patients with PD from a clinical point of view. Since bee venom is a natural toxin, in terms of safety, therapeutic dosage is very important. In our study, the total amount of BEEV per session and total number of treatment sessions applied in our review were 100 µg (in 1 mL of NaCl 0.9%) for 11 sessions [39] and 50 µg (in 1 mL of NaCl 0.9%) for 16 sessions [41], respectively. With regard to safety, attention should be paid to side effects (such as anaphylaxis) when higher doses of BEEV than those reported in this study are applied. In addition to predictable dose-dependent side effects, non-predictable side effects due to individual sensitivity should also be considered.

Interestingly, the combined treatment of sham acupuncture with conventional medicine group (SHAM) was superior to the conventional medicine alone group (CONV). Placebo acupuncture is known to have a larger non-specific effect than other physical and pharmacological placebo modalities [65]. Sham acupuncture is known to be more effective than usual care or wait-list control groups for musculoskeletal diseases, such as non-specific low back pain [66]. Our study suggests that sham acupuncture might also have considerable non-specific effects on degenerative neurological diseases, such as PD. Therefore, a sham acupuncture-controlled design might underestimate the effect of acupuncture treatment. A pragmatic clinical study on comprehensive acupuncture treatment (combining ELEC, MANU, and BEEV) compared to an active control group (such as rehabilitation, medication, qi-gong) might be a more appropriate design to address physicians' questions about which intervention should be added to CM.

4.3. Strengths and Limitations

Our study had several strengths. This is the first NMA acupuncture study for PD in an area that is difficult to conduct clinical trials due to resource limitations and research priorities. We included studies across multiple databases without language restrictions. The assumptions for performing the network meta-analysis were systemically reviewed, and there was a methodological advantage in that a sensitivity analysis was performed to confirm the robustness of the NMA results. We provided the NMA results with MD (not standardized MD) for applicability and interpretability in clinical practice.

However, this study has several limitations. First, the number of included studies and types of acupuncture modalities were relatively small. Heterogeneity exists between acupuncture regimens, even though we adopted a random-effects model. Therefore, further acupuncture RCTs on PD are needed to ensure the robustness of our results. In further NMA studies with more clinical RCTs, we can focus on more specific clinical questions, such as responders to acupuncture treatment in terms of severity, age, sex, disease duration, and accompanying symptoms [67]. In terms of dosage, we could not conduct a subgroup analysis of treatment duration, frequency, or needle retention time due to the lack of relevant studies. Since it is an important factor for the therapeutic effect of acupuncture [68,69], we need further subgroup analysis or meta-regression studies for detailed treatment regimens and dosages in acupuncture treatment. Second, in the sensitivity analysis, although this is largely consistent with the results of the primary analysis, the order of the effect sizes of ELEC and MANU was reversed in some cases. This suggests that it is difficult to differentiate between ELECs and MANUs. Further research is needed on this issue from an academic perspective. However, from a clinical perspective, it is recommended to combine electroacupuncture and MA simultaneously based on CM, as a commercial electroacupuncture device usually covers less than 12 acupuncture points. Third, we excluded combined acupuncture strategies, such as BVA combined with electroacupuncture, to explore the effect of a single acupuncture modality. However, in real-world clinical practice, each acupuncture modality is combined with other types of acupuncture. Therefore, we could not assess the synergetic effects of acupuncture modalities. Moreover, we might have underestimated the effects of acupuncture. Because the number of relevant RCTs was insufficient, further NMA studies are also needed on combined acupuncture modalities in the future. Next, the methodological quality of the included RCTs was relatively poor. Therefore, caution should be exercised when interpreting these results. Caution is also required when interpreting our results, as the reference group (CONV) of NMA had considerable heterogeneity. Finally, we included only CM in the reference (control) group. However, there are various standard treatments, such as surgical intervention and rehabilitation. As we used pharmacologic treatment as a control group, it might provide different results when using non-pharmacological intervention as a control group in the further NMA study.

5. Conclusions

We conducted a PMA and NMA to evaluate the effects of various acupuncture modalities on patients with idiopathic PD. The probability of comparative effectiveness in motor symptoms of patients with idiopathic PD was assumed to be in the order of BEEV, MANU, ELEC, SHAM, and CONV. However, more rigorous RCTs are needed for further NMA, including non-motor symptoms of PD. Along with conventional levodopa therapy, BVA, electroacupuncture, and MA could be more effective in clinical practice than single-drug therapy.

Supplementary Materials: The following are available online at https://www.mdpi.com/article/10.3390/healthcare9111502/s1. Supplemental Digital Content 1. Search strategies used on each database. Supplemental Digital Content 2. Articles excluded after the full text review with reasons. Supplemental Digital Content 3. Risk of bias graph. Supplemental Digital Content 4. Forest plot of PMA (UPDRS-III and UPDRS-II). Supplemental Digital Content 5. Net-split plot: UPDRS-III score. Supplemental Digital Content 6. Sensitivity analysis. Supplemental Digital Content 7. Network plot, forest plot, league table, net-split plot, and funnel plot on the secondary outcome (UPDRS-II).

Author Contributions: Conceptualization, J.L. and T.-h.K.; methodology, M.J.C.; software, J.L.; validation, T.-h.K.; formal analysis, J.L. and M.K.; investigation, M.K.; resources, J.L.; data curation, M.J.C.; writing—original draft preparation, M.K.; writing—review and editing, J.L. and T.-h.K.; visualization, J.L.; supervision, T.-h.K.; project administration, J.L.; funding acquisition, J.L. All authors have read and agreed to the published version of the manuscript.

Funding: This work was supported by a National Research Foundation of Korea (NRF) grant funded by the Korean government (MSIT) (No. NRF-2019R1F1A1059310).

Institutional Review Board Statement: Not Applicable.

Informed Consent Statement: Not applicable.

Data Availability Statement: Data are available on request to the corresponding author. The study protocol is available at the open science platform (https://osf.io/q8n7z/).

Acknowledgments: This article is based on the doctorate thesis of Miri Kwon.

Conflicts of Interest: The authors declare no conflict of interest.

References

1. Armstrong, M.J.; Okun, M.S. Diagnosis and Treatment of Parkinson Disease: A Review. *JAMA* **2020**, *323*, 548–560. [CrossRef]
2. Tolosa, E.; Wenning, G.; Poewe, W. The Diagnosis of Parkinson's Disease. *Lancet Neurol.* **2006**, *5*, 75–86. [CrossRef]
3. Tysnes, O.-B.; Storstein, A. Epidemiology of Parkinson's Disease. *J. Neural Transm.* **2017**, *124*, 901–905. [CrossRef] [PubMed]
4. Abbas, M.M.; Xu, Z.; Tan, L.C.S. Epidemiology of Parkinson's Disease—East Versus West. *Mov. Disord. Clin. Pract.* **2017**, *5*, 14–28. [CrossRef] [PubMed]
5. Armstrong, M.J.; Okun, M.S. Choosing a Parkinson Disease Treatment. *JAMA* **2020**, *323*, 1420. [CrossRef] [PubMed]
6. Schapira, A.H.V.; Chaudhuri, K.R.; Jenner, P. Non-Motor Features of Parkinson Disease. *Nat. Rev. Neurosci.* **2017**, *18*, 435–450. [CrossRef]
7. Freitas, M.E.; Hess, C.W.; Fox, S.H. Motor Complications of Dopaminergic Medications in Parkinson's Disease. *Semin. Neurol.* **2017**, *37*, 147–157. [CrossRef]
8. Sun, B.; Wang, T.; Li, N.; Qiao, J. Analysis of Motor Complication and Relative Factors in a Cohort of Chinese Patients with Parkinson's Disease. *Park. Dis.* **2020**, *2020*, e8692509. [CrossRef] [PubMed]
9. Abosch, A.; Gross, R.E. Surgical Treatment of Parkinson's Disease: Deep Brain Stimulation versus Radiofrequency Ablation. *Clin. Neurosurg.* **2004**, *51*, 296–303.
10. Rossi, M.; Bruno, V.; Arena, J.; Cammarota, Á.; Merello, M. Challenges in PD Patient Management After DBS: A Pragmatic Review. *Mov. Disord. Clin. Pract.* **2018**, *5*, 246–254. [CrossRef]
11. Sveinbjornsdottir, S. The Clinical Symptoms of Parkinson's Disease. *J. Neurochem.* **2016**, *139*, 318–324. [CrossRef] [PubMed]
12. Ghaffari, B.D.; Kluger, B. Mechanisms for Alternative Treatments in Parkinson's Disease: Acupuncture, Tai Chi, and Other Treatments. *Curr. Neurol. Neurosci. Rep.* **2014**, *14*, 451. [CrossRef]
13. Lee, S.-H.; Lim, S. Clinical Effectiveness of Acupuncture on Parkinson Disease: A PRISMA-Compliant Systematic Review and Meta-Analysis. *Medicine* **2017**, *96*, e5836. [CrossRef] [PubMed]
14. Chen, Y.; Feng, W.; Zhang, X. Parkinson's disease combined with overactive bladder syndrome treated with acupuncture and medication. *Chin. Acupunct. Moxibustion* **2012**, *32*, 215–218.
15. Jung, J.; Kim, K.; Park, Y.; Kim, H.; Lee, S.; Chang, D.; Lee, Y. The Study on the Effect of Acupuncture on UPDRS and Heart Rate Variability in the Patients with Idiopathic Parkinson's Disease. *J. Korean Acupunct. Moxibustion Soc.* **2006**, *23*, 143–153.
16. Noh, H.; Kwon, S.; Cho, S.-Y.; Jung, W.-S.; Moon, S.-K.; Park, J.-M.; Ko, C.-N.; Park, S.-U. Effectiveness and Safety of Acupuncture in the Treatment of Parkinson's Disease: A Systematic Review and Meta-Analysis of Randomized Controlled Trials. *Complement. Ther. Med.* **2017**, *34*, 86–103. [CrossRef] [PubMed]
17. Liu, H.; Chen, L.; Zhang, Z.; Geng, G.; Chen, W.; Dong, H.; Chen, L.; Zhan, S.; Li, T. Effectiveness and Safety of Acupuncture Combined with Madopar for Parkinson—s Disease: A Systematic Review with Meta-Analysis. *Acupunct. Med.* **2017**, *35*, 404–412. [CrossRef] [PubMed]
18. Rouse, B.; Chaimani, A.; Li, T. Network Meta-Analysis: An Introduction for Clinicians. *Intern. Emerg. Med.* **2017**, *12*, 103–111. [CrossRef] [PubMed]

19. Pratt, M.; Wieland, S.; Ahmadzai, N.; Butler, C.; Wolfe, D.; Pussagoda, K.; Skidmore, B.; Veroniki, A.; Rios, P.; Tricco, A.C.; et al. A Scoping Review of Network Meta-Analyses Assessing the Efficacy and Safety of Complementary and Alternative Medicine Interventions. *Syst. Rev.* **2020**, *9*. [CrossRef] [PubMed]
20. Kanters, S.; Ford, N.; Druyts, E.; Thorlund, K.; Mills, E.J.; Bansback, N. Use of Network Meta-Analysis in Clinical Guidelines. *Bull. World Health Organ.* **2016**, *94*, 782–784. [CrossRef]
21. Hutton, B.; Salanti, G.; Caldwell, D.M.; Chaimani, A.; Schmid, C.H.; Cameron, C.; Ioannidis, J.P.A.; Straus, S.; Thorlund, K.; Jansen, J.P.; et al. The PRISMA Extension Statement for Reporting of Systematic Reviews Incorporating Network Meta-Analyses of Health Care Interventions: Checklist and Explanations. *Ann. Intern. Med.* **2015**, *162*, 777–784. [CrossRef] [PubMed]
22. Tambasco, N.; Romoli, M.; Calabresi, P. Levodopa in Parkinson's Disease: Current Status and Future Developments. *Curr. Neuropharmacol.* **2018**, *16*, 1239–1252. [CrossRef] [PubMed]
23. Fahn, S.; Oakes, D.; Shoulson, I.; Kieburtz, K.; Rudolph, A.; Lang, A.; Olanow, C.W.; Tanner, C.; Marek, K.; Parkinson Study Group. Levodopa and the Progression of Parkinson's Disease. *N. Engl. J. Med.* **2004**, *351*, 2498–2508. [CrossRef] [PubMed]
24. Ramaker, C.; Marinus, J.; Stiggelbout, A.M.; Hilten, B.J. van Systematic Evaluation of Rating Scales for Impairment and Disability in Parkinson's Disease. *Mov. Disord.* **2002**, *17*, 867–876. [CrossRef]
25. Goetz, C.G.; Fahn, S.; Martinez-Martin, P.; Poewe, W.; Sampaio, C.; Stebbins, G.T.; Stern, M.B.; Tilley, B.C.; Dodel, R.; Dubois, B.; et al. Movement Disorder Society-Sponsored Revision of the Unified Parkinson's Disease Rating Scale (MDS-UPDRS): Process, Format, and Clinimetric Testing Plan. *Mov. Disord. Off. J. Mov. Disord. Soc.* **2007**, *22*, 41–47. [CrossRef] [PubMed]
26. Higgins, J.P.T.; Thomas, J.; Chandler, J.; Cumpston, M.; Li, T.; Page, M.J.; Welch, V.A. *Cochrane Handbook for Systematic Reviews of Interventions*; John Wiley & Sons: Hoboken, NJ, USA, 2019; ISBN 978-1-119-53661-1.
27. Egger, M.; Davey Smith, G.; Schneider, M.; Minder, C. Bias in Meta-Analysis Detected by a Simple, Graphical Test. *BMJ* **1997**, *315*, 629–634. [CrossRef] [PubMed]
28. Borenstein, M.; Hedges, L.V.; Higgins, J.P.T.; Rothstein, H.R. A Basic Introduction to Fixed-Effect and Random-Effects Models for Meta-Analysis. *Res. Synth. Methods* **2010**, *1*, 97–111. [CrossRef] [PubMed]
29. Shim, S.R.; Kim, S.-J.; Lee, J.; Rücker, G. Network Meta-Analysis: Application and Practice Using R Software. *Epidemiol. Health* **2019**, *41*. [CrossRef]
30. Watt, J.; Tricco, A.C.; Straus, S.; Veroniki, A.A.; Naglie, G.; Drucker, A.M. Research Techniques Made Simple: Network Meta-Analysis. *J. Investig. Dermatol.* **2019**, *139*, 4–12.e1. [CrossRef]
31. Biondi-Zoccai, G.; Abbate, A.; Benedetto, U.; Palmerini, T.; D'Ascenzo, F.; Frati, G. Network Meta-Analysis for Evidence Synthesis: What Is It and Why Is It Posed to Dominate Cardiovascular Decision Making? *Int. J. Cardiol.* **2015**, *182*, 309–314. [CrossRef]
32. Tonin, F.S.; Rotta, I.; Mendes, A.M.; Pontarolo, R. Network Meta-Analysis: A Technique to Gather Evidence from Direct and Indirect Comparisons. *Pharm. Pract.* **2017**, *15*, 943. [CrossRef] [PubMed]
33. Rücker, G.; Schwarzer, G. Ranking Treatments in Frequentist Network Meta-Analysis Works without Resampling Methods. *BMC Med. Res. Methodol.* **2015**, *15*, 58. [CrossRef]
34. Higgins, J.P.T.; Jackson, D.; Barrett, J.K.; Lu, G.; Ades, A.E.; White, I.R. Consistency and Inconsistency in Network Meta-Analysis: Concepts and Models for Multi-Arm Studies. *Res. Synth. Methods* **2012**, *3*, 98–110. [CrossRef] [PubMed]
35. Bowden, J.; Davey Smith, G.; Burgess, S. Mendelian Randomization with Invalid Instruments: Effect Estimation and Bias Detection through Egger Regression. *Int. J. Epidemiol.* **2015**, *44*, 512–525. [CrossRef] [PubMed]
36. Lei, H.; Toosizadeh, N.; Schwenk, M.; Sherman, S.; Karp, S.; Sternberg, E.; Najafi, B. A Pilot Clinical Trial to Objectively Assess the Efficacy of Electroacupuncture on Gait in Patients with Parkinson's Disease Using Body Worn Sensors. *PLoS ONE* **2016**, *11*. [CrossRef] [PubMed]
37. Kong, K.H.; Ng, H.L.; Li, W.; Ng, D.W.; Tan, S.I.; Tay, K.Y.; Au, W.L.; Tan, L.C.S. Acupuncture in the Treatment of Fatigue in Parkinson's Disease: A Pilot, Randomized, Controlled, Study. *Brain Behav.* **2017**, *8*. [CrossRef] [PubMed]
38. Li, Z.; Chen, J.; Cheng, J.; Huang, S.; Hu, Y.; Wu, Y.; Li, G.; Liu, B.; Liu, X.; Guo, W.; et al. Acupuncture Modulates the Cerebello-Thalamo-Cortical Circuit and Cognitive Brain Regions in Patients of Parkinson's Disease with Tremor. *Front. Aging Neurosci.* **2018**, *10*. [CrossRef]
39. Hartmann, A.; Müllner, J.; Meier, N.; Hesekamp, H.; van Meerbeeck, P.; Habert, M.-O.; Kas, A.; Tanguy, M.-L.; Mazmanian, M.; Oya, H.; et al. Bee Venom for the Treatment of Parkinson Disease—A Randomized Controlled Clinical Trial. *PLoS ONE* **2016**, *11*, e0158235. [CrossRef]
40. Wang, F.; Sun, L.; Zhang, X.; Jia, J.; Liu, Z.; Huang, X.; Yu, S.; Zuo, L.; Cao, C.; Wang, X.; et al. Effect and Potential Mechanism of Electroacupuncture Add-On Treatment in Patients with Parkinson's Disease. *Evid.-Based Complement. Altern. Med. ECAM* **2015**, *2015*. [CrossRef]
41. Cho, S.-Y.; Shim, S.-R.; Rhee, H.Y.; Park, H.-J.; Jung, W.-S.; Moon, S.-K.; Park, J.-M.; Ko, C.-N.; Cho, K.-H.; Park, S.-U. Effectiveness of Acupuncture and Bee Venom Acupuncture in Idiopathic Parkinson's Disease. *Parkinsonism Relat. Disord.* **2012**, *18*, 948–952. [CrossRef]
42. Xu, Y.; Cai, X.; Qu, S.; Zhang, J.; Zhang, Z.; Yao, Z.; Huang, Y.; Zhong, Z. Madopar Combined with Acupuncture Improves Motor and Non-Motor Symptoms in Parkinson's Disease Patients: A Multicenter Randomized Controlled Trial. *Eur. J. Integr. Med.* **2020**, *34*, 101049. [CrossRef]

43. Kluger, B.M.; Rakowski, D.; Christian, M.; Cedar, D.; Wong, B.; Crawford, J.; Uveges, K.; Berk, J.; Abaca, E.; Corbin, L.; et al. Randomized, Controlled Trial of Acupuncture for Fatigue in Parkinson's Disease. *Mov. Disord.* **2016**, *31*, 1027–1032. [CrossRef]
44. Takeo, M. Treatment Results between Matched Pair of L-Dopa Medication Treatment and Acupuncture Treatment Combination on Parkinson Disease. *Kampo Med.* **2011**, *62*, 691–694. (In Japanese) [CrossRef]
45. Park, Y.-C.; Chang, D.-I.; Lee, Y.-H.; Park, D.-S. The Study on the Effect of Acupuncture Treatment in Patients with Idiopathic Parkinson's Disease. *J. Acupunct. Res.* **2007**, *24*, 43–54.
46. Yong, H.; Ying, Z.; XueMei, J.; AnWu, T.; DongJiang, L.; Ming, S.; ZhouHua, W. Effect of scalp acupuncture on regional cerebral blood flow in Parkinson's disease patients. *China J. Tradit. Chin. Med. Pharm.* **2009**, *24*, 305–308.
47. Ren, X.; Shi, Y.; Song, S.; Hu, X.; Han, Z. Clinical Study on Acupuncture Tonifying Liver and Kidney in the Treatment of Parkinson Disease (in Chinese). *Chin. Arch. Tradit. Chin. Med.* **2011**, *29*, 2470–2473.
48. Gu, K.; Liu, K.; Lu, Z.; Fan, X.; Zong, L. Clinical Observations on Combined Treatment of Parkinson's Disease Using Acupuncture and Medicine. *Shanghai J. Acu-Mox* **2013**, *32*, 993–995.
49. Liu, B. Clinical Study on Acupuncture Treatment of Parkinson's Disease. *China Health Stand. Manag.* **2016**, *7*, 128–129.
50. Lu, Y.-K.; Wang, X.-Z.; Yang, G.-F.; Yang, H.-Y. Clinical Observation of Liver-Calming and Kidney-Nourishing Acupuncture Therapy Combined with Acupuncture at Starting and Ending Points of Muscles in Treating Middle and Late Stages of Parkinson's Disease. *J. Guangzhou Univ. Tradit. Chin. Med.* **2020**, *37*, 1907–1912.
51. Park, H.-J.; Lim, S.; Joo, W.-S.; Yin, C.-S.; Lee, H.-S.; Lee, H.-J.; Seo, J.-C.; Leem, K.; Son, Y.-S.; Kim, Y.-J.; et al. Acupuncture Prevents 6-Hydroxydopamine-Induced Neuronal Death in the Nigrostriatal Dopaminergic System in the Rat Parkinson's Disease Model. *Exp. Neurol.* **2003**, *180*, 93–98. [CrossRef]
52. Park, J.-Y.; Kim, S.-N.; Yoo, J.; Jang, J.; Lee, A.; Oh, J.-Y.; Kim, H.; Oh, S.T.; Park, S.-U.; Kim, J.; et al. Novel Neuroprotective Effects of Melanin-Concentrating Hormone in Parkinson's Disease. *Mol. Neurobiol.* **2017**, *54*, 7706–7721. [CrossRef]
53. Salthun-Lassalle, B.; Hirsch, E.C.; Wolfart, J.; Ruberg, M.; Michel, P.P. Rescue of Mesencephalic Dopaminergic Neurons in Culture by Low-Level Stimulation of Voltage-Gated Sodium Channels. *J. Neurosci.* **2004**, *24*, 5922–5930. [CrossRef]
54. Badawi, H.M.; Abdelsalam, R.M.; Abdel-Salam, O.M.; Youness, E.R.; Shaffie, N.M.; Eldenshary, E.-E.D.S. Bee Venom Attenuates Neurodegeneration and Motor Impairment and Modulates the Response to L-Dopa or Rasagiline in a Mice Model of Parkinson's Disease. *Iran. J. Basic Med. Sci.* **2020**, *23*, 1628–1638. [CrossRef] [PubMed]
55. Huang, J.; Qin, X.; Cai, X.; Huang, Y. Effectiveness of Acupuncture in the Treatment of Parkinson's Disease: An Overview of Systematic Reviews. *Front. Neurol.* **2020**, *11*. [CrossRef] [PubMed]
56. Tan, X.; Pan, Y.; Su, W.; Gong, S.; Zhu, H.; Chen, H.; Lu, S. Acupuncture Therapy for Essential Hypertension: A Network Meta-Analysis. *Ann. Transl. Med.* **2019**, *7*. [CrossRef] [PubMed]
57. Zhang, J.; Liu, Y.; Huang, X.; Chen, Y.; Hu, L.; Lan, K.; Yu, H. Efficacy Comparison of Different Acupuncture Treatments for Functional Dyspepsia: A Systematic Review with Network Meta-Analysis. *Evid.-Based Complement. Altern. Med. ECAM* **2020**, *2020*. [CrossRef] [PubMed]
58. Xu, H.; Shi, Y.; Xiao, Y.; Liu, P.; Wu, S.; Pang, P.; Deng, L.; Chen, X. Efficacy Comparison of Different Acupuncture Treatments for Primary Insomnia: A Bayesian Analysis. *Evid.-Based Complement. Altern. Med. ECAM* **2019**, *2019*. [CrossRef] [PubMed]
59. Shulman, L.M.; Gruber-Baldini, A.L.; Anderson, K.E.; Fishman, P.S.; Reich, S.G.; Weiner, W.J. The Clinically Important Difference on the Unified Parkinson's Disease Rating Scale. *Arch. Neurol.* **2010**, *67*, 64–70. [CrossRef] [PubMed]
60. Hauser, R.A.; Gordon, M.F.; Mizuno, Y.; Poewe, W.; Barone, P.; Schapira, A.H.; Rascol, O.; Debieuvre, C.; Fräßdorf, M. Minimal Clinically Important Difference in Parkinson's Disease as Assessed in Pivotal Trials of Pramipexole Extended Release. *Park. Dis.* **2014**, *2014*, e467131. [CrossRef] [PubMed]
61. Horváth, K.; Aschermann, Z.; Ács, P.; Deli, G.; Janszky, J.; Komoly, S.; Balázs, É.; Takács, K.; Karádi, K.; Kovács, N. Minimal Clinically Important Difference on the Motor Examination Part of MDS-UPDRS. *Parkinsonism Relat. Disord.* **2015**, *21*, 1421–1426. [CrossRef]
62. Sánchez-Ferro, Á.; Matarazzo, M.; Martínez-Martín, P.; Martínez-Ávila, J.C.; Gómez de la Cámara, A.; Giancardo, L.; Arroyo Gallego, T.; Montero, P.; Puertas-Martín, V.; Obeso, I.; et al. Minimal Clinically Important Difference for UPDRS-III in Daily Practice. *Mov. Disord. Clin. Pract.* **2018**, *5*, 448–450. [CrossRef] [PubMed]
63. Zeng, B.-Y.; Zhao, K. Effect of Acupuncture on the Motor and Nonmotor Symptoms in Parkinson's Disease—A Review of Clinical Studies. *CNS Neurosci. Ther.* **2016**, *22*, 333–341. [CrossRef] [PubMed]
64. Cherniack, E.P.; Govorushko, S. To Bee or Not to Bee: The Potential Efficacy and Safety of Bee Venom Acupuncture in Humans. *Toxicon Off. J. Int. Soc. Toxinol.* **2018**, *154*, 74–78. [CrossRef] [PubMed]
65. Linde, K.; Niemann, K.; Meissner, K. Are Sham Acupuncture Interventions More Effective than (Other) Placebos? A Re-Analysis of Data from the Cochrane Review on Placebo Effects. *Complement. Med. Res.* **2010**, *17*, 259–264. [CrossRef] [PubMed]
66. Xiang, Y.; He, J.; Li, R. Appropriateness of Sham or Placebo Acupuncture for Randomized Controlled Trials of Acupuncture for Nonspecific Low Back Pain: A Systematic Review and Meta-Analysis. *J. Pain Res.* **2017**, *11*, 83–94. [CrossRef]
67. Leem, J. Acupuncture for Motor Symptom Improvement in Parkinson's Disease and the Potential Identification of Responders to Acupuncture Treatment. *Integr. Med. Res.* **2016**, *5*, 332–335. [CrossRef] [PubMed]
68. Bauer, M.; McDonald, J.L.; Saunders, N. Is Acupuncture Dose Dependent? Ramifications of Acupuncture Treatment Dose within Clinical Practice and Trials. *Integr. Med. Res.* **2020**, *9*, 21–27. [CrossRef]
69. Leem, J. Does Acupuncture Reduce the Risk of Acute Myocardial Infarction? *Integr. Med. Res.* **2016**, *5*, 165–168. [CrossRef]

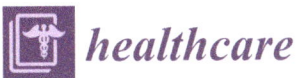

Article

The Use of Traditional Korean Medicine (TKM) by Children: A Correlational Study between Parent's Perception and Their Children's Use Reported by Parents

Jihye Kim [1], Jang-Kyung Park [2], Jung-Youn Park [3], Eun-Jin Lee [4] and Soo-Hyun Sung [4],*

[1] Research Institute of Korean Medicine Policy, The Association of Korean Medicine, Seoul 07525, Korea; jihyekim1217@gmail.com
[2] Department of Obstetrics and Gynecology, College of Korean Medicine, Pusan National University, Yangsan 50612, Korea; vivat314@pusan.ac.kr
[3] Department of Health and Welfare, Yuhan University, Bucheon 14780, Korea; park0625@yuhan.ac.kr
[4] Department of Policy Development, National Development Institute of Korean Medicine, Seoul 04554, Korea; eunjin6434@nikom.or.kr
* Correspondence: koyote10010@nikom.or.kr

Citation: Kim, J.; Park, J.-K.; Park, J.-Y.; Lee, E.-J.; Sung, S.-H. The Use of Traditional Korean Medicine (TKM) by Children: A Correlational Study between Parent's Perception and Their Children's Use Reported by Parents. *Healthcare* **2021**, *9*, 385. https://doi.org/10.3390/healthcare9040385

Academic Editors: Manoj Sharma and Kavita Batra

Received: 17 February 2021
Accepted: 26 March 2021
Published: 1 April 2021

Publisher's Note: MDPI stays neutral with regard to jurisdictional claims in published maps and institutional affiliations.

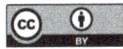

Copyright: © 2021 by the authors. Licensee MDPI, Basel, Switzerland. This article is an open access article distributed under the terms and conditions of the Creative Commons Attribution (CC BY) license (https://creativecommons.org/licenses/by/4.0/).

Abstract: This cross-sectional study investigated the correlation between parents' perception and their children's traditional Korean medicine (TKM) use reported by parents in order to discover policy intervention points and provide a reference for establishing generalized TKM policies. Participant data from a 2017 national survey on TKM usage was divided into two groups based on the children's TKM use reported by parents. The female participants' children had a higher rate of experience in using TKM (8.1%; $p = 0.029$). Additionally, 91.4% of the parent group with a child who used TKM turned out to have used TKM, which was higher than 71.9% of the parents whose children never used TKM ($p < 0.001$). As for the awareness on the use of TKM, 44.0% of the parents with a child who experienced TKM answered they were aware of it, while only 35.3% of the parent group whose child never experienced TKM did so ($p = 0.033$). The present study suggests that parental experience in using TKM could have an impact on the children's TKM use reported by parents. Further study is necessary to assess which parental factor (awareness level, medical disorder to be treated, therapy, therapeutic efficacy, the purpose of visit, sex, age, etc.) has a close relationship with TKM usage experience of their children.

Keywords: traditional Korean medicine (TKM); complementary and alternative medicine (CAM); national survey TKM usage; parents' perception of TKM; children's TKM use

1. Introduction

Complementary and Alternative Medicine (CAM), which is not considered to be part of conventional medicine, is a compilation of knowledge, skills, and practices which are based on the theories, beliefs, and experiences indigenous to different cultures and used for health maintenance and in the prevention, diagnosis, improvement, or treatment of physical and mental illness [1–3]. CAM approaches include natural products (e.g., herbs, vitamins and minerals and probiotics), and mind body practice such as yoga, meditation, chiropractic, acupuncture, relaxation techniques, tai chi, qigong, and hypnotherapy [4]. The use of CAM is increasing in many countries of the world [5]. Approximately 88% of the member states of the World Health Organization (WHO) are using CAM through the development of national policies, laws, regulations, and applied programs [6]. In East-Asian countries such as South Korea and China, traditional medicine has been the form of medical care treating the diseases of the people. Currently, it is still taking a crucial part in health care along with conventional medicine (CM) [7,8]. In East-Asian countries such as China, Korea, and Taiwan, traditional medicine practitioners are considered as doctors, as is the case with the doctors who provide CM [9,10]. Traditional Korean medicine (TKM) doctors use acupuncture, electro-acupuncture, pharmacopuncture, herbal medicine, chuna, cupping, moxibustion, and other forms of intervention to treat their patients [11]. In Korea, 14% of the total population and 7.6% of those in their 20 s or younger, are using TKM, and 10% of the total male population and 18.1% of the total female population visited TKM clinics [12]. The purpose of using TKM was treating a disease (94.1%), improving health (18.4%), and cosmetic purposes (4.0%) [13].

Health in the pediatric or juvenile period has an impact on adulthood health, education, achievement, and economic performance. Therefore, the health of children and teenagers is of paramount importance [14,15]. Additionally, parents' experience with using medical services can have varying effects on their children [16]. Some well-known factors impacting the health and the usage of medical services during pediatric and juvenile periods include respective family structure, parental education level, and their social- status [17–22].

In the field of traditional Chinese medicine (TCM), Loh [23] surveyed 300 parents who visited TCM clinics, and 84.3% of their children used TCM clinics, while 80.3% of them reported that they used both TCM clinics and CM clinics. Yeh [24] used the National Health Insurance data of Taiwan to analyze the overall usage of TCM and reported that about 20% of the children under 20 used TCM clinics. In the field of TKM, Choi [25] conducted a survey of 300 parents who used the TKM clinic and had a child under 19. As a result of the said survey, it was resulted that 81% of the children experienced and visited TKM clinics for the purpose of treating respiratory disease (21.6%) gastrointestinal disease (10.6%,), and skin disease (9.2%). Park [26] surveyed 702 parents who used daycare centres and reported that 55.3% of the children's age from 1 to 13 used TKM clinics, mainly for the purpose of treating respiratory disease (34.5%), gastrointestinal disease (17.2%), and skin disease (13.8%). As such, the previous studies on the usage of traditional medicine among children or adolescents under 20, were mainly conducted as cross-sectional studies. In three studies [23,25,26], the study samples were not representative of the general population of the country. Yeh [24] used the representative data of the general population of Taiwan. However, the study was intended to investigate the usage of TCM in the entire population, including children.

An assessment of TKM usage has been undertaken by Statistics Korea, as a certified national statistic every 3 years since 2008. This assessment covers all household members of the sample families who are at least 19 years old, providing a representative sample of the country [13]. In order to effectively integrate TKM into the healthcare system, it is necessary that policies are developed and implemented based on accurate statistics of TKM. To fulfil this requirement, the national survey on TKM use data from 5000 Korean participants was used in order to examine the correlation between parental awareness of TKM use and the use of TKM by their children.

2. Materials and Methods

2.1. Data Sources

The source data used in this study is from the TKM usage survey of 2017, conducted by the Ministry of Health and Welfare and National Institute of Korean Medicine Development. The survey was reviewed and approved by Korea Statistics (National Certified Statistics Approval Number: 117087). As for the survey data, the researchers made a request for micro-data through the surveys on the traditional herbal medicines consumption and the TKM usage database (https://www.koms.or.kr/main.do, accessed on 18 November 2020) run by the National Institute of Korean Medicine Development (NIKOM). Approval was obtained to use and analyze the data from the NIKOM, which was commissioned by the government to conduct the above-mentioned survey and analyzed the micro-data which was provided by the said organization to conduct this study.

As for the surveys on the traditional herbal medicine consumption and the TKM usage, the survey on the usage of TKM started in 2008 (1st survey), which was followed by the survey on the consumption of traditional herbal medicine (1st survey) in 2009. In 2011, the two separate surveys were integrated into one survey on TKM usage. Since then, the survey has been conducted every 3 years. Among all the data collected over the years, we used the data on the usage of TKM obtained during the 4th survey that took place in 2017.

2.2. Sample Selection

The data used in this study was obtained from 5000 participants selected among the general population during the TKM usage survey in 2017. When the 5000 participants, who were the national survey samples, were selected, they did not enroll both parents from a family. In particular the following selecting questions were used to assess eligibility: Do you have a child who is under 19 (born after September 1998)? (1) Yes [the number of children under 19 is (...)] (2) No. The participants in the survey item or were the parent who was the caregiver of the children. Also, we instructed the participants to tell us the number of children in their family if they answered they had a child under 19. This resulted in the inclusion of 872 participants who chose 'Yes'. Their answers were included for analysis in order to obtain the results on the satisfaction and awareness data, as well as the information regarding their children. The selection process of the participants is shown in Figure 1.

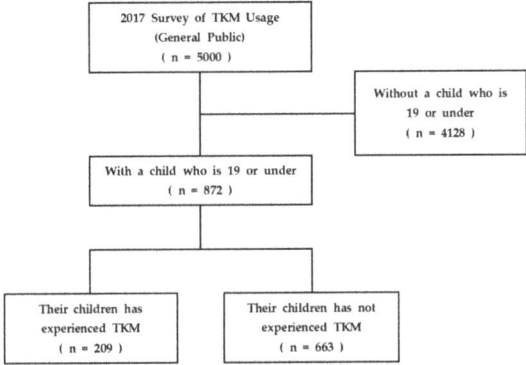

Figure 1. Flow chart of inclusion and exclusion of participants from the 2017 National Survey of Traditional Korean Medicine Usage. TKM: Traditional Korean Medicine.

2.3. Analysis Items

The analysis items included in this study were the participants who answered 'Yes' to the question asking whether they had a child under the age of 19, during the TKM usage survey in 2017, as well as the questions regarding the satisfaction and awareness of their children. Additionally, based on the children's TKM use reported by parents, the relationships between the demographics, the experience of using TKM, their opinion on the use of TKM, and the perception of treatment effects on sixteen diseases, were analyzed. The demographics of the participants (mother or father) were used to examine the relationship between the answers about the children and the characteristics of participants. The answers about the children included the children's experience with TKM, the reason why their children used TKM, the kind of TKM treatment the children experienced, the degree of satisfaction with their children's TKM experience, and cause of dissatisfaction with using TKM. The basic demographic information of the participants included their sex, age group, area of residence, education, employment status, household income, type of healthcare coverage, and subscription status of private medical insurance. The experience of using TKM variables included TKM participation, the reason for choosing to use TKM, participants' experience with TKM, participants' satisfaction with TKM, participants' awareness of TKM, money invested to use TKM, their willingness to use TKM again in the future, and their willingness to recommend TKM to others. Regarding the perception of treatment effects on diseases, variables were used following sixteen diseases: (1) disc related disease (herniation of intervertebral disc, spinal stenosis); (2) osteoarthritis; (3) frozen shoulder shoulder pain;

(4) back pain; (5) sprain; (6) facial nerve paralysis; (7) stroke; (8) hypertension; (9) diabetes mellitus; (10) digestive disease; (11) common cold rhinitis; (12) dementia (13) cancer related pain; (14) infertility; (15) skin disease (atopic dermatitis); (16) genitourinary disease. Also, whether the characteristics of the participants (demographics, their opinion or ideas on TKM, etc.) had an impact on the children's use of TKM and the possible strategies to promote use of TKM in different target groups, were explored.

2.4. Statistical Analysis

In order to better understand the general characteristics of the participants included for analysis, the frequencies and ratios were calculated. Based on the children's TKM use reported by parents, the correlations between variables were analyzed using the chi-square test (χ^2-test), which is a cross-analysis method of the ratios between different groups and is commonly used when analyzing categorized data. IBM SPSS Statistics for Windows, version 25 (IBM Corp., Armonk, NY, USA) was used for all statistical analyses and the significance level was set at 5% ($p < 0.05$).

3. Results

3.1. The Information on and Characteristics of the Children of the Participants

The basic statistics of the 5000 participants (fathers or mothers) from the general population who participated in the survey were obtained based on their answers to the question regarding their children (Table 1). Regarding the question about their children, 872 participants answered that they had a child (or children) under the age of 19, accounting for 17.4% of all participants (Table 1). The majority of these contributors answered that they only had one child that fell into that particular age group ($n = 425$, 48.7%), which was followed by those with two children in the corresponding age group ($n = 393$, 45.1%). When asked whether their children had any experience of using TKM over the past 12-month period, 209 answered they had, while 663 answered none (24.0% and 76.0%, respectively).

Table 1. Information and characteristics of the respondent's children.

Category			n (%)
Existence of chlidren under 19	Yes		872 (17.4)
	No		4128 (85.6)
TKM experience of children reported by parents	Yes		209 (24.0)
	No		663 (76.0)
Number and TKM experiences of children	Number of children	1	425 (48.7)
	TKM experience of children reported by parents	Yes	78 (18.4)
		No	346 (81.6)
	Number of children	2	393 (45.1)
	TKM experience of children reported by parents	Yes	108 (27.5)
		No	285 (72.5)
	Number of children	3	52 (6.0)
	TKM experience of children reported by parents	Yes	22 (42.3)
		No	30 (57.7)
	Number of children	4	2 (0.2)
	TKM experience of children reported by parents	Yes	1 (50.0)
		No	1 (50.0)

TKM: Traditional Korean Medicine.

3.2. The Demographics of the Parents and Their Children's TKM Use Reported by Parents

Differences in the children's demographics were assessed based on their (or their parents) experience with TKM (Table 2). Interestingly, female participants were more likely to have children with experience of using TKM ($p = 0.029$). Furthermore, the chance of having a child with experience of using TKM was higher in Chungcheong ($n = 116$, 13.3%) and Gyeongsang ($n = 225$, 25.8%) areas compared to the capital area ($n = 371$, 42.5%). Participants in their 50 s (50 to 60 years or older) showed a higher value compared to participants that were 40 years old or younger (30 to 40 years or younger) ($p = 0.042$). There was also no difference in employment status in terms of the children's TKM usage reported by parents. No tendency of significance was observed with the household income as well. Participants with higher education levels (university or higher education) were more likely to answer that their children had experienced using TKM. However, the difference was not statistically significant. As for the types of government health care coverage, the groups without a child who experienced using TKM had a higher rate of having workplace health insurance coverage. Similarly, the group with children with experience of using TKM had a higher rate of having private medical insurance. However, these differences were non-statistically significant. Additionally, no significant differences were observed based on household income or area of residence.

Table 2. Characteristics of the study population from the survey with and without traditional Korean medicine (TKM) experience of children.

Category		Existence of TKM Experience of Children		Total n (%)	χ^2 (p)
		Yes n (%)	No n (%)		
Parent Gender	Male	57 (27.3)	235 (35.4)	292 (33.5)	4.765
	Female	152 (72.7)	428 (64.6)	580 (66.5)	($p = 0.029$)
Residence	Metropolitan	78 (37.3)	293 (44.2)	371 (42.5)	
	Chungcheng province	31 (14.8)	85 (12.8)	116 (13.3)	3.793
	Gyeongsang province	55 (26.3)	170 (25.6)	225 (25.8)	($p = 0.285$)
	Jeolla province	45 (21.5)	115 (17.3)	160 (18.3)	
Age	30 s ≤	2 (1.0)	31 (4.7)	33 (3.8)	
	40 s	79 (37.8)	277 (41.8)	356 (40.8)	8.196
	50 s	111 (53.1)	311 (46.9)	422 (48.4)	($p = 0.042$)
	≥60 s	17 (8.1)	44 (6.6)	61 (7.0)	
Job	Yes	139 (66.5)	449 (67.7)	588 (67.4)	0.107
	No	70 (33.5)	214 (32.3)	284 (32.6)	($p = 0.744$)
Household income	Less than 1500 USD	20 (0.5)	7 (1.1)	8 (0.9)	
	1500 USD less than 3000 USD	26 (12.4)	105 (15.8)	131 (15.0)	5.036
	3000 USD less than 4500 USD	79 (37.8)	267 (40.3)	346 (39.7)	($p = 0.284$)
	4500 USD less than 6000 USD	73 (34.9)	218 (32.9)	291 (33.4)	
	No less than 6000 USD	30 (14.4)	66 (10.0)	969 (11.0)	
Academic background	Primary or lower school graduate	1 (0.5)	4 (0.6)	5 (0.6)	
	Middle school graduate	0 (0.0)	8 (1.2)	8 (0.98)	3.034
	High school graduate	62 (29.7)	210 (31.7)	272 (31.2)	($p = 0.386$)
	University or higher school graduate	146 (69.9)	441 (66.5)	587 (67.3)	
Medical security type	Health insurance (district insurance)	63 (37.3)	149 (22.5)	212 (24.3)	5.619
	Health insurance (workplace insurance)	146 (69.9)	512 (77.2)	658 (75.5)	($p = 0.060$)
	Medical care	0 (0.0)	2 (0.3)	2 (0.2)	
Commercial insurance	Subscribed	192 (91.9)	579 (87.3)	771 (88.4)	3.192
	Unsubscribed	17 (8.1)	84 (12.7)	101 (11.6)	($p = 0.074$)

3.3. The Opinion of the Parents on Using TKM and Their Children's TKM Use Reported by Parents

Table 3 shows whether the children's TKM use reported by parents changed depending on the parents' ideas or experience in using TKM. This analysis revealed that the group with a child having experienced using TKM had a higher rate of having experienced TKM themselves, compared with the group without a child who experienced TKM ($p < 0.001$). Overall, the participants' satisfaction with the TKM did not show a significant difference.

Also, parents of the children with experience of using TKM showed a higher level of awareness of TKM ($p = 0.033$). The parents pre-conceived ideas regarding TKM did not result in a statistically significant result. The group with a child who experienced using TKM ($n = 198, 94.7\%$) had a higher number of participants who answered that they were willing to use TKM in the future, compared to children who did not experience using TKM ($n = 565, 85.2\%$) ($p = 0.003$). The group with children with experience of using TKM was more willing to recommend TKM to others ($p < 0.001$).

Table 3. Perception of the survey respondents with and without TKM experience of children.

Variables		Existence of TKM Experience of Children Reported by Parents		Total n (%)	χ2(p)
		Yes n (%)	No n (%)		
Parent's experience on TKM use	Yes	191 (91.4)	477 (71.9)	668 (76.6)	35.220 ($p < 0.001$)
	High school graduate or under	54 (25.8)	154 (23.2)	208 (23.9)	
	University or higher school graduate	137 (65.6)	323 (48.7)	460 (52.8)	
	No	18 (8.6)	186 (28.1)	204 (23.4)	
	High school graduate or under	9 (4.3)	68 (10.3)	77 (8.8)	
	University or higher school graduate	9 (4.3)	118 (17.8)	127 (14.6)	
Parent's satisfaction on TKM treatment	Satisfied	143 (74.9)	369 (77.4)	512 (76.6)	2.925 ($p = 0.712$)
	High school graduate or under	42 (22.0)	119 (24.9)	161 (24.1)	
	University or higher school graduate	101 (52.9)	250 (52.4)	351 (52.5)	
	Average	47 (24.6)	102 (21.4)	149 (22.3)	
	High school graduate or under	12 (6.3)	34 (7.1)	46 (6.9)	
	University or higher school graduate	35 (18.3)	68 (14.3)	103 (15.4)	
	Unsatisfied	1 (0.5)	6 (1.3)	7 (1.0)	
	High school graduate or under	0 (0.0)	1 (0.2)	1 (0.1)	
	University or higher school graduate	1 (0.5)	5 (1.0)	6 (0.9)	
Parent's perception on TKM	Well aware	92 (44.0)	234 (35.3)	326 (37.4)	12.125 ($p = 0.033$)
	High school graduate or under	31 (14.8)	71 (10.7)	102 (11.7)	
	University or higher school graduate	61 (29.2)	163 (24.6)	224 (25.7)	
	Average	72 (34.4)	214 (32.3)	286 (32.8)	
	High school graduate or under	19 (9.1)	68 (10.3)	87 (10.0)	
	University or higher school graduate	53 (25.4)	146 (22.0)	199 (22.8)	
	Not sure	45 (21.5)	215 (32.4)	260 (29.8)	
	High school graduate or under	13 (6.2)	83 (12.5)	96 (11.0)	
	University or higher school graduate	32 (15.3)	132 (19.9)	164 (18.8)	
TKM treatment cost	Expensive	135 (64.6)	386 (58.2)	521 (59.7)	6.055 ($p = 0.301$)
	High school graduate or under	46 (22.0)	129 (19.5)	175 (20.1)	
	University or higher school graduate	89 (42.6)	257 (38.8)	346 (39.7)	
	Average	62 (29.7)	239 (36.0)	301 (34.5)	
	High school graduate or under	14 (6.7)	77 (11.6)	91 (10.4)	
	University or higher school graduate	48 (23.0)	162 (24.4)	210 (24.1)	
	Inexpensive	12 (5.7)	38 (5.7)	50 (5.7)	
	High school graduate or under	3 (1.4)	16 (2.4)	19 (2.2)	
	University or higher school graduate	9 (4.3)	22 (3.3)	31 (3.6)	
Intention of re-visit	Yes	198 (94.7)	565 (85.2)	763 (87.5)	14.195 ($p = 0.003$)
	High school graduate or under	61 (29.2)	189 (28.5)	250 (28.7)	
	University or higher school graduate	137 (65.6)	376 (56.7)	513 (58.8)	
	No	11 (5.3)	98 (14.8)	109 (12.5)	
	High school graduate or under	2 (1.0)	33 (3.8)	35 (4.0)	
	University or higher school graduate	9 (4.3)	65 (9.8)	74 (8.5)	
Intention of recommendation	Yes	178 (85.2)	427 (64.4)	605 (69.4)	33.184 ($p < 0.001$)
	High school graduate or under	55 (26.3)	145 (21.9)	200 (22.9)	
	University or higher school graduate	123 (58.9)	282 (42.5)	405 (46.4)	
	No	31 (14.8)	236 (35.6)	267 (30.6)	
	High school graduate or under	8 (3.8)	77 (11.6)	85 (9.7)	
	University or higher school graduate	23 (11.0)	159 (24.0)	182 (20.9)	

The analysis based on the education levels of the participants showed that, of the 191 participants where all the children and the parents experienced TKM, the proportion of those with higher education was higher than the proportion of the same among the participants where either of or all of the parents of the children had not experienced TKM. A similar trend could be observed in the answers to the question whether they are willing to revisit a TKM clinic or recommend it to others.

3.4. Perception of the TKM Effectiveness for Diseases and Their Children's TKM Use Reported by Parents

Table 4 shows the analysis result on the perception of the treatment effectiveness for 16 diseases by the parents based on the children's TKM use reported by parents. The group in which the children experienced TKM in 14 out of the 16 diseases showed a higher level of perception on the treatment effect for each of the diseases. Of these, the group where the children experienced TKM for two diseases showed a perception level on the treatment effect that was higher by 10% compared to the group in which the children never experienced TKM. The said difference was statistically significant (Common cold rhinitis: $p = 0.011$, skin disease: $p = 0.002$).

Table 4. Perception of the TKM effectiveness of diseases of survey respondents with and without TKM experience of children.

Category		Existence of TKM Experience of Children Reported by Parents		Total n (%)	χ^2 (p)
		Yes n (%)	No n (%)		
Disc related disease (herniation of intervertebral disc, spinal stenosis)	Effective	157 (75.1)	480 (72.4)	637 (73.1)	2.364 ($p = 0.307$)
	Ineffective	38 (18.2)	115 (17.3)	153 (17.5)	
	No idea	14 (6.7)	68 (10.3)	82 (9.4)	
Osteoarthritis	Effective	158 (75.6)	474 (71.5)	632 (72.5)	1.754 ($p = 0.416$)
	Ineffective	36 (17.2)	124 (18.7)	160 (18.3)	
	No idea	15 (7.2)	65 (9.8)	80 (9.2)	
Frozen shoulder shoulder pain	Effective	180 (86.1)	550 (83.0)	730 (83.7)	1.221 ($p = 0.543$)
	Ineffective	17 (8.1)	69 (10.4)	86 (9.9)	
	No idea	12 (5.7)	44 (6.6)	56 (6.4)	
Back pain	Effective	191 (91.4)	568 (85.7)	759 (87.0)	5.166 ($p = 0.076$)
	Ineffective	9 (4.3)	58 (8.7)	67 (7.7)	
	No idea	9 (4.3)	37 (5.6)	46 (5.3)	
Sprain	Effective	189 (90.4)	559 (84.3)	748 (85.8)	5.170 ($p = 0.075$)
	Ineffective	11 (5.3)	65 (9.8)	76 (8.7)	
	No idea	9 (4.3)	39 (5.9)	48 (5.5)	
Facial nerve paralysis	Effective	152 (72.7)	480 (72.4)	632 (72.5)	0.112 ($p = 0.946$)
	Ineffective	37 (17.7)	123 (18.6)	160 (18.3)	
	No idea	20 (9.6)	60 (9.0)	80 (9.2)	
Stroke	Effective	132 (63.2)	412 (62.1)	544 (62.4)	0.560 ($p = 0.756$)
	Ineffective	52 (24.9)	180 (27.1)	232 (26.6)	
	No idea	25 (12.0)	71 (10.7)	96 (11.0)	
Hypertension	Effective	58 (27.8)	190 (28.7)	248 (28.4)	0.079 ($p = 0.961$)
	Ineffective	109 (52.2)	339 (51.1)	448 (51.4)	
	No idea	42 (20.1)	134 (20.2)	176 (20.2)	
Diabetes mellitus	Effective	55 (26.3)	157 (23.7)	212 (24.3)	0.699 ($p = 0.705$)
	Ineffective	111 (53.1)	358 (54.0)	469 (53.8)	
	No idea	43 (20.6)	148 (22.3)	191 (21.9)	
Digestive disease	Effective	128 (61.2)	361 (54.4)	489 (56.1)	4.261 ($p = 0.119$)
	Ineffective	59 (28.2)	199 (30.0)	258 (29.6)	
	No idea	22 (10.5)	103 (15.5)	125 (14.3)	

Table 4. Cont.

Category		Existence of TKM Experience of Children Reported by Parents		Total n (%)	χ² (p)
		Yes n (%)	No n (%)		
Common cold rhinitis	Effective	124 (59.3)	315 (47.5)	439 (50.3)	9.073 (p = 0.011)
	Ineffective	63 (30.1)	249 (37.6)	312 (35.8)	
	No idea	22 (10.5)	99 (14.9)	121 (13.9)	
Dementia	Effective	52 (24.9)	160 (24.1)	212 (24.3)	1.205 (p = 0.548)
	Ineffective	113 (54.1)	339 (51.1)	452 (51.8)	
	No idea	44 (21.1)	164 (24.7)	208 (23.9)	
Cancer related pain	Effective	44 (21.1)	149 (22.5)	193 (22.1)	1.461 (p = 0.482)
	Ineffective	116 (55.5)	337 (50.8)	453 (51.9)	
	No idea	49 (23.4)	177 (26.7)	226 (25.9)	
Infertility	Effective	72 (34.4)	217 (32.7)	289 (33.1)	0.241 (p = 0.887)
	Ineffective	92 (44.0)	296 (44.6)	388 (44.5)	
	No idea	45 (21.5)	150 (22.6)	195 (22.4)	
Skin disease (atopic dermatitis)	Effective	107 (51.2)	250 (37.7)	357 (40.9)	12.043 (p = 0.002)
	Ineffective	68 (32.5)	282 (42.5)	350 (40.1)	
	No idea	34 (16.3)	131 (19.8)	165 (18.9)	
Genitourinary disease	Effective	70 (33.5)	188 (28.4)	258 (29.6)	2.104 (p = 0.349)
	Ineffective	92 (44.0)	321 (48.4)	413 (47.4)	
	No idea	47 (22.5)	154 (23.2)	201 (23.1)	

4. Discussion

In this study, which was based on the assumption that the experience, opinion, or ideas of parents may influence the use of TKM by their children, the participants were divided into groups based on whether their children had experienced using TKM or not; comparisons were made to evaluate whether these groups showed any differences in terms of the characteristics, awareness, or satisfaction of the parents. This analysis was done for the purpose of developing policies and identifying the ideal time for intervention by understanding the differences in satisfaction and awareness between the two groups.

The initial analysis regarding the participant's children showed that, out of the 5000 participants, 17.4% (n = 872) had a child under the age of 19. Of these, 24% (n = 209) answered that their children experienced the use of TKM. In previous studies, it was reported that 55.3% of the target population had a child with TKM use experience [26], and in another, 81% [25]. However, caution should be practiced when interpreting these results as the target populations were from a daycare center within a self-governing district or the outpatients of a TKM clinic who were familiar with TKM pediatric practices. Especially, the value of 81% provided in Choi [25] was in contrast with the result of this study, where the proportion of the children who experienced TKM was 17.4%. It is believed to be because of the bias in the selection of the participants, who were selected from the patients who used the TKM clinic of the researcher. In this study, certified national statistics were used and thus based on a representative, standard sample of Korea's general public; therefore, it is believed that the result can be generalized. Also, this study supports the findings in some preceding studies [25,26] that TKM clinics are used to treat the respiratory disease and skin disease in children. However, the said study could not cover the analysis on the purpose for the parents to use TKM clinics due to the limitations of the questions in the questionnaire, making it necessary to use caution in interpreting these findings, as it was assumed using the perception of treatment effect by parents based on the children's TKM use reported by parents.

The reason why the children in Chungcheong and Gyeongsang regions are more likely to use TKM compared to those in the Capital area is attributed to the shortage of mainstream medical institutions (e.g., CM institutions and TKM institutions) and the demographics of these areas. These two regions are some of the most representative examples of a combination of urban and rural areas in the same region [27]. Also, the demographics of these areas are heavily leaning toward the older population compared to children [27].

The results of the analysis were used to observe whether there was a difference in the characteristics of the parents depending on the experience of their children with TKM showed that 8.1% more females (mothers) answered that their children had experienced using TKM. Also, as the participants grew older, being in their 50 s or older, the rate of answering that their children had experienced using TKM, tended to be higher. This supports the existing study result, where females were more likely to use TKM, and 61.8% of the users of TKM were at least 45 or older [28]. However, this study does not clarify the factors and correlations. Therefore, care is needed as one attempts to interpret it. Future studies are needed to investigate what is the true tendency of female and people in their 50 s or older in their use of TKM and what are the factors that contribute to such a result. Based on such findings, it would be possible to employ a more detailed approach to the use of TKM by the children.

On the other hand, the fact that those in their 30 s or 40 s were less likely to use TKM, compared to those in their 50 s or older, can be attributed to the fact that the younger group corresponds with the prime age of workers, namely those aged 25 to 49 [29], a time when individuals are the most active in terms of economic activities. In addition, if both parents of the children are working, it would be more likely that they would experience time or money obstacles, when trying to seek out using TKM. The findings of this study suggest that if the accessibility to TKM is improved for individuals in their 50 s, the younger parents in their 30 s to 40 s, and females, it would be possible to improve accessibility for their children. Also, in the group where the children had experienced TKM, the proportion of those with a higher level of education was higher among those who gave positive answers concerning the experience of the parents, intent to use in the future, and willingness to recommend. This can be interpreted to be because of the financial resources, desire to be healthy, and interest among these higher-education groups. However, further study is needed in order to clarify this correlation.

About 60% of the participants answered that TKM treatments were more expensive, which is related to the reimbursement ratio of the health care insurance of Korea. As of 2019, the reimbursement coverage rate by the health care insurance over the entirety of medical institutions in Korea was 64.2%, while the rate for TKM clinics was 54% and TKM hospitals was 28.7% [30]. This is based on the national policy that the health care insurance coverage is to be provided for the treatments with a clear scientific basis to treat severe diseases. While CM treatments have accumulated scientific evidence all over the world, CAM treatments and traditional treatments differ between countries, making it difficult to build up scientific evidence. Therefore, it is necessary to accumulate scientific evidence for the treatment effectiveness and safety by means of exchange and harmonization of traditional medicine and CAM with international organizations such as the World Health Organization taking the leading role. If such a worldwide basis of evidence is built, it could be possible to integrate traditional medicine and CAM treatments into the healthcare coverage, eventually contributing to the improvement of the health of the public.

Children of parents with an experience of using TKM were more likely to use TKM, compared with children whose parents had no experience with using TKM. Of the children whose parents experienced using TKM, 91.4% used TKM (n = 191) themselves, while 71.9% of the children whose parents never used TKM used it (n = 477) (p < 0.001). This indicates that the parents' experience with using TKM had a significant impact (20%) on the use of TKM by their children. The Ministry of Health and Welfare developed the TKM health promotion program for toddlers and infants in 2016 [31], which has gradually been implemented through community health centers [32]. As such, in order for the State to maximize the effectiveness of childhood health management, mainly via TKM, a policy-based approach is needed such that the parents of these children may be provided with health management programs through TKM, as well.

In the group of parents whose children experienced using TKM, the rate of answering that they were willing to revisit a TKM clinic was higher by 9.5%, while the rate of answering that they were willing to recommend to others was higher by 20.8% ($p = 0.003$). This indicates that the perception of the parents impacted the use of TKM by their children, and the improvement of the perception of these parents may have an impact on the use of TKM by their children. It is necessary to conduct further studies in order to clarify these correlations.

The limitations of this study were as follows: first, due to the limitations in the data gathered for this study, it was not possible to clarify the correlations between the parents' experience, awareness, and satisfaction with the use of TKM or the use of TKM by their children. Additional studies are needed in order to clarify which variables among the parents' awareness, the purpose of visit, sex, or age, etc., had an impact on the use of TKM by their children. Second, the data obtained through the survey was based on the memories of parents, who were the participants of the survey. Therefore, it is still possible that they answered incorrectly when asked about their children's experience with TKM. Third, the age group of the children of the participants could have had an impact on the experience of using a TKM clinic. However, it was not possible to obtain information on the age of the children. That is, younger children were more likely to have not experienced TKM, which could have contributed to the outcome. Lastly, due to the limitations in the questionnaires, it was not possible to identify the type of treatment the participating patients received. Among the CAM treatments [5,33], vitamins and minerals, probiotics, yoga, qigong, meditation, tai chi, relation techniques, and hypnotherapy are rarely used in TKM clinics, and health insurance coverage of TKM treatment [11] includes acupuncture, electro-acupuncture, pharmacopuncture, herbal medicine, chuna, cupping, and moxibustion. Therefore, it is difficult to compare the usage status and perception of TKM and CAM at the same level and generalize the results of this study.

The strength of this study is that it was conducted using data that is representative of the general Korean population, making the study more generalizable so that the study results can be used as a resource for the government to develop relevant policies. Also, it would be necessary to conduct an in-depth analysis on the decision-makers who decide which medical services to be used, as it is likely that the selection of the medical services used by a child is influenced by parental decisions.

In the future, the following strategies will be needed for the popularization of TKM. First, it is necessary to obtain precise statistical data on the factors and usage of TKM by improving the questionnaire items for the national survey in the future. Based on this study, it was possible to understand that the awareness of the family members on TKM could have an impact on the use of TKM by other members. However, due to the limitations in the question items in the questionnaire, we had difficulties in the analysis of correlations and factors. During the subsequent round of the national survey, the following supplementations are believed to be necessary: (1) Add questions regarding the experience of talking with a family physician or the experience of actually using the TKM for a disease or symptoms; (2) add more question items to ask whether the parents' jobs were related to health care or they were actually healthcare professional, and if so, what type of healthcare professionals; (3) add more question items regarding awareness, the intent of use in the future, intent of the recommendation, and an item regarding the preference toward TKM; (4) more survey items for the children, regarding their age, education, and treated interventions and diseases; and (5) if questions are asked about the use of TKM by the children, conduct a face-to-face interview of the parents and the children at the same time. If the above-mentioned items are supplemented, it would be possible to clarify the point of intervention through policies by means of statistical analyses. Second, government-level standardization is required for the Clinical Practice Guideline (CPG) and the Clinical Pathway (CP) centered around the diseases for which TKM has an advantage over CM. Choose the diseases for which TKM has an advantage in different stages of the life cycle and develop corresponding CPGs and CPs (e.g., children; atopic dermatitis, females; dysmenorrhea, adults; back pain, seniors; osteoarthritis). With the policies to include these into the coverage of health care, it would have an impact on the family members of TKM users, contributing to popularization. In particular, the use and awareness of TKM by a female parent is likely to have an impact on her child. Therefore, it is necessary to survey the diseases in more details when it comes to female participants (e.g., menstruation, sub-fertility, post-natal management, climacterium, and menopause).

5. Conclusions

The present study investigated the correlation between parents' perception and the existence of children's experience with TKM by analyzing the 2017 national survey of TKM usage. The results indicate that the parents' experience of using TKM and their awareness contributed to the differences in their children's experience of using TKM. Our study suggests that the parent's experience of using TKM could have an impact on the children's experience of using TKM. In the future, policy-based interventions would have to be considered for the parents when establishing TKM policies for their children.

Author Contributions: Conceptualization, J.K. and S.-H.S.; methodology, J.K., J.-K.P. and S.-H.S.; software, J.K.; validation, J.K. and J.-Y.P.; formal analysis, J.K.; investigation, J.K.; resources, J.K.; data curation, J.K.; writing—original draft preparation, J.K. and S.-H.S.; writing—review and editing, J.-Y.P., E.-J.L. and S.-H.S.; visualization, J.K.; supervision, S.-H.S.; project administration, S.-H.S.; funding acquisition, S.-H.S. All authors have read and agreed to the published version of the manuscript.

Funding: This work was supported by the Project of Traditional Korean Medicine Community Care Monitoring and Evaluation funded by the Ministry of Health &Welfare.

Institutional Review Board Statement: Not applicable.

Informed Consent Statement: Not applicable.

Data Availability Statement: The data will be made available upon reasonable request.

Conflicts of Interest: The authors declare that there are no conflicts of interest regarding the publication of this paper.

References

1. World Health Organization. *WHO Traditional Medicine Strategy: 2014–2023*; World Health Organization: Geneva, Switzerland, 2013; Available online: https://www.who.int/medicines/publications/traditional/trm_strategy14_23/en/ (accessed on 12 December 2020).
2. Abuduli, M.; Ezat, W.P.; Aljunid, S. Role of traditional and complementary medicine in universal coverage. *Malays. J. Public Health Med.* **2011**, *11*, 1–5.
3. Kristoffersen, A.E.; Stub, T.; Broderstad, A.R.; Hansen, A.H. Use of traditional and complementary medicine among Norwegian cancer patients in the seventh survey of the Tromsø study. *BMC Complement. Altern. Med.* **2019**, *19*, 341. [CrossRef] [PubMed]
4. National Center for Complementary and Integrative Health. Complementary, Alternative, or Integrative Health: What's in a Name? 2015. Available online: https://www.nccih.nih.gov/health/complementary-alternative-or-integrative-health-whats-in-a-name (accessed on 12 December 2020).
5. Ding, A.; Patel, J.P.; Auyeung, V. Understanding the Traditional Chinese Medicine (TCM) consultation: Why do patients adhere to treatment? *Complement. Ther. Clin. Pract.* **2020**, *39*, 101139. [CrossRef]
6. World Health Organization. *WHO Global Report on Traditional and Complementary Medicine 2019*; World Health Organization: Geneva, Switzerland, 2019; Available online: http://www.who.int/publications/i/item/978924151536 (accessed on 12 December 2020).
7. Huang, C.W.; Tran, D.N.H.; Li, T.F.; Sasaki, Y.; Lee, J.A.; Lee, M.S.; Chen, F.P. The utilization of complementary and alternative medicine in Taiwan: An internet survey using an adapted version of the international questionnaire (I-CAM-Q). *J. Chin. Med. Assoc.* **2019**, *82*, 665–671. [CrossRef] [PubMed]
8. Na-Bangchang, K.; Karbwang, J. Traditional herbal medicine for the control of tropical diseases. *Trop. Med. Health* **2014**, *42*, 3–13. [CrossRef]

9. Ko, C.R.; Ku, N.P.; Seol, S.S. A Comparative Study on the Traditional Medicine Policies between Korea and China: Focused on the Second Korean Medicine Development Plan and the 12.5 Traditional Chinese Medicine Development Plan. *J. Korea Technol. Innov. Soc.* **2014**, *17*, 421–447.
10. Park, H.L.; Lee, H.S.; Shin, B.C.; Liu, J.P.; Shang, Q.; Yamashita, H.; Lim, B. Traditional medicine in China, Korea, and Japan: A brief introduction and comparison. *Evid.-Based Complement. Altern. Med.* **2012**, *2012*, 429103. [CrossRef] [PubMed]
11. Kim, H.T.; Hwang, E.H.; Heo, I.; Cho, J.H.; Kim, K.W.; Ha, I.H.; Shin, B.C. Clinical practice guidelines for the use of traditional Korean medicine in the treatment of patients with traffic-related injuries: An evidence-based approach. *Eur. J. Integr. Med.* **2018**, *18*, 34–41. [CrossRef]
12. Suh, N.K.; Kang, T.W.; Heo, S.I.; Lee, H.J.; Kim, D.S.; Lim, B.M.; Jang, S.R.; Hong, K.M.; Jung, S.H.; Oh, Y.H. *The Korean Health System Based on Healthcare Indicators*; Korea Institute for Health and Social Affairs: Sejong, Korea, 2016.
13. Ministry of Health and Welfare; National Development Institute of Korean Medicine; Gallup Korea. *2017 Years National Survey for Traditional Korean Medicine (TKM) Usage*; National Development Institute of Korean Medicine: Seoul, Korea, 2018; Available online: https://www.koms.or.kr/board/researchReport/view.do?post_no=45&menu_no=21 (accessed on 17 December 2020).
14. Kim, J.W.; Choi, J.S. An analysis of family structure on children's medical utilization. *Korean J. Soc. Welf.* **2016**, *68*, 5–27.
15. Blackwell, D.L.; Hayward, M.D.; Crimmins, E.M. Does childhood health affect chronic morbidity in later life? *Soc. Sci. Med.* **2001**, *52*, 1269–1284. [CrossRef]
16. Larsson, I.; Svedberg, P.; Arvidsson, S.; Nygren, J.M.; Carlsson, M. Parents' experiences of an e-health intervention implemented in pediatric healthcare: A qualitative study. *BMC Health Serv. Res.* **2019**, *19*, 800. [CrossRef]
17. An, J.S.; Kim, H.J. A study on the determinants of children and adolescents' health Inequality in Korea. *Stud. Korean Youth* **2013**, *24*, 205–231.
18. Lee, Y.W. Family Income and child health gradient in Korea. *Health Soc. Welf. Rev.* **2014**, *34*, 7–32.
19. Case, A.; Lubotsky, D.; Paxson, C. Economic status and health in childhood: The origins of the gradient. *Am. Econ. Rev.* **2002**, *92*, 1308–1334. [CrossRef]
20. Currie, J. Healthy, wealthy, and wise: Socioeconomic status, poor health in childhood, and human capital development. *J. Econ. Lit.* **2009**, *47*, 87–122. [CrossRef]
21. Basu, A.M.; Stephenson, R. Low levels of maternal education and the proximate determinants of childhood mortality: A little learning is not a dangerous thing. *Soc. Sci. Med.* **2005**, *60*, 2011–2023. [CrossRef]
22. Braveman, P.; Gottlieb, L. The social determinants of health: It's time to consider the causes of the causes. *Public Health Rep.* **2014**, *129*, 19–31. [CrossRef]
23. Loh, C.H. Use of traditional chinese medicine in singapore children: Perceptions of parents and paediatricians. *Singap. Med. J.* **2009**, *50*, 1162–1168.
24. Yeh, Y.H.; Chou, Y.J.; Huang, N.; Pu, C.; Chou, P. The trends of utilization in traditional chinese medicine in taiwan from 2000 to 2010: A population-based study. *Medicine* **2016**, *95*, e4115. [CrossRef]
25. Choi, Y.J.; Kim, J.H. Survey on outpatients' perception and use of pediatric herbal medicine. *J. Korea Inst. Orient. Med. Inform.* **1995**, *1*, 1–24.
26. Park, Y.J.; Lee, S.J.; Yoon, J.Y.; Myoung, S.M. A survey on parent's recognition and utilization patterns of oriental medical care of preschool students in Seong-Dong district. *J. Pediatr. Korean Med.* **2011**, *25*, 90–110. [CrossRef]
27. Kim, E.S.; Kim, J.; Kim, B.; Park, K. Classification of regional age structure based on dynamic age structure model and an analysis of association among regional population, economy, education and welfare environment. *Korea J. Popul. Stud.* **2019**, *42*, 83–113.
28. Kim, D.S. Study on Factors Related to the Use of Oriental Medical Service among Outpatient. Ph.D. Thesis, Yonsei University, Seoul, Korea, 2013.
29. Choi, Y.S.; Kim, M.Y.; Lim, U. The effects of local labor market characteristics on migration of prime-age workers in Korea. *J. Korea Plan. Assoc.* **2015**, *50*, 25–42. [CrossRef]
30. National Health Insurance Service. *2019 Years Survey on the Benefit Coverage Rate of National Health Insurance*; National Health Insurance Service: Wonju, Korea, 2020.
31. Park, H.M.; Lee, S.D.; Sung, H.K.; Min, D.L.; Park, S.J.; Sung, D.M. *Development of Traditional Korean Medicine Health Promotion Program for Infants and Children*; Ministry of Health and Welfare: Sejong, Korea, 2016.
32. Korea Health Promotion Institute. 2021 Integrated Community Health Promotion Program: Traditional Korean Medicine (TKM) Health Promotion. 2020. Available online: https://www.khealth.or.kr/kps/publish/view?menuId=MENU00890&page_no=B2017003&board_idx=10454 (accessed on 13 January 2021).
33. Rodrigues, J.M.; Mestre, M.; Fredes, L.I. Qigong in the treatment of children with autism spectrum disorder: A systematic review. *J. Integr. Med.* **2019**, *17*, 250–260. [CrossRef] [PubMed]

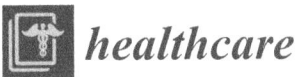

Article

Korean Medicine Clinical Practice Guidelines for Lumbar Herniated Intervertebral Disc in Adults: Based on Grading of Recommendations Assessment, Development and Evaluation (GRADE)

Bonhyuk Goo [1,†], Min-gi Jo [1,†], Eun-Jung Kim [2], Hyun-Jong Lee [3], Jae-Soo Kim [3], Dongwoo Nam [4], Jung Won Kang [4], Tae-Hun Kim [5], Yeon-Cheol Park [4], Yong-Hyeon Baek [4], Sang-Soo Nam [4], Myeong Soo Lee [6] and Byung-Kwan Seo [4,*]

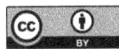

Citation: Goo, B.; Jo, M.-g.; Kim, E.-J.; Lee, H.-J.; Kim, J.-S.; Nam, D.; Kang, J.W.; Kim, T.-H.; Park, Y.-C.; Baek, Y.-H.; et al. Korean Medicine Clinical Practice Guidelines for Lumbar Herniated Intervertebral Disc in Adults: Based on Grading of Recommendations Assessment, Development and Evaluation (GRADE). Healthcare 2022, 10, 246. https://doi.org/10.3390/healthcare10020246

Academic Editors: Manoj Sharma and Kavita Batra

Received: 25 December 2021
Accepted: 24 January 2022
Published: 27 January 2022

Publisher's Note: MDPI stays neutral with regard to jurisdictional claims in published maps and institutional affiliations.

Copyright: © 2022 by the authors. Licensee MDPI, Basel, Switzerland. This article is an open access article distributed under the terms and conditions of the Creative Commons Attribution (CC BY) license (https://creativecommons.org/licenses/by/4.0/).

1 Department of Acupuncture & Moxibustion, Kyung Hee University Hospital at Gangdong, Seoul 05278, Korea; goobh99@naver.com (B.G.); turtlessam@naver.com (M.-g.J.)
2 Department of Acupuncture & Moxibustion Medicine, College of Oriental Medicine, Dongguk University, Gyeongju-si 38066, Korea; hanijjung@naver.com
3 Department of Acupuncture & Moxibustion Medicine, College of Korean Medicine, Daegu Haany University, Daegu 42158, Korea; whiteyyou@hanmail.net (H.-J.L.); jaice@daum.net (J.-S.K.)
4 Department of Acupuncture & Moxibustion Medicine, College of Korean Medicine, Kyung Hee University, Seoul 02447, Korea; hanisanam@daum.net (D.N.); doctorkang@naver.com (J.W.K.); icarus08@hanmail.net (Y.-C.P.); byhacu@khu.ac.kr (Y.-H.B.); dangun66@gmail.com (S.-S.N.)
5 Korean Medicine Clinical Trial Center, Department of Korean Medicine, Korean Medicine Hospital, Kyung Hee University, Seoul 02447, Korea; rockandmineral@gmail.com
6 KM Science Research Division, Korea Institute of Oriental Medicine, Daejeon 34054, Korea; drmslee@gmail.com
* Correspondence: seohbk@hanmail.net
† These authors contributed equally to this work.

Abstract: A significant number of individuals suffer from low back pain throughout their lifetime, and the medical costs related to low back pain and disc herniation are gradually increasing in Korea. Korean medicine interventions have been used for the treatment of lumbar intervertebral disc herniation. Therefore, we aimed to update the existing Korean medicine clinical practice guidelines for lumbar intervertebral disc herniation. A review of the existing guidelines for clinical treatment and analysis of questionnaires targeting Korean medicine doctors were performed. Subsequently, key questions on the treatment method of Korean medicine used for disc herniation in actual clinical trials were derived, and drafts of recommendations were formed after literature searches using the Grading of Recommendations, Assessment, Development and Evaluation. An expert consensus was reached on the draft through the Delphi method and final recommendations were made through review by the development project team and the monitoring committee. Fifteen recommendations for seven interventions for lumbar disc herniation were derived, along with the grade of recommendation and the level of evidence. The existing Korean medicine clinical practice guidelines for lumbar intervertebral disc herniation have been updated. Continuous updates will be needed through additional research in the future.

Keywords: clinical practice guideline; Korean medicine; lumbar intervertebral disc herniation; grading of recommendations assessment; development and evaluation

1. Introduction

With the ageing of the intervertebral disc, the compression force increases, squeezing out the nucleus pulposus through the fissure and resulting in the mechanical pressure on the spinal nerve that causes low back pain (LBP) and radiating pain, known as lumbar intervertebral disc herniation (LHIVD) [1].

In Korea, the overall annual incidence rate for spinal disease was a median of 16,387 per 100,000 individuals in 2016. The incidence rate and annual costs per patient increased by 7.6% and 14.7%, respectively, over the period from 2012 to 2016. The incidence and medical expenses of LHIVD were the highest in patients aged under 60 years [2].

Several clinical practice guidelines (CPGs) with a focus on Western medicine are available for LHIVD, such as CPGs for the diagnosis and treatment of LHIVD with radiculopathy (North American Spine Society, 2012) [3]. In Korea, several Korean medicine (KM) treatments are used to treat low back pain. As a result of a survey on low back pain patients conducted by the Ministry of Health and Welfare in 2017, 83.1% of outpatients and 90.3% of inpatients answered that they thought KM was effective, indicating a high level of trust in KM treatment [4].

In 2015, the Korea Institute of Oriental Medicine (KIOM) developed guidelines for LHIVD based on an acknowledgment of the need to amend the CPG evaluation instrument using the Appraisal of Guidelines for Research and Evaluation (AGREE) II [5]. We aimed to update the outdated 2015 KM CPGs for LHIVD and use Grading of Recommendations Assessment, Development and Evaluation (GRADE) to provide appropriate recommendations and address the key clinical questions about LHIVD in adults for KM doctors.

2. Materials and Methods

2.1. Planning of CPG Development

We collected and analyzed new data with previous data that was used as evidence in the latest KM CPGs for LHIVD [6], which was developed by KIOM in 2015. To establish a revision strategy, a questionnaire was developed to investigate KM doctors' current utilization and opinions about KM CPGs for LHIVD. The survey was conducted by sending an email to all KM doctors. The survey items included awareness, utilization, accessibility, understanding, usability for explanation, usability for clinical decisions, and improvement points of the existing guidelines. To reflect the opinions of the clinicians, the frequency of intervention, demand for clinical trials, and use of herbal medicines were also investigated [7].

2.2. Development Process

A development committee analyzed previously developed CPGs for LHIVD and selected the key clinical questions with the results of the questionnaire survey. The Korean Acupuncture and Moxibustion Medicine Society, Society of Korean Medicine Rehabilitation, Association of the Spine and Joint Korean Medicine, and related experts reviewed and approved the key questions. After screening, quality evaluation, and synthesis of the retrieved literature, the recommendations were drafted. Expert consensus was reached on the draft using the Delphi method. After an internal review, an external review by the Korean Medical Standard Clinical Practice Guideline Project Group and the monitoring committee was conducted. Subsequently, the CPGs were reviewed and certified by the relevant group.

2.3. Establishment of the Expert Committee

The expert committee consisted of a working group and a review committee. The working group collected evidence on the key clinical questions and drafted the CPGs. The multidisciplinary experts, including economic evaluators, clinical experts, methodology experts, and guide users, participated in this activity. The review committee group reviewed the draft version and decided on the final recommendations.

2.4. Key Clinical Question

Acupuncture, pharmacopuncture, herbal medicine, Tuina manual therapy, moxibustion, thread-embedding acupuncture (TEA), and cupping were evaluated as KM interventions. The effects of single treatment, combination treatment, and differences in the effect according to the technique of the same treatment method were set for each intervention as three categories of clinical questions.

In the comparative intervention, the active control group included all interventions actually used for therapeutic purposes in Western medicine, and the category of conventional treatments applied as a combination therapy encompassed all the current KM and Western medicine interventions actually used for therapeutic purposes.

2.5. Search Strategy

The following international databases were used: PubMed, EMBASE, Cochrane Library, China National Knowledge Infrastructure, Citation Information by NII, and J-stage. The following Korean databases were used: KoreaMed, Korean Medical Database, Korean Studies Information Service System, National Digital Science Library, Korea Institute of Science and Technology Information, and Oriental Medicine Advanced Searching Integrated System. The search process was performed by setting the search period until May 2019, including the data from the last CPGs. Details regarding the search strategy and PICO approach are shown in the Supplementary Materials S1.

2.6. Selection of Study

Two independent reviewers performed the screening procedure. Duplicate articles were excluded, and the selection and exclusion processes through the title, abstract, and full-text review were performed sequentially. The preferred reporting items for systematic reviews and meta-analyses (PRISMA) were adopted.

Randomized controlled clinical trial studies (RCTs) adopting the following three designs and including adult patients with LHIVD were selected based on the PICO approach:

(1) KM treatment vs. active control.
(2) KM treatment + conventional treatment vs. conventional treatment.
(3) Specific technique of KM treatment vs. another technique of same KM intervention

The exclusion criteria were as follows:

1. Non-RCTs, such as literature reviews, case reports, observational studies, and animal experiments.
2. Unclear presentation of the evaluation tool or method.
3. In the case of an intervention that cannot be used in the clinical field or an intervention that cannot be viewed as a medical practice.
4. When the specific effect of the intervention alone cannot be confirmed due to the design problems of the experimental group and the control group.

2.7. Quality Assessment of the Studies

The Cochrane Risk of Bias Evaluation tool [8] was used for RCTs included in this study. All the evaluations were performed by two independent researchers. In case of disagreement, an agreement was reached with the aid of the supervisor.

2.8. Analysis and Synthesis of Evidence

The evidence gathered for each clinical question was synthesized and analyzed through a meta-analysis. The analysis was conducted using RevMan 5.3, provided by Cochrane.

The evidence was synthesized for each evaluation index of the evidence documents included in each clinical question. For a continuous variable, the mean difference (MD) was derived, and for a nominal variable, the risk ratio (RR) was derived to evaluate the magnitude and significance of the effect.

The magnitude and significance of the effect were used to establish a basic grade at the level of evidence and evaluate non-precision. The sample size of the data synthesized for each indicator was applied to the imprecision evaluation, and the heterogeneity data (I^2) derived during the evidence synthesis process was applied to the inconsistency item when evaluating the level of evidence.

2.9. Classification of the Level of Evidence

We used the GRADE, developed by the Cochrane GRADE working group, to determine the level of evidence and the grade of recommendation [9]. In the GRADE, the level of evidence is preferentially determined according to the study design. RCTs are categorized as having a high level of evidence while observational studies are categorized as having a low level of evidence. If there is a risk of bias, inconsistency, indirectness, imprecision, or publication bias through the evaluation of evidence in a systematic literature review, the level of evidence is lowered by the first or second grade. If the effect size is large, the confounding variable reduces the effect size or if there is a dose–response relationship, the level of evidence can be increased.

The GRADE categorizes the level of evidence into four categories: high, moderate, low, and very low [10]. In the past, the definition of the level of evidence meant the possibility of change according to future research; however, since further research is not always possible, it has been revised to be the level of confidence now. In our CPGs, the classification of the classical text-based (CTB) level of evidence was also applied. The levels of evidence and definitions are provided in Table 1.

Table 1. GRADE level of evidence.

Level of Evidence	Definition
High	We are very confident that the true effect lies close to that of the estimate of the effect.
Moderate	We are moderately confident of the effect estimate; the true effect is likely to be close to the estimate of the effect; however, there is a possibility that it is substantially different.
Low	Our confidence in the effect estimate is limited: The true effect may be substantially different from the estimate of the effect.
Very low	We have very little confidence in the effect estimate; the true effect is likely to be substantially different from the estimate of the effect.
Classical text-based	Although there is evidence recorded in the classical texts, such as traditional Korean medicine books, evidence studies using modern research methodology have not been conducted.

2.10. Development and Agreement of Recommendations

2.10.1. Principles of Creating Recommendations

Recommendations were prepared according to the following principles:

(1) The recommendations should contain a specific and accurate description of what management is appropriate for a particular situation and patient based on the evidence.
(2) The key recommendations should be easily identifiable.
(3) The recommendations and the supporting evidence should be linked.
(4) The level of recommendation should be properly expressed.
(5) The patients or population targeted for the recommendation and the recommended intervention should be specified in as much detail as possible.

2.10.2. Recommendation Grade

The level of recommendation was determined by the magnitude of the benefit or harm. Based on the level of evidence, focusing on the level of confidence in the effect, comparison between the desired and unwanted effects, reliability of values and preferences, and use of resources was conducted.

When the benefit outweighs the harm, the use of the intervention is recommended and the recommendation grade A is assigned. According to the degree, grades B, C, and D are assigned separately.

If the CTB level of evidence is derived based on the textbook of KM prescribed by the Ministry of Health and Welfare and the Ministry of Food and Drug Safety and textbooks of the KM College, the utilization in the clinical field is evaluated and the Good Practice Point (GPP) grade was assigned through the expert consensus process of the development committee. An external consensus was conducted using the Delphi technique. The definitions and notations of the recommendation grades are summarized in Table 2.

Table 2. GRADE definitions and notations.

Grade	Definition	Notation
A	It is recommended when the benefits are clear, and utilization is high in the clinical field.	Is recommended
B	It is given when the benefit is reliable, and the utilization is high or moderate in the real-world practice or when the clinical benefit is obvious even though the evidence from the research related to the evidence of the recommendation is insufficient.	Should be considered
C	It is given when the benefit is not reliable; however, the utilization is high or moderate in the treatment field.	May be considered
D	Benefits are unreliable and can cause harmful consequences.	Is not recommended
Good Practice Point	It is recommended on the basis of a group of experts based on bibliographic evidence or clinical utilization.	Is recommended based on the expert group consensus

2.11. AGREEII

According to the 23 main items of AGREE II, [11] the contents of CPGs was reviewed. Some points of errors, Such as Instances of essential content omission, non-specific content descriptions, descriptions of inappropriate contents were pointed out. A repeated feedback process was performed by adding and revising the inappropriate points.

3. Results

Our CPGs confirmed 15 recommendations based on the 7 types of KM treatments containing interventions, comparators, level of evidence, and grade of recommendation for the key clinical questions (Table 3). PRISMA flow charts and the GRADE data including the outcome measures, risk of bias, inconsistency, indirectness, imprecision, and other considerations are summarized in the Supplementary Materials S2. The details of recommendation and clinical findings, including the number of patients, number of studies, and pooled relative effect with p values extracted from all the included studies, are summarized in the Supplementary Materials S3.

Table 3. Interventions, comparators, and level of evidence/grade of recommendation for the key clinical questions.

Key Clinical Question	Intervention (I)	Comparator (C)	Grade of Recommendation/Level of Evidence/
Acupuncture			
CQ1. Is acupuncture treatment helpful to improve the overall symptoms in adult patients with lumbar intervertebral disc herniation compared to usual conventional treatment (UCT)?	Acupuncture	UCT	A/High
CQ2. Is acupuncture treatment with UCT helpful to improve the pain and overall symptoms in adult patients with lumbar intervertebral disc herniation compared to UCT?	Acupuncture + UCT	UCT	A/Moderate
CQ3. Is electro-acupuncture, fire needling, or warm needling treatment helpful to improve the overall symptoms in adult patients with lumbar intervertebral disc herniation compared to acupuncture?	Electro-acupuncture, fire needling, or warm needling	Acupuncture	A/High
CQ4. Is the deep-injection acupuncture treatment helpful to improve the overall symptoms in adult patients with lumbar intervertebral disc herniation compared to superficial-injection acupuncture?	Deep-injection acupuncture	Superficial-injection acupuncture	B/Moderate

Table 3. Cont.

Key Clinical Question	Intervention (I)	Comparator (C)	Grade of Recommendation/Level of Evidence/
Moxibustion			
CQ5. Is moxibustion treatment helpful to improve the overall symptoms in adult patients with lumbar intervertebral disc herniation compared to UCT?	Moxibustion	UCT	GPP/Very low
CQ6. Is a combination treatment or moxibustion with acupuncture or Tuina manual therapy treatment helpful to improve the overall symptoms in adult patients with lumbar intervertebral disc herniation compared to acupuncture or Tuina monotherapy?	Moxibustion + acupuncture or moxibustion + Tuina manual therapy	Acupuncture or Tuina manual therapy	A/High
CQ7. Is moxibustion treatment that suspends deqi sensation helpful in improving the overall symptoms in adult patients with lumbar intervertebral disc herniation compared to moxibustion treatment that does not cause deqi sensation?	Moxibustion with deqi sensation	Moxibustion without deqi sensation	C/Low
Herbal medicine			
CQ8. Is herbal medicine monotherapy helpful to improve the overall symptoms in adult patients with lumbar intervertebral disc herniation compared to UCT?	Herbal medicine	UCT	B/Moderate
CQ9. Is herbal medicine with UCT helpful to improve the overall symptom in adult patients with lumbar intervertebral disc herniation compared to UCT?	Herbal medicine + UCT	UCT	A/High
Pharmacopuncture			
CQ10. Is pharmacopuncture treatment with UCT helpful to improve the overall symptoms in adult patients with lumbar intervertebral disc herniation compared to UCT?	Pharmacopuncture + UCT	UCT	B/Moderate
Tuina manual therapy			
CQ11. Is Tuina manual therapy helpful to improve the overall symptoms in adult patients with lumbar intervertebral disc herniation compared to UCT?	Tuina manual therapy	UCT	A/High
CQ12. Is Tuina manual therapy with UCT helpful to improve the overall symptoms in adult patients with lumbar intervertebral disc herniation compared to UCT?	Tuina manual therapy + UCT	UCT	A/Moderate
Thread-embedding acupuncture			
CQ13. Is thread-embedding acupuncture monotherapy helpful to improve the overall symptoms in adult patients with lumbar intervertebral disc herniation compared to UCT?	Thread-embedding acupuncture	UCT	B/Moderate
CQ14. Is thread-embedding acupuncture therapy with UCT helpful to improve the overall symptoms in adult patients with lumbar intervertebral disc herniation compared to UCT?	Thread-embedding acupuncture + UCT	UCT	B/Moderate
Cupping			
CQ15. Is cupping with UCT helpful to improve the overall symptoms in adult patients with lumbar intervertebral disc herniation compared to UCT?	Cupping + UCT	UCT	B/Moderate

UCT: usual conventional treatment.

3.1. Acupuncture

3.1.1. Acupuncture vs. Active Control Treatment

The level of evidence and recommendations were derived based on 24 RCTs [12–35] comparing acupuncture for LHIVD and the active control treatment in terms of pain, function, and overall symptom improvement.

Acupuncture, electroacupuncture, and warm needle acupuncture were compared with active control treatments, such as Western medicine, injection, and physical therapy. The meta-analysis showed that acupuncture was more effective in improving overall symptoms (RR: 1.20, 95% confidence interval [CI]: 1.16–1.25, $p < 0.001$), pain (MD, 1.86, 95% CI: -1.91–-1.81, $p < 0.001$), and function (MD, 4.48, 95% CI: 3.93–5.03, $p < 0.001$) than active control treatment.

In conclusion, acupuncture is recommended for improving the overall symptoms of LHIVD(A/High).

3.1.2. Acupuncture + Usual Conventional Therapy vs. Usual Conventional Therapy

The level of evidence and recommendations were derived based on 15 RCTs [20,36–49] that observed the combined effect of acupuncture and conventional treatment for LHIVD in terms of pain, function, and overall symptom improvement.

As a result of the meta-analysis, acupuncture combined with conventional treatments, such as moxibustion, herbal medicine, Western medicine, injection, and physical therapy, was more effective than usual conventional therapy in improving the overall symptoms (RR: 1.21, 95% CI: 1.16–1.28, $p < 0.001$), pain (MD, -1.03, 95% CI: -1.16–-0.90, $p < 0.001$), and function (ODI: MD, -3.27, 95% CI: -3.86–-2.68, $p < 0.001$; JOA: MD, 4.00, 95% CI: 3.48–4.52, $p < 0.001$). However, the heterogeneity (I2 = 80%) between studies was high; therefore, the level of evidence was evaluated at one level lower due to inconsistency.

Acupuncture has been reported to have a low clinical risk in safety-related studies [50] and in the utilization survey of experts, it has been shown to be a highly useful treatment method [51].

In conclusion, acupuncture in combination with conventional treatment is recommended for improving the overall symptoms of LHIVD (A/Moderate).

3.1.3. Electro-Acupuncture, Fire Needling, or Warm Needling vs. Acupuncture

The level of evidence and recommendations were derived based on seven RCTs [22,52–57] that observed the effect of additional thermal or electrical stimulation in acupuncture for LHIVD in terms of pain, function, and overall symptom improvement.

As a result of the meta-analysis, the addition of thermal stimulation or electrical stimulation during acupuncture was effective in improving the overall symptoms (RR: 1.16, 95% CI: 1.09–1.23, $p < 0.001$), pain (MD, -0.58, 95% CI: -0.76–-0.39, $p < 0.001$), and function (ODI: MD, -0.71, 95% CI: -1.29–-0.13, $p < 0.05$) compared to acupuncture monotherapy.

In conclusion, the addition of thermal stimulation or electrical stimulation during acupuncture is recommended for improving the overall symptoms of LHIVD (A/High).

3.1.4. Deep-Insertion Acupuncture vs. Superficial-Insertion Acupuncture

The level of evidence and recommendations were derived based on eight RCTs [58–65] that observed the effect of the difference in the depth of insertion with respect to the pain and overall symptom improvement in acupuncture for LHIVD.

The meta-analysis showed that deep-insertion acupuncture was more effective in improving the overall symptoms (RR: 1.31, 95% CI: 1.23–1.39, $p < 0.001$) than superficial-insertion acupuncture. However, the level of evidence was evaluated to be one level lower due to inconsistency owing to the high heterogeneity (I2 = 88%) observed between studies. There was no significant difference in pain improvement (MD, -1.66, 95% CI: -3.97–0.65, $p = 0.16$).

In conclusion, deep-insertion acupuncture should be considered for improving the overall symptoms of LHIVD (B/Moderate).

3.2. Moxibustion

3.2.1. Moxibustion vs. Active Control Group

As a result of a search for RCTs comparing moxibustion and active control treatment for LHIVD, one study [66] was found, but a sufficient sample size was not secured. There were no significant differences in terms of the effect (RR: 1.15, 95% CI: 0.97–1.36, $p = 0.10$).

In the classical literature contained in the textbooks of the College of KM [67], moxibustion is applied for cold back pain among the 10 classes of LBP. In the classical literature of Singugyeonglon, moxibustion is presented for waist and knee pain, which is similar to LBP and radiating pain. In addition, Donguibogam offers moxibustion for LBP, including when the waist cannot be bent or stretched with LBP.

In a questionnaire study that surveyed the treatment status of LHIVD among KM doctors, 102 of 373 respondents (27.3%) answered that they used moxibustion [7]. Additionally, in a survey on the current status of moxibustion for musculoskeletal disorders in KM doctors in Seoul, 135 of 234 respondents (57.7%) answered that they used moxibustion for LBP, indicating that the utilization of moxibustion in actual clinical practice is high [68].

The clinical evidence for the effect of moxibustion for LHIVD was found to be insufficient. However, based on the evidence from classical literature according to the development strategy of our guidelines, the level of evidence was assessed to be CTB. Considering the high utilization of moxibustio, the GPP grade was assigned through a clinical expert consensus process.

In conclusion, moxibustion is recommended for improving pain with LHIVD based on the consensus of the expert group (CTB/GPP).

3.2.2. Moxibustion + Usual Conventional Therapy vs. Usual Conventional Therapy

The level of evidence and recommendations were derived based on five RCTs [47,57,69–71] that observed the combination effect of "moxibustion and acupuncture" or "moxibustion and Tuina manual therapy" for LHIVD in terms of pain, function, and overall symptom improvement.

As a result of the meta-analysis, the combination of moxibustion and conventional treatments, such as acupuncture and Tuina manual therapy, was more effective in improving the overall symptoms (RR: 1.22, 95% CI: 1.12–1.32, $p < 0.001$), pain (MD, -1.40, 95% CI: -1.85–-0.95, $p < 0.001$), and function (MD, 4.10, 95% CI: 3.42–4.77, $p < 0.001$) than usual conventional therapy, such as acupuncture or Tuina monotherapy.

In conclusion, moxibustion in combination with conventional treatment is recommended for improving the overall symptoms of LHIVD(A/High).

3.2.3. Moxibustion Causing Deqi Sensation vs. Moxibustion Not Causing Deqi Sensation

The level of evidence and recommendations were derived based on four RCTs [72–75] that observed the effect of moxibustion for LHIVD in terms of function and overall symptom improvement.

The meta-analysis showed that moxibustion causing deqi sensation was effective in improving the overall symptoms (RR: 1.19, 95% CI: 1.06–1.33, $p < 0.01$) and function (MD, -2.66, 95% CI: -4.02–-1.30), $p < 0.001$) compared to moxibustion not causing deqi sensation. However, due to the lack of quality of the supporting literature and the number of subjects included, the level of evidence was evaluated at two levels lower due to the risk of bias and imprecision.

In conclusion, moxibustion treatment causing deqi sensation may be considered for improving the overall symptoms of LHIVD (C/Low).

3.3. Herbal Medicine

3.3.1. Herbal Medicine vs. Active Control Treatment

The level of evidence and recommendations were derived based on seven RCTs [76–82] comparing herbal medicine and active control treatment for LHIVD in terms of pain, function, and overall symptom improvement.

The results of the meta-analysis showed that herbal medicine was more effective in improving the overall symptoms (RR: 1.19, 95% CI: 1.11–1.28, $p < 0.001$), pain (MD, −0.55, 95% CI: −0.70--−0.40, $p < 0.001$), and function (ODI: MD, −3.86, 95% CI: −4.71--−3.10, $p < 0.001$; JOA: MD, 1.46, 95% CI: 0.95–1.97, $p < 0.001$) than active control treatments, such as Western medicine and traction treatment.

Although the level of evidence was high in terms of overall symptom improvement, inconsistency and imprecision were observed in terms of pain and function improvement (VAS, I2 = 78%; ODI, I2 = 85%); therefore, the level of evidence was lowered by two grades.

In conclusion, herbal medicine should be considered to improve the overall symptoms of LHIVD (B/Moderate).

3.3.2. Herbal Medicine + Usual Conventional Therapy vs. Usual Conventional Therapy

The level of evidence and recommendations were derived based on 22 RCTs [40,83–103] that observed the combination effect of herbal medicine and conventional treatment for LHIVD in terms of pain, function, and overall symptom improvement.

As a result of the meta-analysis, the combination of conventional herbal medicine with usual conventional treatments, such as acupuncture, pharmacopuncture, Tuina manual therapy, Western medicine, injection, physical therapy, and integrated treatment, was more effective in improving the overall symptoms (RR: 1.32, 95% CI: 1.26–1.37, $p < 0.001$), pain (MD, −1.51, 95% CI: −1.57--−1.46, $p < 0.001$), and function (ODI: MD, −5.25, 95% CI: −8.33--−2.17, $p < 0.001$; JOA: MD, 5.89, 95% CI: 5.31–6.46, $p < 0.001$) than usual conventional therapy.

In conclusion, herbal medicine in combination with conventional treatment is recommended for improving the overall symptoms of LHIVD (A/High).

3.4. Pharmacopuncture

Pharmacopuncture + Usual Conventional Therapy vs. Usual Conventional Therapy

The level of evidence and recommendations were derived based on eight RCTs [97,104–110] that observed the combined effect of pharmacopuncture and conventional treatment for LHIVD in terms of pain, function, and overall symptom improvement.

The meta-analysis showed that the combination of pharmacopuncture with conventional treatments, such as acupuncture and Tuina manual therapy, was more effective in improving the overall symptoms (RR: 1.19, 95% CI: 1.07–1.32, $p < 0.001$), pain (MD, −1.65, 95% CI: 1.70--−1.61, $p < 0.001$), and function (ODI: MD, −8.39, 95% CI: −10.50--−6.28, $p < 0.001$; ODI change: MD, 6.22, 95% CI: 3.10–9.33, $p < 0.001$; JOA: MD, 9.00, 95% CI: 7.89–10.11, $p < 0.001$) than usual conventional therapy. Since the overall number of evidence documents and the number of subjects included in studies was small, the level of evidence was lowered by one grade due to imprecision.

In conclusion, the combination of pharmacopuncture with conventional treatment should be considered for improving the overall symptoms of LHIVD (B/Moderate).

3.5. Tuina Manual Therapy

3.5.1. Tuina Manual Therapy vs. Active Control Treatment

The level of evidence and recommendations were derived based on 10 RCTs [48,111–120] that compared Tuina manual therapy and active control treatment for LHIVD in terms of pain, function, and overall symptom improvement.

As a result of the meta-analysis, Tuina manual therapy was effective in improving the overall symptoms (RR: 1.17, 95% CI: 1.12–1.23, $p < 0.001$), pain (MD, 1.09, 95% CI: 1.32--−0.86, $p < 0.001$), and function (ODI: MD, 9.87; 95% CI: 15.68- −4.06; $p < 0.001$; JOA: MD, 4.85, 95% CI: 3.87–5.83, $p < 0.001$) compared to active control treatments, such as Western medicine, injection, and traction treatment.

In conclusion, Tuina manual therapy is recommended for improving the overall symptoms of LHIVD (A/High).

3.5.2. Tuina Manual Therapy + Usual Conventional Therapy vs. Usual Conventional Therapy

The level of evidence and recommendations were derived based on 32 RCTs [36,39,46,89,99,121–147] that observed the combined effect of Tuina manual therapy and conventional treatment for LHIVD in terms of pain, function, and overall symptom improvement.

As a result of the meta-analysis, the combination of Tuina manual therapy with conventional treatments, such as acupuncture, herbal medicine, injection, and traction therapy, was more effective in improving the overall symptoms (RR: 1.25, 95% CI: 1.22–1.29, $p < 0.001$), pain (MD, −1.08, 95% CI: 1.21−−0.95, $p < 0.001$), and function (ODI: MD, 2.93, 95% CI: 3.38−−2.49, $p < 0.001$; JOA: MD, 4.86, 95% CI: 4.19–5.53, $p < 0.001$) than conventional treatment. However, the heterogeneity ($I2 = 76\%$) between studies was high; therefore, the level of evidence was evaluated at one level lower due to inconsistency.

In conclusion, a combination of Tuina manual therapy and conventional treatment is recommended for improving the overall symptoms of LHIVD (A/Moderate).

3.6. TEA

3.6.1. TEA vs. Active Control Treatment

The level of evidence and recommendations were derived based on 12 RCTs [148–159] that compared TEA and active control treatment for LHIVD in terms of pain, function, and overall symptom improvement.

As a result of the meta-analysis, TEA was more effective in improving the overall symptoms (RR: 1.14, 95% CI: 1.10–1.19, $p < 0.001$), pain (MD, 0.40, 95% CI: 0.54−−0.26, $p < 0.001$), and function (ODI: MD, 1.30, 95% CI: 2.42−−0.18, $p < 0.05$; JOA: MD, 2.03, 95% CI: 0.30–3.76, $p < 0.05$) than active control treatments, including acupuncture and complex treatment. However, in terms of overall symptom improvement, the risk of bias was high; therefore, the level of evidence was lowered by one grade.

In conclusion, TEA should be considered to improve the overall symptoms of LHIVD (B/Moderate).

3.6.2. TEA + Usual Conventional Therapy vs. Usual Conventional Therapy

The level of evidence and recommendations were derived based on seven RCTs [160–166] that observed the combined effect of TEA and conventional treatment in terms of pain, function, and overall symptom improvement for LHIVD

As a result of the meta-analysis, the combination of TEA and conventional treatments, such as acupuncture, herbal medicine, and traction treatment, was more effective in improving the overall symptoms (RR: 1.15, 95% confidence interval [CI] 1.09–1.21, $p < 0.001$), pain (MD, −2.00, 95% CI: -2.46−−1.54, $p < 0.001$), and function (ODI: MD, 21.07, 95% CI: 27.18−−14.96, $p < 0.001$; JOA: MD, 2.37, 95% CI: 0.78–3.96, $p < 0.001$) compared to usual conventional therapy. However, in the area of overall symptom improvement, heterogeneity ($I2 = 80\%$) between studies was observed, and the level of evidence was lowered by one level due to inconsistency.

In conclusion, TEA in combination with conventional treatment should be considered for improving the overall symptoms of LHIVD (B/Moderate).

3.7. Cupping

Cupping + Usual Conventional Therapy vs. Usual Conventional Therapy

The level of evidence and recommendations were derived based on five RCTs [167–171] that observed the combined effect of cupping and conventional treatment for LHIVD in terms of pain, function, and overall symptom improvement.

As a result of the meta-analysis, the combination of cupping and conventional treatment had a significant effect on the overall symptom improvement (RR: 1.43, 95% CI: 1.27–1.62, $p < 0.001$) compared to conventional therapy without cupping. However, there was no significant difference in pain improvement (MD, −1.08, 95% CI: −2.24–0.08, $p = 0.07$); therefore, the level of evidence was evaluated as very low due to the high imprecision.

In conclusion, cupping treatment should be considered in combination with conventional treatment for improving the overall symptoms of LHIVD (B/Moderate).

4. Discussion

CPGs are systematically developed statements to assist practitioners and patient decisions about the appropriate healthcare for specific clinical circumstances.

Among the several standard methods used to develop CPGs, we mainly used the GRADE to assess the quality of evidence.

We applied seven types of interventions to the clinical question. In a preliminary study, it was found that the studied interventions were used frequently in the actual clinical field [7]. The studied interventions are often used alone or in combination with other treatments.

When the intervention was applied alone, acupuncture and Tuina manual therapy were evaluated as A grade, herbal medicine and TEA were evaluated as B grade, and moxibustion was evaluated as GPP grade. Each single treatment was compared to active control treatments, including drugs, injection therapy, and physical therapy. This comparison showed that KM treatment can be used as an alternative to conventional treatment.

For herbal medicine, the level of evidence was lowered by two grades due to the inconsistency and imprecision observed in terms of pain and function improvement. For TEA, the level of evidence was lowered by one grade due to the risk of bias. Further research is required to expand the evidence.

When intervention was applied as combination therapy, the combination of acupuncture with active control treatment, combination of moxibustion with acupuncture or Tuina manual therapy, combination of herbal medicine with active control treatment, and combination of Tuina manual therapy with active control treatment were evaluated as A grade, and the combination of pharmacopuncture with active control treatment, combination of TEA with active control treatment, and combination of cupping treatment with active control treatment were evaluated as B grade. Conventional therapies include Western medicine and KM treatments. This comparison showed that KM treatment can be used as a complementary treatment to conventional treatments.

Regarding the combination of pharmacopuncture with active control treatment, the level of evidence was lowered by one grade due to imprecision because the overall number of evidence documents and the number of subjects included in the studies were small. For the combination of Tuina manual therapy with active control treatment and combination of TEA with active control treatment, the level of evidence was evaluated as one level lower due to the inconsistency owing to the high heterogeneity between studies. Further research is required to expand the evidence.

In actual clinical practice, KM techniques have different treatment techniques. Among them, we developed recommendations for the depth of acupuncture, thermal and electrical stimulation with acupuncture, and deqi sensation caused by moxibustion. Additional heat or electrical stimulation during acupuncture was classified as grade A. Deep-insertion acupuncture was evaluated as B grade, and moxibustion causing deqi sensation was evaluated as C grade. For deep-insertion acupuncture, the level of evidence was evaluated as one level lower due to inconsistency owing to the high heterogeneity between studies. Regarding moxibustion that causes deqi sensation, the level of evidence was evaluated at two levels lower due to the risk of bias and imprecision owing to the lack of quality of the supporting data and the number of subjects included. Further research is required to expand the evidence.

4.1. Limitations of the Present Guidelines

Our CPGs have several limitations. First, there are limitations in the search strategy. Since the terms were not the same for each treatment intervention, it was difficult to present a standardized method for selecting a search word, and there were limitations in establishing a consistent level of search strategy due to the different terms by country.

Second, there are some qualitative limitations that include cases where bias risk evaluation factors were not presented, cases that were not blinded, and cases where there were limitations in the design of the study. Moreover, some studies had limitations, such as study inconsistency and imprecision, and a lack of evaluation indicators, such as segmentation, safety, and economics.

Finally, there are methodological limitations that do not reflect the diversity of KM treatment techniques. Few studies have compared and analyzed the detailed elements of KM treatments. There may be some disparity from the actual clinical practice in the method of synthesizing KM treatments, including various detailed attributes, into a certain category and arriving at a conclusion. Except for the diagnosis of LHIVD, there is insufficient evidence to consider clinical variables, such as severity.

4.2. Recommendation for Further Guidelines

To overcome the limitations of our CPGs, a number of clinical studies are needed to accumulate evidence. In addition, to acquire data on stability and provide recommendations that can be realistically applied in the clinical field, it is necessary to expand the scope to case reports and observational studies while using RCTs as supporting literature in CPGs. A close review of more clinical experts is necessary to prevent the deterioration of quality.

Supplementary Materials: The following are available online at https://www.mdpi.com/article/10.3390/healthcare10020246/s1, Supplementary Materials S1–S5.

Author Contributions: Conceptualization, B.-K.S.; Funding acquisition: B.-K.S.; methodology: E.-J.K., H.-J.L., J.-S.K., D.N., T.-H.K., Y.-C.P., Y.-H.B., S.-S.N., M.S.L. and B.-K.S.; project administration: B.G., M.-g.J., E.-J.K., H.-J.L., J.-S.K., D.N., T.-H.K. and B.-K.S.; supervision: B.-K.S.; writing—original draft: B.G. and M.-g.J.; writing—review and editing: E.-J.K., H.-J.L., J.-S.K., D.N., J.W.K., T.-H.K., Y.-C.P., Y.-H.B., S.-S.N., M.S.L. and B.-K.S. All authors have read and agreed to the published version of the manuscript.

Funding: This research was funded by a grant of the Korea Health Technology R&D Project through the Korea Health Industry Development Institute (KHIDI), supported by the Ministry of Health & Welfare, Republic of Korea (grant number: HI20C1405, HB16C0061). Funding did not affect the content of the CPGs.

Institutional Review Board Statement: Not applicable.

Informed Consent Statement: Not applicable.

Data Availability Statement: All relevant data are included in this manuscript and Supplementary Materials.

Conflicts of Interest: The authors declare no conflict of interest.

References

1. Deyo, R.A.; Loeser, J.D.; Bigos, S.J. Herniated lumbar intervertebral disk. *Ann. Intern. Med.* **1990**, *112*, 598–603. [CrossRef] [PubMed]
2. Lee, C.H.; Chung, C.K.; Kim, C.H.; Kwon, J.W. Health care burden of spinal diseases in the republic of Korea: Analysis of a nationwide database from 2012 through 2016. *Neurospine* **2018**, *15*, 66–76. [CrossRef] [PubMed]
3. Kreiner, D.S.; Hwang, S.W.; Easa, J.E.; Resnick, D.K.; Baisden, J.L.; Bess, S.; Cho, C.H.; Depalma, M.J.; Dougherty, P.; Fernand, R.; et al. An evidence-based clinical guideline for the diagnosis and treatment of lumbar disc herniation with radiculopathy. *Spine J.* **2014**, *14*, 180–191. [CrossRef] [PubMed]
4. *Ministry of Health and Welfare Report of Survey on Korean Medical Use Status*; Version 2017; Ministry of Health and Welfare: Sejong, Korea, 2017.
5. Choi, T.Y.; Choi, J.; Lee, J.A.; Jun, J.H.; Park, B.; Lee, M.S. The quality of clinical practice guidelines in traditional medicine in Korea: Appraisal using the AGREE II instrument. *Implement. Sci.* **2015**, *10*, 104. [CrossRef] [PubMed]
6. Jun, J.H.; Cha, Y.; Lee, J.A.; Choi, J.; Choi, T.Y.; Park, W.; Chung, W.; Shin, B.C.; Lee, M.S. Korean medicine clinical practice guideline for lumbar herniated intervertebral disc in adults: An evidence based approach. *Eur. J. Integr. Med.* **2017**, *9*, 18–26. [CrossRef]
7. Goo, B.; Seo, B.K. Strategies to revise the Korean Medicine Clinical Practice Guideline for lumbar herniated intervertebral disc—A web based approach. *Eur. J. Integr. Med.* **2020**, *37*, 101169. [CrossRef]

8. Sterne, J.A.C.; Higgins, J.P.T.; Altman, D.G. *Cochrane Handbook for Systematic Reviews of Interventions*; Version, 5.1.0; Higgins, J.P.T., Green, S., Eds.; Wiley-Blackwell: Chichester, UK; Hoboken, NJ, USA, 2011; Available online: https://handbook-5-1.cochrane.org (accessed on 24 December 2021).
9. Guyatt, G.H.; Oxman, A.D.; Vist, G.E.; Kunz, R.; Falck-Ytter, Y.; Alonso-Coello, P.; Schünemann, H.J. GRADE: An emerging consensus on rating quality of evidence and strength of recommendations. *BMJ* **2008**, *336*, 924–926. [CrossRef]
10. Balshem, H.; Helfand, M.; Schünemann, H.J.; Oxman, A.D.; Kunz, R.; Brozek, J.; Vist, G.E.; Falck-Ytter, Y.; Meerpohl, J.; Norris, S.; et al. GRADE guidelines: 3. Rating the quality of evidence. *J. Clin. Epidemiol.* **2011**, *64*, 401–406. [CrossRef]
11. Brouwers, M.C.; Kho, M.E.; Browman, G.P.; Burgers, J.S.; Cluzeau, F.; Feder, G.; Fervers, B.; Graham, I.D.; Grimshaw, J.; Hanna, S.E.; et al. AGREE II: Advancing guideline development, reporting and evaluation in health care. *Can. Med. Assoc. J.* **2010**, *182*, 839–842. [CrossRef]
12. Chen, M.R.; Wang, P.; Cheng, G.; Guo, X.; Wei, G.W.; Cheng, X.H. The warming acupuncture for treatment of sciatica in 30 cases. *J. Tradit. Chin. Med.* **2009**, *29*, 50–53. [CrossRef]
13. Du, Z.; Shao, P.; He, Y.H.; Dai, Q.P.; Qiu, M.L.; Zheng, X.; Xin, Z.P. Clinical Observation on 32 Cases of Lumber Intervertebral Disc Herniation Treated by Electro-acupuncture on Huatuo Jiaji Points. *J. Tradit. Chin. Med.* **2009**, *50*, 617–619. (In Chinese)
14. Liu, D.M. Study on the Rehabilitation Effect of Acupuncture and Moxibustion Therapy for Patients with Lumbar Disc Herniation. *Contemp. Med.* **2018**, *24*, 89–91. (In Chinese)
15. Tuzun, E.H.; Gildir, S.; Angin, E.; Tecer, B.H.; Dana, K.O.; Malkoc, M. Effectiveness of dry needling versus a classical physiotherapy program in patients with chronic low-back pain: A single-blind, randomized, controlled trial. *J. Phys. Ther. Sci.* **2017**, *29*, 1502–1509. [CrossRef] [PubMed]
16. Yin, Q. Effect of acupuncture and moxibustion for prolapse of lumbar intervertebral disc. *Contemp. Med. Symp.* **2018**, *16*, 8–9. (In Chinese)
17. Zhang, J.H.; Fan, J.Z.; Qi, Z.Q. The clinical and neuroelectrophysiological study of electronic acupuncture on acute lumbar disc herniation. *Chin. J. Rehabil. Med.* **2004**, *19*, 647–649. (In Chinese)
18. Feng, H.; Zhang, Y.F.; Ding, M. Analysis of therapeuttic effect of lower limb sensation disorder after lumbar disc herniation operation treated with plum-blossom needle along meridians. *Chin. Acupunct. Moxibustion* **2012**, *32*, 129–132. (In Chinese with English abstract)
19. Geng, X.; Leng, E.R.; Feng, T.Z. Clinical Observation on the Treatment of 56 Cases of Lumbar Intervertebral Disc Protrusion by Electroacupuncture at Jiaji Points and Traction. *Shanxi J. Tradit. Chin. Med.* **2009**, *25*, 36–37. (In Chinese)
20. Hou, S.B. Curative Effect Observation on 30 Cases of Lumbar Intervertebral Disc Protrusion Treated by Warming Needle Moxibustion and Western Medicine. *Hebei J. Tradit. Chin. Med.* **2009**, *31*, 588–589. (In Chinese)
21. Wang, X.G. Clinical analysis of 52 cases of lumbar intervertebral disc herniation treated with acupuncture and moxibustion. *Asia-Pac. Tradit. Med.* **2008**, *4*, 39–40. (In Chinese)
22. Wu, Y.C.; Zhang, B.R. Clinical Observations on Electroacupuncture Treatment of Lumbar Intervertebral Disc Protrusion. *Shanghai J. Acupunct. Moxibustion* **2004**, *23*, 15–17. (In Chinese)
23. Zhang, B.M.; Wu, Y.C.; Shao, P.; Shen, J.; Jiu, R.F. Electro-acupuncture therapy for lumbar intervertebral disc protrusion: A randomized controlled study. *J. Clin. Rehabil. Tssue Eng. Res.* **2008**, *12*, 353–355. (In Chinese)
24. Li, Y.Q.; Liu, Y.Q. Therapeutic effect of acupuncture on postoperative recovery of prolapse of lumbar intervertebral disc. *Chin. Acupunct. Moxibustion* **2006**, *26*, 566–568. (In Chinese with English abstract)
25. Huang, C.H.; Xue, X.R. Observation on Therapeutic Effect of Acupuncture and Moxibustion for Treatment of Lumbar Intervertebral Disc Protrusion. *Chin. J. Misdiagnostics* **2007**, *7*, 745–746. (In Chinese)
26. Tang, S.D.; Chen, G.H.; Lu, Z.M. Study of Efficacy on Intervertebral Lumbar Disc Protrusion Treated by Abdominal Acupuncture. *World J. Integr. Tradit. West. Med.* **2009**, *4*, 572–573. (In Chinese)
27. Gao, H.; Zhu, H.L. Acupuncture Treatment of 120 Cases of Lumbar Intervertebral Disc Protrusion. *Mod. Med. J. China* **2007**, *9*, 71. (In Chinese)
28. Ma, L.X. Observation on Therapeutic Effect of Acupuncture on 106 Cases of Lumbar Intervertebral Disc Protrusion. *China Foreign Med. Treat.* **2010**, *12*, 33. (In Chinese)
29. Shan, Y.L. Observation on therapeutic effect of electroacupuncture at Jiaji (EX-B 2) and points of bladder meridian mainly for lumbar disc herniation. *Chin. Acupunct. Moxibustion* **2011**, *31*, 987–990. (In Chinese)
30. Ding, W.C. Observing the Curative Effect of 75 Cases of Balance Acupuncture in Treating Lumbar Intervertebral Disc Protrusion Caused Back Pain. *Mod. Tradit. Chin. Med.* **2014**, *34*, 48–50. (In Chinese)
31. Lu, W.; Xiong, D.J.; Jiang, J.; Hao, J.H.; Chai, W.; Zhang, M. Clinical study on treatment of lumbar vertebral disc herniation with lumber Du channel electrical acupuncture. *Chin. J. Tissue Eng. Res.* **2002**, *6*, 1164–1165. (In Chinese)
32. Xia, S.Y. Acupuncture and Moxibustion in the Treatment of Postoperative Pain of Lumbar Intervertebral Disc Herniation for 55 Cases. *Guangming J. Chin. Med.* **2018**, *33*, 1446–1448. (In Chinese)
33. Fan, Y.; Xue, L.F.; Meng, X.F. Effect Analysis of Warming Acupuncture Treatment on Lumbar IntervertebraI Disc Herniation. *Chin. Med. Mod. Distance Educ. China* **2009**, *7*, 114–115. (In Chinese)
34. Hu, J.Z. Clinical analysis of acupuncture and moxibustion for treatment of lumbar intervertebral disc pain. *Nei Mong. J. Tradit. Chin. Med.* **2014**, 68–69. (In Chinese) [CrossRef]

35. Li, L.X.; Lin, G.H.; Zhang, H.L.; Liu, X.R. The clinical observation of herniation of internertebral disk treated by the electric acupuncture. *J. Clin. Acupunct. Moxibustion* **2006**, *22*, 36–37. (In Chinese)
36. Guo, J.G.; Liu, Y.; Chen, B.Q.; Hu, D.M.; Li, Y.F.; Liao, H.L.; Li, Y.F.; Xu, N.Y. Clinical research of balance acupuncture combined with Long's bonesetting massage treating lumbar disc herniation. *China Mod. Med.* **2013**, *20*, 110–112. (In Chinese)
37. Hu, Y. Comparison of Curative Effect Observation of Acupuncture Add Massage Manipulation with Traction and Manipulation of Massage with Traction on Treating Prolapse of Lumbar Intervertebral Disc. *J. Sichuan Tradit. Chin. Med.* **2013**, *31*, 137–139. (In Chinese)
38. Liu, X. Clinical Observation on Treatment of Lumbar Intervertebral Disc Protrusion Mainly by Warming Needle. *Mod. J. Integr. Tradit. Chin. West. Med.* **2009**, *18*, 641–658. (In Chinese)
39. Xiong, J.; Fang, J.B.; Chen, X.; Jiang, L.Y.; Zhou, D.Y. Evaluation of the clinical efficacy of three programs: Single acupuncture, single massage, and acupuncture combined with massage for the treatment of lumbar disc herniation. *Guid. China Med.* **2013**, *11*, 300–301. (In Chinese)
40. Liu, L.; Liu, L.G.; Lu, M.; Ran, W.J. Observation on therapeutic effect of electroacupuncture combined with Chinese herbs for treatment of prolapse of lumbar intervertebral disc of yang deficiency and cold coagulation type. *Chin. Acupunct. Moxibustion* **2009**, *29*, 626–628, (In Chinese with English abstract)
41. Yang, Y.J.; Wang, Y.; Zeng, Y.Y. Randomized Parallel Controlled Study on the Treatment of Lumbar Intervertebral Disc Herniation (Fenghan Shibi) with Traditional Chinese Medicine Rehuangbao plus Electroacupuncture combined with Diclofenac Sodium. *J. Pract. Tradit. Chin. Intern. Med.* **2018**, *32*, 49–52. (In Chinese)
42. Ji, X.L.; Li, D.; Huo, Z.J.; Cheng, T. Comparison of therapeutic effects in treating lumbar disc herniation in prone traction combined with acupuncture and supine traction. *J. Basic Chin. Med.* **2015**, *21*, 1043–1045. (In Chinese)
43. Qu, M.; Ding, X.N.; Liu, H.B.; Liu, Y.Q. Clinical observation on acupuncture combined with nerve block for treatment of lumbar disc herniation. *Chin. Acupunct. Moxibustion* **2010**, *30*, 633–636. (In Chinese with English abstract)
44. Guo, R. Randomized Parallel Controlled Study of Warming Acupuncture combined with Yaotong Ning for Treating Lumbar Disc Herniation. *J. Pract. Tradit. Chin. Intern. Med.* **2018**, *32*, 43–45. (In Chinese)
45. Chen, X.H.; Huang, J.H.; Liu, J.H. Effect of electroacupuncture on rehabilitation of patients with sciatica caused by lumbar disc herniation. *Chin. J. Inf. Tradit. Chin. Med.* **2006**, *13*, 81–82. (In Chinese)
46. Chen, Y.; Ran, Q.F. Curative effect observation of protrusion of lumbar intervertebral disc treated by massage combined with acupuncture. *Beijing J. Tradit. Chin. Med.* **2010**, *29*, 543–544. (In Chinese)
47. Ma, S.; Ma, J.; Pan, J.N.; Zhang, X.S. Comparative research of lumbar disc herniation treated with acupuncture and snake moxibustion. *Chin. Acupunct. Moxibustion* **2010**, *30*, 563–566. (In Chinese with English abstract)
48. Chen, R.H.; Chen, S.R. Observation on Therapeutic Effect of Acupuncture and Massage for Treatment of Lumbar Intervertebral Disc Protrusion. *Mod. Rehabil.* **2000**, *4*, 766. (In Chinese)
49. Fu, X.S. Comparative Study on the Efficacy of 240 Cases of Lumbar Disc Herniation Treated with Acupuncture and Chinese Massage. *World J. Integr. Tradit. West. Med.* **2011**, *6*, 1058–1060. (In Chinese)
50. Kim, M.; Shin, J.; Lee, J.; Lee, Y.J.; Ahn, Y.; Park, K.B.; Lee, H.D.; Lee, Y.; Kim, S.G.; Ha, I. Safety of Acupuncture and Pharmacopuncture in 80,523 Musculoskeletal Disorder Patients: A Retrospective Review of Internal Safety Inspection and Electronic Medical Records. *Medical* **2016**, *95*, e3635. [CrossRef]
51. Shin, Y.; Shin, J.; Lee, J.; Lee, Y.J.; Kim, M.; Ahn, Y.; Park, K.B.; Shin, B.; Lee, M.S.; Kim, J.; et al. A survey among Korea Medicine doctors (KMDs) in Korea on patterns of integrative Korean Medicine practice for lumbar intervertebral disc displacement: Preliminary research for clinical practice guidelines. *BMC Complement. Altern. Med.* **2015**, *15*, 432. [CrossRef]
52. Jung, S.H.; Sung, H.J.; Lim, S.J.; Lee, E.Y.; Lee, C.K. The Comparative Study on the Effect of Fire Needling Therapy and General Acupuncture with Other Korean Traditional Medical Treatment for the Patient with Lumbar Herniated Intervertebral Disc: A Randomized Assessor Blinded Two Arm Trial. *J. Acupunct. Res.* **2015**, *32*, 29–36. [CrossRef]
53. Wang, Y.L. Observation on the therapeutic effect of lumbar disc herniation treated with different acupuncture therapies. *Chin. Acupunct. Moxibustion* **2013**, *33*, 605–608, (In Chinese with English abstract).
54. Zhang, J.L.; Zhang, Z.G.; Yang, L.J.; Sheng, X.Y. Clinical Observations on Zhen's "Warming and Unblocking Acupuncture" for Lumbar Intervertebral Disc Herniation. *Shanghai J. Acupunct. Moxibustion* **2018**, *37*, 937–940. (In Chinese)
55. Du, X.Z.; Bao, C.L.; Dong, G.R. Observation on therapeutic effect of Tongluo Guben needling method for lumbar disc herniation. *Chin. Acupunct. Moxibustion* **2011**, *31*, 204–208. (In Chinese)
56. Yang, G.S. Treatment of 45 Cases of Lumbar Intervertebral Disc Protrusion by Electroacupuncture. *Nei Mong. J. Tradit. Chin. Med.* **2017**, *36*, 138–144. (In Chinese)
57. He, X.W.; Huang, J.H.; Zeng, L.Y. Observation on the therapeutic effect of warming needle moxibustion on prolapse of lumbar intervertebral disc. *Chin. Acupunct. Moxibustion* **2007**, *27*, 264–266. (In Chinese with English abstract)
58. Itoh, K.; Katsumi, Y. Effect of Acupuncture Treatment on Chronic Low Back Pain with Leg Pain in Aged Patients: A Controlled Trial about Short-term Effects of Trigger Point Acupuncture. *Zen Nihon Shinkyu Gakkai zasshi. J. Japan. Acupunct. Moxibustion Soc.* **2005**, *55*, 530–537. [CrossRef]
59. Hong, J.Y. Observation on Therapeutic Effect of Deep Jiaji Acupuncture on Lumbar Intervertebral Disc Herniation. *J. Clin. Acupunct. Moxibustion* **2005**, *21*, 33–34. (In Chinese)

60. Jiang, Y.Q. Clinical Observation on the Relationship between Acupuncture Depth and Curative Effect of Lumbar Disc Herniation. *J. Clin. Acupunct. Moxibustion* **2005**, *21*, 2–3. (In Chinese)
61. She, R.P. Observation on therapeutic effect of deeply needling Qiangji 4 points on prolapse of lumbar intervertebral disc. *Chin. Acupunct. Moxibustion* **2008**, *28*, 341–344. (In Chinese with English abstract)
62. Wu, H.H. Observation on 100 Cases of Treatment of Lumbar Intervertebral Disc Protrusion by Deep Needling. *J. Pract. Tradit. Chin. Med.* **2013**, *29*, 1047. (In Chinese)
63. Xing, Y.H.; Fan, Y.Y. Clinical Observation on Treatment of Lumbar Intervertebral Disc Protrusion by Deep Needing at Dachangshu and Guanyuanshu. *Tradit. Chin. Med. J.* **2004**, *3*, 30–31. (In Chinese)
64. Xiong, J.F. Clinical Study on Shu-point Acupuncture in Predominant for Lumbar Intervertebral Disc Herniation. *Shanghai J. Acupunct. Moxibustion* **2012**, *31*, 166–167. (In Chinese)
65. Xue, P.W. Clinical observation on deeply needling Ciliao (BL 32) for treatment of prolapse of lumbar intervertebral disc. *Chin. Acupunct. Moxibustion* **2007**, *27*, 182–184, (In Chinese with English abstract).
66. Tang, F.Y. Clinical Study of Moxibustion at Heat Sensitive Points on Lumbar Disc Herniation. *J. Jiangxi Univ. Tradit. Chin. Med.* **2009**, *21*, 25–27. (In Chinese)
67. *Journal of Korean Acupuncture & Moxibustion Society Textbook Compilation Committee Acupuncture Medicine*; Hanmimedical: Seoul, Korea, 2016.
68. Young-Rye, L.; Eun-Jung, K.; Hyun-Seok, C.; Seung-Deok, L.; Kap-Sung, K.; Kyung-Ho, K. Interview Survey Methods for Moxibustion Treatment of Knee pain, Neck Pain and Back Pain: Subject to Oriental Doctors in Seoul. *J. Acupunct. Res.* **2011**, *28*, 1–11.
69. Xu, Q.; Xiong, Z.F.; Xie, C.X.; Li, S.J. Therapeutic Observation of Bai Xiao Moxibustion plus Electroacupuncture for Lumbar Intervertebral Disc Herniation. *Shanghai J. Acupunct. Moxibustion* **2018**, *37*, 316–319. (In Chinese with English abstract)
70. Wang, G.S.; Zhang, X.L.; Li, C.S.; Huang, W. Observations on the Efficacy of Electroacupuncture plus Indirect Moxibustion Treating Lumbar Intervertebral Disc Herniation. *Shanghai J. Acupunct. Moxibustion* **2017**, *36*, 1466–1468. (In Chinese)
71. Xu, C.H.; Yu, N.T.; Lu, J.; Xiong, S.B.; Liu, Y.D. Observations on Efficacy of Spreading Medicinal Moxibustion on Ginger plus Massotherapy for Lumbar Intervertebral Disc Herniation. *Shanghai J. Acupunct. Moxibustion* **2018**, *37*, 1059–1062. (In Chinese)
72. Chen, M.; Chen, R.; Xiong, J.; Chi, Z.; Sun, J.; Su, T.; Zhou, M.; Yi, F.; Zhang, B. Evaluation of different moxibustion doses for lumbar disc herniation: Multicentre randomised controlled trial of heat-sensitive moxibustion therapy. *Acupunct. Med.* **2012**, *30*, 266–272. [CrossRef]
73. Chen, R.; Chen, M.; Xiong, J.; Su, T.; Zhou, M.; Sun, J.; Chi, Z.; Zhang, B.; Xie, D. Influence of the deqi sensation by suspended moxibustion stimulation in lumbar disc herniation: Study for a multicenter prospective two arms cohort study. *Evidence-Based Complement. Altern. Med.* **2013**, *2013*, 718593. [CrossRef]
74. Tang, F.Y.; Huang, C.J.; Chen, R.X.; Xu, M.; Liu, B.X.; Liang, Z. Observation on therapeutic effect of moxibustion on temperature-sensitive points for lumbar disc herniation. *Chin. Acupunct. Moxibustion* **2009**, *29*, 382–384. (In Chinese with English abstract)
75. Tang, F.Y.; Liang, Z.; Wang, J.; Liang, D.B.; Tang, H.W. Treatment of 60 Cases of Lumbar Intervertebral Disc Protrusion by Heat-sensitive Moxibustion. *Jiangxi J. Tradit. Chin. Med.* **2011**, *42*, 53–55. (In Chinese)
76. He, J.L.; Wang, W.; Li, C.G. Short-term Effect Observation of Chushi Tongbi Decoction Combined with Traction Treatment on Limbar Disc Herniation. *Chin. J. Exp. Tradit. Med. Formulae* **2016**, *22*, 186–189. (In Chinese)
77. Seo, B.K. Clinical research on the efficacy and safety of Bosinji on low back pain and radiculopathy by herniated intervertebral disc of lumbar spine; A multicenter, randomized, controlled, clinical trial. *Clin. Res. Inf. Serv.* **2018**, *97*, e13684.
78. Zhang, H.; Liu, T. Clinical observation on the treatment of lumbar disc herniation with Shenjinhuoxue decoction and Wei's fumigation. *Shanxi Med. J.* **2018**, *47*, 135–137. (In Chinese)
79. Chen, H.W.; Zhu, J.; Li, Y.W. Clinical Observation on the Treatment of Lumbar Intervertebral Disc Protrusion by Modified Churong Niuxie Decoction. *Hebei J. Tradit. Chin. Med.* **2017**, *39*, 1650–1652. (In Chinese)
80. Li, B.J.; He, W.R. Treatment of 64 Cases of Prolapse of Lumbar Intervertebral Disc with Modified Duhuojii Decoction. *Mod. J. Integr. Tradit. Chin. West. Med.* **2009**, *18*, 3319–3320. (In Chinese)
81. Xu, M.; Jiang, H. The clinical efficacy and prognosis of Duhuo Jisheng decoction in the treatment of cold dampness type lumbar intervertebral disc herniation. *Shanxi J. Tradit. Chin. Med.* **2018**, *39*, 157–159. (In Chinese)
82. Bao, C.Y.; Ma, C.J. Clinical observation on the curative effect of Duhuo Jisheng decoction on the treatment of lumbar disc herniation. *J. Tradit. Chin. Orthop. Traumatol.* **2010**, *22*, 11–12. (In Chinese)
83. Wang, Z.J.; Zhang, R.J.; Gao, S.R. Clinical observation of acupuncture combined with Bushen-tongluo formula on lumbar disc herniation with kidney deficiency and blood stasis type. *Hebei J. Tradit. Chin. Med.* **2017**, *39*, 1239–1242. (In Chinese)
84. Wang, J.; Chu, C.Y.; Liang, W.W.; Wang, F.; Zhang, J.H.; Dong, X.P.; Ding, Y.Y. Clinical Observation on the Treatment of Prolapse of Lumbar Intervertebral Disc with the Method of Promoting Blood Circulation and Dredging Collaterals. *Chin. Tradit. Pat. Med.* **2015**, *37*, 2798–2800. (In Chinese)
85. Wu, Y.J. Buyang Huanwu decoction combined with functional exercise in the treatment of posterior longitudinal ligament rupture type lumbar disc herniation. *Shanxi J. Tradit. Chin. Med.* **2017**, *38*, 638–640. (In Chinese)
86. Lin, X.M.; Wu, Q.M.; Yang, Z.H.; Fu, L. Treatment of 43 Cases of Lumbar Intervertebral Disc Protrusion with Acupuncture and Duhuojii Decoction. *J. Clin. Acupunct. Moxibustion* **2008**, *24*, 15–16. (In Chinese)

87. Chen, Y.F. Clinical Observation of Duhuojii Decoction Combined with Massage for Treatment of Lumbar Intervertebral Disc Herniation. *Jilin Med. J.* **2011**, *32*, 5262–5263. (In Chinese)
88. Lin, K.L.; Sun, X.D. Observation on 60 Cases of Lumbar Intervertebral Disc Protrusion Treated by Tuina Traction and Modified Duhuojii Decoction. *J. Pract. Tradit. Chin. Med.* **2011**, *27*, 446. (In Chinese)
89. Meng, D.Y. Clinical Observation of Oral Administration of Chinese Medicine and Massage for Prolapse of Lumbar Intervertebral Disc. *China Pract. Med.* **2010**, *5*, 143–144. (In Chinese)
90. Guo, X.Y.; Li, X.F. Treatment of 52 Cases of Prolapse of Lumbar Intervertebral Disc with Modified Duhuojijie Decoction. *Xinjiang J. Tradit. Chin. Med.* **2011**, *29*, 26–27. (In Chinese)
91. Li, Z.; Wen, J.; Li, G.X.; Wu, Z.Q.; Yu, L.M.; Li, J.Y. Clinical observation in the treatment of 100 cases of LIDP with combination of traditional Chinese and western medicine. *China Med. Her.* **2010**, *7*, 61–62. (In Chinese)
92. Li, S.F. Clinical Observation on Treatment of 65 Cases of Prolapse of Lumbar Intervertebral Disc with Duhuojii Decoction Combined with Traction Physiotherapy. *Guangming J. Chin. Med.* **2009**, *24*, 1326–1328. (In Chinese)
93. He, X.L.; Yan, S. Observation on Therapeutic Effect of 500 Cases of Lumbar Intervertebral Disc Protrusion Treated by Combination of Chinese and Western Methods. *Chin. Community Dr.* **2007**, *5*, 71. (In Chinese)
94. Zhang, Z.Y.; Zhu, Q.; Huang, J.F. Evaluation of Clinical Effect of Infrared Acupoint Irradiation Combined with Bushen Huoxue Decoction for Treatment of Lumbar Intervertebral Disc Protrusion. *Hebei J. Tradit. Chin. Med.* **2018**, *40*, 65–67. (In Chinese)
95. Liu, S.B.; Zhao, F.C. Comprehensive treatment of 36 cases of lumbar intervertebral disc herniation. *Yunnan J. Tradit. Chin. Med. Mater. Med.* **2008**, *29*, 66–67. (In Chinese)
96. Zheng, Y.J.; Guo, X. Clinical Observation on the Treatment of 91 Cases of Lumbar Intervertebral Disc Protrusion. *Henan Tradit. Chin. Med.* **2004**, *24*, 55–56. (In Chinese)
97. Zhao, M.X.; Dong, Y.J.; Tian, W.M.; Gao, Y.X. Clinical Observation on Treatment of Lumbar Prolapse with Acupoint Injection and Qutong Decoction. *Chongqing Med.* **2015**, *44*, 4153–4156. (In Chinese)
98. Gao, Y.H. Effect of Duhuojii Decoction on Lumbar Intervertebral Disc Herniation of Liver and Kidney Deficiency and Qi and Blood Insufficiency. *Chin. Community Dr.* **2019**, *35*, 97–99. (In Chinese)
99. Wen, D.D. Clinical observation of four-step massage combined with traditional Chinese medicine in the treatment of non-spinal lumbar disc herniation. *Guid. J. Tradit. Chin. Med. Pharmacol.* **2010**, *16*, 55–56. (In Chinese)
100. Xie, Y.S.; Wu, G.B.; Yang, B.; Deng, Z. Clinical study of Duhuo Jisheng decoction combined with traction-manipulation on herniated lumbar disc. *J. Tradit. Chin. Med. Univ. Hunan* **2011**, *31*, 61–63. (In Chinese)
101. Miao, L.H. Clinical Study on the Effect of Xiaosui Huahe Decoction on Reabsorption after Lumbar Intervertebral Disc Herniation. *Chin. Foreign Med. Res.* **2018**, *16*, 59–60. (In Chinese)
102. Cao, G.Y. Clinical Observation on Comprehensive Treatment of Lumbar Intervertebral Disc Herniation. *Jilin J. Chin. Med.* **2006**, *26*, 30–31. (In Chinese)
103. Chang, H. The Clinical Observation of Lumbar Intervertebral Disc Herniation Treated with Traditional Chinese Medicine for Oral Administration in Combination with Radiofrequency Ozone Intervention. *Henan Tradit. Chin. Med.* **2018**, *38*, 414–416. (In Chinese)
104. Chung, W.-S.; Lee, J.-S.; Chung, S.-H.; Kim, S.-S. The Effect of Bee Venom Acupuncture on Patient with Herniation of Nucleus Pulposus of Lumbar Spine. *J. Orient. Rehab. Med.* **2003**, *13*, 87–101.
105. Zou, R.; Xu, Y.; Zhang, H.X. Evaluation on analgesic effect of electroacupuncture combined with acupoint-injection in treating lumbar intervertebral disc herniation. *China J. Orthop. Traumatol.* **2009**, *22*, 759–761. (In Chinese with English abstract)
106. Jun, B.-C.; Kim, E.-S.; Kim, D.; Kim, T.-H.; Kim, J. Effectiveness of ShinBaro Pharmacopuncture on Lumbar Spinal Herniated Intervertebral Disc: A Randomized Controlled Trial. *J. Korea Chuna Man. Med. Spine Nerves* **2011**, *6*, 109–119. (In Korean with English abstract)
107. Lee, S.H.; Kang, M.W.; Lee, H.; Lee, S.Y. Effectiveness of Bee-venom Acpuncture and Ouhyul Herbal Acpuncture in Herniation of Nucleus Pulposus-comparison with Acpuncture Therapy Only. *J. Korean Acupunct. Moxib. Soc.* **2007**, *24*, 197–205. (In Korean with English abstract)
108. Song, H.; Choi, J.; Kang, J.; Lee, H. The Effect of the Acupuncture Therapy in Combination with Soyeom Pharmacopuncture Therapy on the Improvement of the Symptoms of the Patients with Herniated Intervertebral Disk of L-spine in His Initial Stage of Hospitalization. *J. Korean Pharmacopunct. Inst.* **2009**, *12*, 111–118. (In Korean with English abstract) [CrossRef]
109. Yu, S.M.; Lee, J.Y.; Kwon, K.R.; Lee, H.S. Comparative Study of Acupuncture, Bee Venom Acupuncture, and Bee venom Pharmacopuncture on the Treatment of Herniation of Nucleus Pulpous. *J. Korean Acupunct. Moxib. Soc.* **2006**, *23*, 39–54. (In Korean with English abstract)
110. Cha, J.; Jeong, S.; Kim, G.; Kim, G.; Kim, N. The Comparison of Effectiveness between Acupuncture and Its Cotreatment with Bee venom Acua-Acupuncture Therapy on the Treatment of Herniation of Nucleus Pulpous. *J. Korean Acupunct. Moxib. Soc.* **2004**, *21*, 149–158, (In Korean with English abstract).
111. Chen, J.H.; Sun, B.; Wu, Y.D.; Li, L.P.; Wang, Z.Q.; Shi, G.T.; Huang, S.R.; Wu, X.Z. Clinical study on lumbar disc herniation treated by Luwen's traditional Chinese manipulation. *China J. Orthop. Traumatol.* **2006**, *19*, 705–707. (In Chinese)
112. Dong, T. Clinical Study on the Treatment of Lumbar Intervertebral Disc Protrusion with Special Massage Manipulation. *Mod. Med. Healthc.* **2010**, *26*, 1393–1395. (In Chinese)

113. Gu, F.; Lv, Q.; Liu, K.P.; Wei, M.; Zheng, L.; Hu, B.L.; Zhang, C.; Huang, Y. Popularization and application of Three-steps Massage Therapy for treating lumbar disc herniation in communities. *Shanghai J. Tradit. Chin. Med.* **2013**, *47*, 60–62. (In Chinese)
114. Hu, G.X.; Liu, Z.G.; Xia, Z. Clinical Research on Three-step Massage in Treatment of Lumbar Intervertebral Disc Protrusion. *Chin. J. Tradit. Med. Traumatol. Orthop.* **2009**, *17*, 41–43. (In Chinese)
115. Tang, X.Z.; Ding, H.T.; Yang, F.; Chen, J. Observation on the clinical effect of treating lumbar disc herniation by three postures and eight steps layer by layer Tuina method. *China J. Tradit. Chin. Med. Pharm.* **2012**, *27*, 1464–1466. (In Chinese)
116. Weng, W.S.; Lin, Y.F.; Wang, H.L.; Dong, J.Q.; Zhao, J.L.; Li, Z.Q. Observation on Therapeutic Effect of Chiropractic and Massage for Treatment of Lumbar Intervertebral Disc Protrusion. *Chin. Manip. Rehabil. Med.* **2008**, *24*, 2–3. (In Chinese)
117. Zhang, L.; Zhang, L.; Fan, H.T. Observation on Therapeutic Effect of Massage for Treatment of Lumbar Intervertebral Disc Protrusion. *Med. J. Natl. Defending Forces Northwest China* **2012**, *33*, 675–676. (In Chinese)
118. Zhang, Q.M.; Zhu, Q.G.; Fang, M.; Liu, Y.M.; Gong, L.; Wu, J.R.; Yan, Z. Clinical Analysis of Modified Three-Step Massage Therapy for Prolapse of Lumbar Intervertebral Discs. *Acad. J. Shanghai Univ. Tradit. Chin. Med.* **2008**, *22*, 27–28. (In Chinese)
119. Li, J. Influence of Massage on Hemorheology in Patients with Lumbar Intervertebral Disc Herniation. *Shandong J. Tradit. Chin. Med.* **2010**, *29*, 545–546. (In Chinese)
120. Lin, X.; Yuan, W.A.; He, T.X. Clinical Research on Tuina Therapy in Treating Lumbar Intervertebral Disc Protrusion. *J. Liaoning Univ. Tradit. Chin. Med.* **2008**, *10*, 129–130. (In Chinese)
121. Zhang, P.T. Clinical Observation on TuiNa and Rotatory Manual Reduction in Treating Lumbar Disc Herniation. *West. J. Tradit. Chin. Med.* **2012**, *25*, 98–100. (In Chinese)
122. Shi, L. Traction Combination with Manual Massage for Treating Lumbar Discherniation. *J. Liaoning Univ. Tradit. Chin. Med.* **2010**, *12*, 163–165. (In Chinese)
123. Zhu, J. Evaluation of the Efficacy of Traction Combined with Massage on Lumbar Intervertebral Disc Herniation. *Chin. J. Clin. Med.* **2005**, *12*, 864–865. (In Chinese)
124. Chen, Z.L. Clinical Obsevation of Bonesetting Massage Combined with EA JIAJI in the Treatment of Lumbar Disc Herniation. *Mod. Hosp.* **2013**, *13*, 33–34. (In Chinese)
125. Gao, X.D.; Li, T.J.; Yu, Z.G. Observation on the clinical curative effect of massage combined with warm needling on lumbar intervertebral disc herniation. *J. Aerosp. Med.* **2010**, *21*, 1740. (In Chinese)
126. He, Q.; Pan, X.L.; Wu, Z.R.; Li, J.; Huang, Z.H.; Wang, L.J.; Liu, C.F.; Zhou, J.Y. Clinical Study on Treatment of Lumbar Intervertebral Disc Protrusion by Acupuncture and Massage. *Asia-Pac. Tradit. Med.* **2007**, *3*, 61–62. (In Chinese)
127. He, Z.D.; Tan, W.; Chen, Z.B. A Controlled Observation on the Treatment of Lumbar Intervertebral Disc Protrusion by Massage Combined with Jiaji Electroacupuncture. *J. Clin. Acupunct. Moxibustion* **2009**, *25*, 21–23. (In Chinese)
128. Xiang, K.W.; Cui, Z.; Peng, K.Z. Study on the clinical efficacy and biochemical mechanism of intradermal acupuncture combined with massage in the treatment of lumbar intervertebral disc herniation. *J. Sichuan Tradit. Chin. Med.* **2008**, *26*, 107–109. (In Chinese)
129. Xu, B.J.; Tan, W.Z. Clinical analysis of the treatment of lumbar disc herniation with massage of lumbar back muscles and Jiaji electroacupuncture. *Nei Mong. J. Tradit. Chin. Med.* **2013**, *17*, 76. (In Chinese)
130. Zeng, R.; Hong, W.; Tang, J.L. Observation on therapeutic effect of electro-acupuncture combined with tuina on lumbar intervertebral disc. *China Pract. Med.* **2009**, *4*, 17–18. (In Chinese)
131. Ding, X.Y. Analysis of the effect of treatment of lumbar intervertebral disc herniation with bone setting massage combined with intervertebral foramina block. *Guid. China Med.* **2013**, *11*, 147–148. (In Chinese)
132. Lu, C.P.; Ou, Y.; Chen, C. Observation of Therapeutic Effect of Epidural Block and Tuina Therapy on Lumbar Intervertebral Disc Herniation. *J. Huaihai Med.* **2013**, *31*, 412–413. (In Chinese)
133. Yan, Q. Treatment of lumbar intervertebral disc protrusion by lumbar paravertebral or sacral canal injection in combination withorthopaedic spinal massage. *Jiangxi Med. J.* **2005**, *40*, 375–377. (In Chinese)
134. Feng, L.G. Clinical Observation on Treatment of Lumbar Intervertebral Disc Protrusion by Traction and Massage. *Contemp. Med.* **2011**, *17*, 2–3. (In Chinese)
135. Xie, T.J. Clinical Observation of Massage Combined with Traction on Lumbar Intervertebral Disc Protrusion. *Shanxi J. Tradit. Chin. Med.* **2012**, *28*, 32–33. (In Chinese)
136. Yuan, H.C. Clinical Observation on the Efficacy of Traction and Massage in Treating Prolapse of Waist Intervertebral Disc. *Hebei Med.* **2010**, *16*, 149–152. (In Chinese)
137. Zeng, S.P.; Peng, J.M. Observation on Therapeutic Effect of Traction Combined with Suspended Pulling Massage on Lumbar Disc Herniation. *J. Pract. Tradit. Chin. Med.* **2002**, *18*, 26. (In Chinese)
138. Zhang, J.P.; Zhao, J.P.; Zhou, J. Therapeutic Evaluation on PLID with Traction Combining with Tuina and Traction Simply. *Chin. Arch. Tradit. Chin. Med.* **2009**, *27*, 2419–2420. (In Chinese)
139. Zhang, S.Y.; Wu, J. Observation of Therapeutic Effect on Lumbar Disc Herniation Treated by Traction Combined with Chinese Massage. *J. Pract. Tradit. Chin. Med.* **2010**, *26*, 176–177. (In Chinese)
140. Zhang, X.W. Traction and Massage Treat Prolapse of Waist Intervertebral Disc. *J. Zhejiang Chin. Med. Univ.* **2008**, *32*, 243–244. (In Chinese)
141. Yang, T.H.; Zhu, Y.F. Three Dimensional Traction Combined Masssge treating of Lumbar Disc Hemiations:clinical research. *J. Liaoning Univ. Tradit. Chin. Med.* **2008**, *10*, 75–76. (In Chinese)

142. He, Q.; Xu, L.H.; Wu, W.F.; Huang, Z.H.; Wu, Z.R.; Li, J.; Pan, X.L.; Wang, L.J.; Liu, C.F.; Cao, Y.F. Clinical Observation on Acupuncture Combined with Massage for Treatment of Lumbar Intervertebral Disc Protrusion. *J. Guangzhou Univ. Tradit. Chin. Med.* **2010**, *27*, 242–245. (In Chinese)
143. Hong, D.F. The effect of acupuncture at the lumbar Jiaji points combined with four-finger spine adjustment on the pain index of patients with lumbar disc herniation. *J. Emerg. Tradit. Chin. Med.* **2013**, *22*, 318–319. (In Chinese)
144. Huang, C.J.; Zhou, X.P. Effect of Acupuncture and Long's Manipulation on Pain Improvement of Lumbar Intervertebral Disc Herniation. *J. Emerg. Tradit. Chin. Med.* **2011**, *20*, 306–307. (In Chinese)
145. Xu, Z.Y. Efficacy Observation of Acupuncture at Baliao Points plus Tuina for L5-S1 Intervertebral Disc Herniation. *Shanghai J. Acupunct. Moxibustion* **2018**, *37*, 941–945. (In Chinese)
146. Zhang, Y.Q.; Yang, Z.L.; Tong, B.; Zuo, Q. Clinical Observation on Treatment of Lumbar Intervertebral Disc Protrusion with Tuina and Epidural Infusion. *Jiangxi J. Tradit. Chin. Med.* **2005**, *36*, 40–41. (In Chinese)
147. Ku, H.N.; Lin, G.H. *Clinical Observation of Acupoint Catgut Embedding Therapy for Lumbar Disc Herniation*; Guangzhou University of Chinese Medicine: Guangzhou, China, 2012.
148. Xie, H.Y.; Zhang, J.W. Clinical Observation on the Treatment of Lumbar Intervertebral Disc Protrusion by Catgut Embedding at Acupoint. *J. New Chin. Med.* **2012**, *44*, 122–123. (In Chinese)
149. Wang, D.; Lin, X.J. Clinical Observation on Lumbar Disc Herniation Treated with Acupoint Catgut Embedding. *Henan Tradit. Chin. Med.* **2009**, *29*, 1116–1117. (In Chinese)
150. Zhou, W.P. 52 Cases of Lumbar Intervertebral Disc Protrusion Treated by Catgut Embedding at Acupoint. *China Pract. Med.* **2006**, *1*, 60–61. (In Chinese)
151. Zhang, Y.B.; Xu, P.C.; Geng, C.F. Randomized Parallel Controlled Study of Acupoint Catgut Embedding in Treating Lumbar Disc Herniation Due(Qizhi Xueyu/). *J. Pract. Tradit. Chin. Intern. Med.* **2018**, *32*, 65–68. (In Chinese)
152. Zhang, Z.Q.; He, X.J.; Bai, W.J.; He, Y.F. Clinical study on the treatment of lumbar intervertebral disc herniation with catgut embedding at acupoint. *China Med. Eng.* **2013**, *21*, 95–96. (In Chinese)
153. Liu, J. Clinical Observation on Lumbar Disc Herniation Treated by Catgut Embedding Therapy. *Shanghai J. Acupunct. Moxibustion* **2011**, *30*, 22–23. (In Chinese)
154. Sun, Z.D.; Wang, J.J. Observations on the Efficacy of New Medicated Thread Embedding Therapy for Lumbar Intervertebral Disc Herniation. *Shanghai J. Acupunct. Moxibustion* **2009**, *28*, 652–654. (In Chinese)
155. Xia, F.X.; Lim, L.X.; Sun, X.Y. Controlled observation on catgut implantation at acupoint for treatment of prolapse of lumbar intervertebral disc. *Chin. Acupunct. Moxibustion* **2006**, *26*, 195–197. (In Chinese)
156. Ye, L.H.; Hu, Y.M.; Zhang, S.L.; Zuo, L.H. Clinical study on treatment of prolapse of lumbar intervertebral disc with hypodermic catgut embedding therapy. *Chin. Acupunct. Moxibustion* **2004**, *24*, 245–247. (In Chinese)
157. Zhu, S.X.; Tang, B.F.; Zhang, Y.D. Clinical Observation on 200 Cases of Lumbar Intervertebral Disc Protrusion Treated by Catgut Embedding at Jiaji Points. *Hunan J. Tradit. Chin. Med.* **2014**, *30*, 74–75. (In Chinese)
158. Li, P. Clinical Study on Acupoint Thread Embedding and Subcutaneous Thread Embedding in Treatment of Lumbar Intervertebral Disc Herniation. *J. Clin. Acupunct. Moxibustion* **2007**, *23*, 46–47. (In Chinese)
159. Lee, Y.H.; Zhuang, L.X. *Clinical Observation on Treatment of Acupuncture Combined with Catgut Implantation at Acupoint Treatment of Vertebral Disc Herniation*; Guangzhou University of Chinese Medicine: Guangzhou, China, 2010.
160. Seo, B.K. Clinical research on the efficacy and safety of thread-embedding acupuncture for treatment of herniated intervertebral disc of the lumbar spine: A multicenter, randomized, patient-assessor blinded, controlled, parallel, clinical trial. *Clin. Res. Inf. Serv.* **2018**, *19*, 484.
161. Chen, Z.X. Sequential Treatment of 54 Cases of Lumbar Intervertebral Disc Protrusion by Electroacupuncture at Acupoints. *Shanxi J. Tradit. Chin. Med.* **2004**, *25*, 744–745. (In Chinese)
162. Huang, D.W. Therapeutic Observation of Acupoint Thread-embedding plus Acupuncture for Lumbar Intervertebral Disc Herniation. *Shanghai J. Acupunct. Moxibustion* **2014**, *33*, 254–255. (In Chinese)
163. Li, Y.Q.; Lv, L.; Chen, X.L.; Xu, J.L. Observation on Therapeutic Effect of Acupotomy Combined with Acupoint Thread Embedding in Treating Lumbar Intervertebral Disc Protrusion. *Chin. Acupunct. Moxibustion* **2010**, *30*, 30–32. (In Chinese)
164. Xie, H.Y.; Lan, W.H.; Chen, L.P.; Zhang, J.W. Clinical Observation on Acupoint Thread-Embedding Combined with Tendon-relaxing and Lumber-strengthening Decoction in Treatment of 43 Lumbar Disc Herniation Cases. *Mod. Tradit. Chin. Med. Mater. Med.-World Sci. Technol.* **2014**, *16*, 416–420. (In Chinese)
165. Chen, L.Y. Observation on the curative effect of 103 cases of lumbar intervertebral disc herniation treated with minimally invasive thread embedding and traction. *J. Guangxi Med. Univ.* **2015**, *32*, 835–837. (In Chinese)
166. Chen, Y.L.; Liu, X.L.; Xia, J.Z. Clinical Observation on 30 Cases of Blood Stasis Type Lumbar Intervertebral Disc Protrusion Treated with Blood Stasis Type Lumbar Intervertebral Disc Protrusion Treated by Blood Stasis Type Cupping. *Jiangsu J. Tradit. Chin. Med.* **2008**, *40*, 47–48. (In Chinese)
167. Li, J.J.; Li, D.; Liu, H. Three-step Acupuncture and Cupping in Acute Lateral Prolapse of Lumber Intervertebral Disc and Its Effect on Nailfold Microcirculation. *Chin. Gen. Pract.* **2009**, *12*, 1341–1343. (In Chinese)
168. Lu, J.; Wang, Y. Clinical observations of curative effect of lumbar disc prolapse by acupuncture combined with punctural cupping. *J. Clin. Acupunct. Moxibustion* **2007**, *23*, 16–17. (In Chinese)

169. Tao, Q.; Lu, H.X. Observation on the curative effect of electroacupuncture and cupping blood pricking in treatment of lumbar protrusion related abdominal aortic calcification. *J. Clin. Acupunct. Moxibustion* **2007**, *23*, 46–47. (In Chinese)
170. Zhang, Q.L.; Fu, X.H. Observation on the curative effect of flocculation cupping combined with electroacupuncture in the treatment of blood stasis type lumbar disc herniation. *Acta Chin. Med. Pharmacol.* **2009**, *37*, 79–80. (In Chinese)
171. Institute of Medicine. *Clinical Practice Guidelines: Directions for a New Program*; Field, M.J., Lohr, K.N., Eds.; The National Academies Press: Washington, DC, USA, 1990; ISBN 9780309043465.

MDPI
St. Alban-Anlage 66
4052 Basel
Switzerland
Tel. +41 61 683 77 34
Fax +41 61 302 89 18
www.mdpi.com

Healthcare Editorial Office
E-mail: healthcare@mdpi.com
www.mdpi.com/journal/healthcare

www.ingramcontent.com/pod-product-compliance
Lightning Source LLC
LaVergne TN
LVHW070617100526
838202LV00012B/669